The *Essential* Handbook of
Memory Disorders for Clinicians

The *Essential* Handbook of Memory Disorders for Clinicians

Edited by

Alan D. Baddeley
Department of Psychology, University of York, UK

Michael D. Kopelman
*University Department of Psychiatry and Psychology,
St Thomas' Hospital (Institute of Psychiatry and King's College London),
London, UK*

and

Barbara A. Wilson
MRC Cognition and Brain Sciences Unit, Cambridge, UK

John Wiley & Sons, Ltd

Other Wiley Editorial Offices

John Wiley & Sons, Inc., 111 River Street, Hoboken, NJ 07030, USA

Jossey-Bass, 989 Market Street, San Francisco, CA 94103-1741, USA

Wiley-VCH Verlag GmbH, Boschstr. 12, D-69469 Weinheim, Germany

John Wiley & Sons Australia, Ltd., 33 Park Road, Milton, Queensland 4064, Australia

John Wiley & Sons (Asia) Pte Ltd., 2 Clementi Loop #02-01, Jin Xing Distripark, Singapore 129809

John Wiley & Sons Canada, Ltd., 22 Worcester Road, Etobicoke, Ontario, Canada M9W 1L1

Wiley also publishes its books in a variety of electronic formats. Some content that appears
in print may not be available in electronic books.

Library of Congress Cataloging-in-Publication Data

The essential handbook of memory disorders for clinicians / edited by
Alan D. Baddeley, Michael D. Kopelman, Barbara A. Wilson.
  p.   cm.
Rev. ed. of: Handbook of memory disorders. 2nd ed. New York : J. Wiley, c2002
Includes bibliographical references and indexes.
ISBN 0-470-09141-X (pbk.: alk. paper)
1. Memory disorders. 2. Memory.   3. Amnesia.   I. Baddeley, Alan D., 1934-
II. Kopelman, Michael D.   III. Wilson, Barbara, A., 1941-   IV. Handbook of memory disorders.
RC394.M46 E85   2004
616.8′4—dc22   2003026697

British Library Cataloguing in Publication Data

A catalogue record for this book is available from the British Library

ISBN 10: 0-470-09141-X (P/B)
ISBN 13: 978-0-470-09141-8 (P/B)

Typeset in 10/12 pt Times by TechBooks, New Delhi, India
Printed and bound in Great Britain by Antony Rowe Ltd, Chippenham, Wiltshire, UK
This book is printed on acid-free paper responsibly manufactured from sustainable forestry
in which at least two trees are planted for each one used for paper production.

Contents

About the Editors

Alan D. Baddeley, *Department of Psychology, University of York, Heslington, York, YO10 5DD, UK*

Alan Baddeley was Director of the Medical Research Council Applied Psychology Unit in Cambridge, UK for over 20 years. He is now at the University of York. He is a cognitive psychologist with broad interests in the functioning of human memory under both normal conditions and conditions of brain damage and stress.

Michael D. Kopelman, *Neuropsychiatry and Memory Disorders Clinic, St Thomas' Hospital, Lambeth Palace Road, London SE1 7EH, UK*

Michael Kopelman is Professor of Neuropsychiatry in the Institute of Psychiatry based at St Thomas' Hospital, King's College, London. He holds qualifications in both neuropsychiatry and neuropsychology, and has particular interest and expertise in a wide range of memory disorders, both neurological and psychogenic. He runs a neuropsychiatry and memory disorders clinic at St Thomas's Hospital.

Barbara A. Wilson, *MRC Cognition and Brain Sciences Unit, 15 Chaucer Road, Cambridge CB2 2EF, UK*

Barbara Wilson is a senior scientist at the MRC Cognition and Brain Sciences Unit and is Director of Research at the Oliver Zangwill Centre for Neuropsychological Rehabilitation, Ely, UK. She is a clinical psychologist with particular interests in the impact of neuropsychological memory deficits on everyday functioning and improving methods of neurorehabilitation. She was awarded an OBE in 1998 for services to medical rehabilitation, and is Editor-in-Chief of the journal *Neuropsychological Rehabilitation*.

Contributors

Alan D. Baddeley, *Department of Psychology, University of York, Heslington, York YO10 5DD, UK*

James T. Becker, *UPMC Health System, Western Psychiatric Institute and Clinic, Neuropsychology Research Program, Suite 830, 3501 Forbes Avenue, Pittsburgh, PA 15213-3323, USA*

Jason Brandt, *Department of Psychiatry and Behavioral Sciences, Johns Hopkins University School of Medicine, 600 North Wolfe Street/Meyer 218, Baltimore, MD 21287-7218, USA*

Linda Clare, *Sub-department of Clinical Health Psychology, University College London, Gower Street, London WC1E 6BT, UK*

Elizabeth L. Glisky, *Department of Psychology, University of Arizona, PO Box 210068, Tucson, AZ 85721, USA*

Gerri Hanten, *Departments of Physical Medicine and Rehabilitation, Neurosurgery and Psychiatry, and Behavioral Sciences, Baylor College of Medicine, Houston, TX 77030, USA*

Diane B. Howieson, *Department of Neurology, Oregon Health Sciences University, 3181 SW Sam Jackson Park Road, Portland, OR 97201-3098, USA*

Narinder Kapur, *Wessex Neurological Centre, Southampton General Hospital, Southampton SO16 6YD, UK*

Michael D. Kopelman, *Neuropsychiatry and Memory Disorders Clinic, St Thomas' Hospital, Lambeth Palace Road, London SE1 7EH, UK*

Harvey S. Levin, *Departments of Physical Medicine and Rehabilitation, Neurosurgery and Psychiatry, and Behavioral Sciences, Baylor College of Medicine, Houston, TX 77030, USA*

Muriel D. Lezak, *Department of Neurology, Oregon Health Sciences University, 3181 SW Sam Jackson Park Road, Portland, OR 97201-3098, USA*

Judith A. Middleton, *Oxford Department of Clinical Neuropsychology, Radcliffe Hospitals NHS Trust, The Russell Cairns Unit, The Radcliffe Infirmary, Woodstock Road, Oxford OX2 6HE, UK*

Cynthia A. Munro, *Department of Psychiatry and Behavioral Sciences, Johns Hopkins University School of Medicine, 600 North Wolfe Street/Meyer 218, Baltimore, MD 21287-7218, USA*

Margaret O'Connor, *Beth Israel Deaconess Medical Center, 330 Brookline Avenue, Boston, MA 02215, USA*

Amy A. Overman, *UPMC Health System, Western Psychiatric Institute and Clinic, Neuropsychology Research Program, 502 Iroquois Building, 3600 Forbes Avenue, Pittsburgh, PA 15213-3418, USA*

Robyn L. Tate, *Rehabilitation Studies Unit, Department of Medicine, University of Sydney, PO Box 6, Ryde, NSW 1680, Australia*

Christine M. Temple, *Department of Psychology, Developmental Neuropsychology Unit, University of Essex, Wivenhoe Park, Colchester CO4 3SQ, UK*

Mieke Verfaellie, *Memory Disorders Research Center (151-A), Boston VA Medical Center, 150 South Huntington Avenue, Boston, MA 02130, USA*

Barbara A. Wilson, *MRC Cognition and Brain Sciences Unit (CBU), Addenbrooke's Hospital, Box 58, Hills Road, Cambridge CB2 2QQ, UK*

Bob Woods, *Dementia Services Development Centre, University of Wales, Normal Site, Holyhead Road, Bangor LL57 2PX, UK*

Preface

In editing the first edition of *The Handbook of Memory Disorders*, our principal aim was to inform practicing clinicians about the extensive developments that had occurred in the study of memory and its disorders. We were pleased to discover in due course that the resulting handbook also proved to be very useful to non-clinicians with interests in both research and teaching in the field of human memory. When the opportunity to revise the handbook was offered, we opted to respond to this extended range of readers by increasing the scope of the handbook, including a wider field of topics, not all of which were equally likely to be of direct interest to the busy clinician. This resulted in a much more comprehensive handbook, as we had hoped, but also in a heftier and more expensive book, which might well be seen as less directly relevant to clinical practice. For that reason, it was suggested that a more clinically focused selection from the original 35 chapters might be desirable, decreasing the weight and cost, and resulting in a greater probability of reaching our initial target readership of forward-looking practising clinicians. The selection of chapters was made with this in mind. Authors were given the opportunity to make modifications, although the time constraints discouraged the possibility of major re-writing. We were pleased to find that all the authors were happy to agree to republication in this form, which we have titled *The* Essential *Handbook of Memory Disorders for Clinicians*. We are grateful to Vivien Ward for suggesting this revised edition and to Ruth Graham for making its prompt publication possible.

ADB
MDK
BAW

CHAPTER 1

The Psychology of Memory

Alan D. Baddeley
Department of Psychology, University of York, UK

In this chapter I will try to provide a brief overview of the concepts and techniques that are most widely used in the psychology of memory. Although it may not appear to be the case from sampling the literature, there is in fact a great deal of agreement as to what constitutes the psychology of memory, much of it developed through the interaction of the study of normal memory in the laboratory and of its breakdown in brain-damaged patients. A somewhat more detailed account can be found in Parkin & Leng (1993) and Baddeley (1999), while a more extensive overview is given by Baddeley (1997), and within the various chapters comprising the *Handbook of Memory* (Tulving & Craik, 2000).

THE FRACTIONATION OF MEMORY

The concept of human memory as a unitary faculty began to be seriously eroded in the 1960s with the proposal that long-term memory (LTM) and short-term memory (STM) represent separate systems. Among the strongest evidence for this dissociation was the contrast between two types of neuropsychological patient. Patients with the classic amnesic syndrome, typically associated with damage to the temporal lobes and hippocampi, appeared to have a quite general problem in learning and remembering new material, whether verbal or visual (Milner, 1966). They did, however, appear to have normal short-term memory (STM), as measured for example by digit span, the capacity to hear and immediately repeat back a unfamiliar sequence of numbers. Shallice & Warrington (1970) identified an exactly opposite pattern of deficit in patients with damage to the perisylvian region of the left hemisphere. Such patients had a digit span limited to one or two, but apparently normal LTM. By the late 1960s, the evidence seemed to be pointing clearly to a two-component memory system. Figure 1.1 shows the representation of such a system from an influential model of the time, that of Atkinson & Shiffrin (1968). Information is assumed to flow from the environment through a series of very brief sensory memories, that are perhaps best regarded as part of the perceptual system, into a limited capacity short-term store. They proposed that the longer an item resides in this store, the greater the probability of its transfer to LTM. Amnesic patients were assumed to have a deficit in the LTM system, and STM patients in the short-term store.

The Essential *Handbook of Memory Disorders for Clinicians.* Edited by A.D. Baddeley, M.D. Kopelman and B.A. Wilson.
© 2004 John Wiley & Sons, Ltd. ISBN 0-470-09141-X.

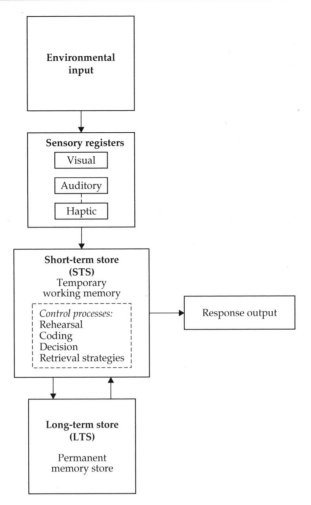

Figure 1.1 The model of human memory proposed by Atkinson & Shiffrin. Reproduced from Atkinson & Shiffrin (1968)

By the early 1970s, it was clear that the model had encountered at least two problems. The first of these concerned the learning assumption. Evidence suggested that merely holding an item in STM did not guarantee learning. Much more important was the processing that the item underwent. This is emphasized in the *levels-of-processing* framework proposed by Craik & Lockhart (1972). They suggested that probability of subsequent recall or recognition was a direct function of the *depth* to which an item was processed. Hence, if the subject merely noted the visual characteristics of a word, for example whether it was in upper or lower case, little learning would follow. Slightly more would be remembered if the word were also processed acoustically by deciding, for example, whether it rhymed with a specified target word. By far the best recall, however, followed semantic processing, in which the subject made a judgement about the meaning of the word, or perhaps related it to a specified sentence, or to his/her own experience.

This levels of processing effect has been replicated many times, and although the specific interpretation proposed is not universally accepted, there is no doubt that a word or experience that is processed in a deep way that elaborates the experience and links it with prior knowledge, is likely to be far better retained than one that receives only cursory analysis. The effect also occurs in the case of patients with memory deficits, making it a potentially useful discovery for those interested in memory rehabilitation, although it is important to remember that cognitive impairment may hinder the processes necessary for such elaboration. Indeed, it was at one point suggested that failure to elaborate might be at the root of the classic amnesic syndrome, although further investigation showed this was not the case (see Baddeley, 1997, for further discussion).

A second problem for the Atkinson & Shiffrin model was presented by the data on STM patients that had initially appeared to support it. Although such patients argued strongly for a dissociation between LTM and STM, the Atkinson & Shiffrin model assumed that STM was necessary, indeed crucial, for long-term learning, and indeed for many other cognitive activities. In fact, STM patients appeared to have normal LTM, and with one or two minor exceptions, such as working out change while shopping, had very few everday cognitive problems.

This issue was tackled by Baddeley & Hitch (1974), who were explicitly concerned with the relationship between STM and LTM. A series of experiments attempted to block STM in normal subjects by requiring them to recite digit sequences while performing other tasks, such as learning, reasoning or comprehending, that were assumed to depend crucially upon STM. Decrement occurred, with the impairment increasing with the length of the digit sequence that was being retained, suggesting that STM and LTM *did* interact. However, the effect was far from dramatic, again calling into question the standard model. Baddeley & Hitch proposed that the concept of a simple unitary STM be replaced by a more complex system which they termed "*working memory*", so as to emphasize its functional importance in cognitive processing. The model they proposed is shown in Figure 1.2.

Working memory is assumed to comprise an attentional controller, the *central executive*, assisted by two subsidiary systems, the *phonological loop* and the *visuospatial sketchpad*. The phonological (or articulatory) loop is assumed to comprise a store that holds memory traces for a couple of seconds, combined with a subvocal rehearsal process. This is capable of maintaining the items in memory using subvocal speech, which can also be used to convert nameable but visually presented stimuli, such as letters or words, into a phonological code. STM patients were assumed to have a deficit in this system, whereas the remainder of working memory was assumed to be spared (Vallar & Baddeley, 1984). Subsequent research, based on STM patients, normal children and adults, and children with specific language impairment, suggest that the phonological loop system may have evolved for the purpose of language acquisition (Baddeley et al., 1998). A more detailed account of this system and its breakdown is given by Vallar & Papagno (2002).

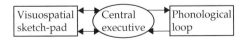

Figure 1.2 The Baddeley & Hitch model of working memory. Reproduced from Baddeley & Hitch (1974)

The visuospatial sketchpad (or scratchpad) is assumed to allow the temporary storage and manipulation of visual and spatial information. Its function can be disrupted by concurrent visuospatial activity and, as in the case of the phonological loop, our understanding has been advanced by the study of neuropsychological patients. More specifically, there appear to be separate visual and spatial components, which may be differentially disrupted. A more detailed account of this system and the relevant neuropsychological evidence is given by Della Sala & Logie (2002).

The third component of the model, the central executive, was assumed to provide an attentional control system, both for the subsystems of working memory and for other activities. Baddeley (1986) suggested that a good account of it might be provided by the *supervisory attentional system* (SAS) proposed by Norman & Shallice (1986) to account for the attentional control of action. They assume that much activity is controlled by well-learned habits and schemata, guided by environmental cues. Novel actions that were needed to respond to unexpected situations, however, depended upon the intervention of the limited-capacity SAS. This was assumed to be capable of overriding habits so as to allow novel actions in response to new challenges. Slips of action, such as driving to the office rather than the supermarket on a Saturday morning, were attributed to the failure of the SAS to override such habits. The problems in action control shown by patients with frontal lobe damage were also attributed to failure of the SAS; hence, perseverative activity might reflect the failure of the SAS to break away from the domination of action by environmental cues (Shallice, 1988).

Both Shallice himself and others have extended their account to include a range of potentially separable executive processes, hence providing an account of the range of differing deficits that may occur in patients with frontal lobe damage (Baddeley, 1996; Duncan, 1996; Shallice & Burgess, 1996). Given the far from straightforward mapping of anatomical location onto cognitive function, Baddeley & Wilson (1988) suggested that the term "frontal lobe syndrome" be replaced by the more functional term, "*dysexecutive syndrome*". For a recent review of this area, see Roberts et al. (1998) and Stuss & Knight (2002).

The implications of frontal lobe function and executive deficit for the functioning of memory are substantial, since the executive processes they control play a crucial role in the selection of strategy and stimulus processing that has such a crucial influence in effective learning. (See Baddeley et al., 2002a, Chapters 15, 16 and 17 for further discussion of these issues.)

More recently, a fourth component of WM has been proposed, the *episodic buffer*. This is assumed to provide a multimodal temporary store of limited capacity that is capable of integrating information from the subsidiary systems with that of LTM. It is assumed to be important for the *chunking* of information in STM (Miller, 1956). This is the process whereby we can take advantage of prior knowledge to package information more effectively and hence to enhance storage and retrieval. For example, a sequence of digits that comprised a number of familiar dates, such as 1492 1776 1945, would be easier to recall then the same 12 digits in random order. The episodic buffer is also assumed to play an important role in immediate memory for prose, allowing densely amnesic patients with well-preserved intelligence and/or executive capacities to show apparently normal immediate, although not delayed, recall of a prose passage that would far exceed the capacity of either of the subsidiary systems (Baddeley & Wilson, 2002). It seems unlikely that the episodic buffer will reflect a single anatomical location, but it is probable that frontal areas will be crucially involved. For a more detailed account, see Baddeley (2000).

LONG-TERM MEMORY

As in the case of STM, LTM has proved to be profitably fractionable into separate components. Probably the clearest distinction is that between *explicit* (or *declarative*) and *implicit*
(or *non-declarative*) memory. Once again, neuropsychological evidence has proved crucial.
It has been known for many years that densely amnesic patients are able to learn certain
things; for example, the Swiss psychiatrist Claparède (1911) pricked the hand of a patient
while shaking hands one morning, finding that she refused to shake hands the next day
but could not recollect why. There was also evidence that such patients might be able to
acquire motor skills (Corkin, 1968). Probably the most influential work, however, stemmed
from the demonstration by Warrington & Weiskrantz (1968) that densely amnesic patients
were capable of showing learning of either words or pictures, given the appropriate test
procedure. In their initial studies, patients were shown a word or a line drawing, and subsequently asked to identify a degraded version of the item in question. Both patients and
control subjects showed enhanced identification of previously presented items, to a similar degree. This procedure, which is typically termed *priming*, has since been investigated
widely in both normal subjects and across a wide range of neuropsychologically impaired
patients (for review, see Schacter, 1994).

   It has subsequently become clear that a relatively wide range of types of learning may
be preserved in amnesic patients, ranging from motor skills, through the solution of jigsaw
puzzles (Brooks & Baddeley, 1976) to performance on concept formation (Kolodny, 1994)
and complex problem-solving tasks (Cohen & Squire, 1980); a review of this evidence is
provided by Squire (1992). The initial suggestion, that these may all represent a single
type of memory, now seems improbable. What they appear to have in common is that
the learning does *not* require the retrieval of the original learning episode, but can be
based on implicit memory that may be accessed indirectly through performance, rather
than depending on recollection. Anatomically, the various types of implicit memory appear
to reflect different parts of the brain, depending upon the structures that are necessary for
the relevant processing. While pure amnesic patients typically perform normally across the
whole range of implicit measures, other patients may show differential disruption. Hence
Huntington's disease patients may show problems in motor learning while semantic priming
is intact, whereas patients suffering from Alzheimer's disease show the opposite pattern (see
Chapters 6 and 7, this volume).

   In contrast to the multifarious nature and anatomical location of implicit memory systems, explicit memory appears to depend crucially on a system linking the hippocampi
with the temporal and frontal lobes, the so-called Papez circuit. Tulving (1972) proposed
that explicit memory itself can be divided into two separate systems, *episodic* and *semantic* memory, respectively. The term "episodic memory" refers to our capacity to recollect
specific incidents from the past, remembering incidental detail that allows us in a sense
to relive the event or, as Tulving phrases it, to "travel back in time". We seem to be able
to identify an individual event, presumably by using the context provided by the time and
place it occurred. This means that we can recollect and respond appropriately to a piece
of information, even if it is quite novel and reflects an event that is inconsistent with many
years of prior expectation. Learning that someone had died, for example, could immediately
change our structuring of the world and our response to a question or need, despite years
of experiencing them alive.

Episodic memory can be contrasted with "semantic memory", our generic knowledge of the world; knowing the meaning of the word "salt", for example, or its French equivalent, or its taste. Knowledge of society and the way it functions, and the nature and use of tools are also part of semantic memory, a system that we tend to take for granted, as indeed did psychologists until the late 1960s. At this point, attempts by computer scientists to build machines that could understand text led to the realization of the crucial importance of the capacity of memory to store knowledge. As with other areas of memory, theory has gained substantially from the study of patients with memory deficits in general, and in particular of semantic dementia patients (see Snowden, 2002).

While it is generally accepted that both semantic and episodic memory comprise explicit as opposed to implicit memory systems, the relationship between the two remains controversial. One view suggests that semantic memory is simply the accumulation of many episodic memories for which the detailed contextual cue has disappeared, leaving only the generic features (Squire, 1992). Tulving, on the other hand, suggests that they are separate. He regards the actual experience of recollection as providing the crucial hallmark of episodic memory (Tulving, 1989). It is indeed the case that subjects are able to make consistent and reliable judgements about whether they "remember" an item, in the sense of recollecting the experience of encountering it, or simply "know" that it was presented, and that "remember" items are sensitive to variables such as depth of processing, which have been shown to influence episodic LTM, while "know' responses are not (for review, see Gardiner & Java, 1993). If one accepts Tulving's definition, then this raises the further question of whether there are other types of non-episodic but explicit memory.

Once again, neuropsychological evidence is beginning to accumulate on this issue, particularly from the study of developmental amnesia, a rather atypical form of memory deficit that has recently been discovered to occur in children with hippocampal damage (Vargha-Khadem et al., 2002; Baddeley et al., 2001). Such evidence, combined with a reanalysis of earlier neuropsychological data, coupled with evidence from animal research and from neuroimaging, makes the link between semantic and episodic memory a particularly lively current area of research (see Baddeley et al., 2002b, for a range of recent papers on this topic).

Despite considerable controversy over the details, Figure 1.3 shows what would rather broadly be accepted as reflecting the overall structure of long-term memory. It should be

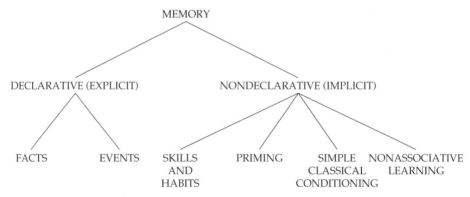

Figure 1.3 The fractionation of long-term memory proposed by Squire. Reproduced from Squire (1992)

adequate for navigating through the subsequent chapters. If you are unfamiliar with memory research, however, there are one or two other things that you might find useful, which are discussed in the sections below.

STAGES OF MEMORY

It is often useful to separate out three aspects of any memory system: *encoding*, the processes whereby information is registered; *storage*, the maintenance of information over time; and *retrieval*, which refers to the accessing of the information by recognition, recall or implicitly by demonstrating that a relevant task is performed more efficiently as a result of prior experience. Encoding is typically studied by varying the nature of the material and/or the way that it is processed during learning. The effect of levels of processing is a good example of this, where processing the visual characteristics of a word leads to a much poorer subsequent recall or recognition than processing it in terms of meaning.

Storage is measured through forgetting. Somewhat surprisingly, although learning is influenced by a wide range of factors that compromise brain function temporarily or permanently, rate of loss of information from memory appears to be relatively insensitive to either patient type, or encoding procedures (Kopelman, 1985). While there have been suggestions that patients whose amnesia stems from damage to the temporal lobes forget at a different rate from those with hippocampal damage (e.g. Huppert & Piercy, 1979), this has not been borne out by subsequent research (Greene et al. 1996; Kopelman, 1985), although it would certainly be premature to conclude that patients never forget more rapidly (see e.g. Kapur *et al.*, 1997).

Given that information has been stored, if it is to be used then it must be retrieved, directly in the case of explicit memory, or indirectly in the case of implicit memory, to have an impact on subsequent performance. The two principal methods of memory retrieval involve recall, in which case the subject is required to reproduce the stimulus items, or recognition. This requires the subject to say whether a given item was presented or not (yes/no recognition) or to choose the previously presented item from a set of two or more alternatives (forced-choice recognition). Yes/no recognition performance will be influenced by the degree of caution the subject applies. By saying "yes" to everything he/she can, of course, correctly categorize all the previously presented targets while not necessarily indicating any memory. Such a subject would of course be discounted, but more subtle differences in the level of caution applied in deciding on whether an item was presented before ("old"), or has just been presented ("new") may also markedly influence performance.

There are a number of procedures for dealing with different degrees of caution among subjects. One is to apply a *guessing correction*, which assumes that the subject guesses on a proportion of the items that are not remembered. On the assumption that the guess is equally likely to be right or wrong, there are likely to be as many items correctly guessed ("hits") as those erroneously classed as "old" ("false alarms"). A guessing correction can then be applied by simply deducting the total number of false alarms from the total hit score. An alternative and slightly more complex way of dealing with the criterion is to utilize *signal detection theory*, which yields two measures, one representing the hypothetical strength of the memory trace, and the other the criterion of degree of caution employed by that subject (Lockhart, 2000). With forced-choice procedures, all subjects are *required always* to choose one item from each set, with the result that degree of caution does not become relevant. In general, recognition is assumed to place a less heavy load on the retrieval processes than recall, where it is necessary not only to discriminate "new" and "old" items but also to produce them.

Probably the simplest recall measure is *free recall*, in which a sequence of items, typically words, is presented, and the subject is required to recall as many as possible in any order he/she wishes. When recall is immediate, the probability of a word being recalled correctly is typically highly dependent on its serial position during presentation, with the first one or two words enjoying a modest advantage (the *primacy effect*), the middle items showing a relatively flat function, and the final words showing the best recall (the *recency effect*). Even though recall is immediate, apart from the recency effect, overall performance in free recall is principally dependent on LTM, with variables such as the imageability, frequency and semantic associability of the words all influencing performance.

A frequent variant of free recall is to use groups of words from the same semantic category; e.g. a 16-item list might have four animals, four flowers, four colours and four professions. Even when they are presented in scrambled order, subjects tend to recall the words in semantic clusters, indicating that they are using meaning as a basis for encoding and retrieval. Such effects become stronger when the same list is repeated for several trials. Indeed, even totally unrelated words will tend to be chunked into clusters that are seen as meaningfully related to the person learning (Tulving and Patkau, 1962). In the case of prose, initial level of recall performance tends to be set in terms of the number of word clusters or chunks, rather than the absolute number of words recalled (Tulving, 1962).

The recency effect tends to follow a very different pattern, being insensitive to a wide range of variables that typically enhance LTM, but to be very sensitive to disruption by a brief subsequent delay filled by an activity such as counting (Glanzer, 1972). The recency effect was, and in some models still is, regarded as representing STM. However, recency effects that broadly follow the same principles can occur over periods of minutes or even days or weeks, as for example in the recall of rugby games played, or parking locations over multiple visits to a laboratory (Baddeley & Hitch, 1977; da Costa Pinto & Baddeley, 1991). It is also the case that a concurrent STM task, such as digit span, leaves the recency effect intact, again suggesting the need for a more complex model (Baddeley & Hitch, 1974). One view is that recency represents an implicit priming mechanism which may operate across a range of different stores, some involving STM, others LTM (for discussion of this view, see Baddeley & Hitch, 1993).

A slightly more complex LTM task involves serial recall, whereby the subject is presented with a sequence of items, typically well beyond memory span, and required to recall them in the order of presentation, with testing continuing either for a standard number of trials or until the subject has completely mastered the sequence. The serial position curve in this case tends to be bowed, with maximum errors somewhere just beyond the middle. This method was used extensively in the 1940s and 1950s, but is less common now.

A popular method of testing LTM is through *paired associate learning*, whereby the subject is required to link together a number of word pairs (e.g. "cow–tree") and is tested by being presented with the stimulus word "cow" and required to produce the response "tree". This technique forms a part of many clinical memory tests, which may contain pairs that fit together readily, such as "cow–milk", together with more arbitrary pairs, such as "dog–cloud". A particular variant of this of course is involved in learning a new vocabulary word in one's own (e.g. "lateen", a kind of sail), or a second language (e.g. "hausrecker", grasshopper). Finally, more complex and realistic material may be used, as in the recall of prose passages or complex visual scenes. These have the advantage of being closer to the environment in which a patient might typically need to use memory. This leads on to a final topic, namely that of everyday memory.

EVERYDAY MEMORY

For over 100 years there has been a tendency for memory research to be pulled in two somewhat different directions. Ebbinghaus (1885) initially demonstrated that memory can be studied objectively by simplifying the remembering task to that of rapidly repeating back sequences of unfamiliar pseudowords, *nonsense syllables*. On the other hand, a more naturalistic approach to psychology was advocated by Galton (1883) and subsequently developed by Bartlett (1932), who required his subjects to recall complex prose passages, often involving unfamiliar material, such as legends from North American Indian culture. Open conflict between these two approaches surfaced more recently with the claim by Neisser (1978) that none of the interesting aspects of memory were being studied by psychologists, evoking a counter-blast from Banaji & Crowder (1989), who claimed that most studies of everday memory were trivial and uninformative. To some extent the controversy was an artificial one, as unfortunately they often are in contemporary psychology. There is no doubt that investigating the detailed nature of memory and producing precise testable models is most readily pursued within the laboratory, with its degree of experimental control. On the other hand, the everyday world and the clinic provide a fruitful source of problems, and a way of testing the generality of laboratory-based theories. A model that can elegantly predict which of two simple responses the subject will make in the laboratory may be of interest to the modelling enthusiast, but unless it can be generalized to more ambitious and important questions, it is unlikely to advance the study of memory. On the other hand, merely observing complex and intriguing phenomena is equally unlikely to generate constructive scientific theory.

There have been two constructive responses to the real world–laboratory dilemma, one being to attempt to generalize laboratory findings to complex real-world situations, and the other being to identify phenomena in everyday life that are not readily accounted for by current memory models. Examples of the first type include the previously described work studying recency effects in the recall of parking locations or rugby games. The attempt to extend laboratory-based recall studies from lists of unrelated words to the oral tradition of memory for songs and poems is another such example (Rubin, 1995).

A good example of identifying a problem in the world that requires solution is that of *prospective memory*, our capacity to remember to do something at a given time or place. It is typically when we forget to do things that we complain that our memories are terrible. But despite its practical importance, it is far from clear how prospective memory works. It certainly does require memory, since amnesic patients tend to be appallingly bad at it, but young intelligent people are often not particularly good at remembering to do things at the right time either. There is clearly an element of motivation, and almost certainly one of strategy, in successful prospective memory. Elderly people tend to forget fewer appointments than the young, partly because they know their memory is vulnerable and find ways to support it, e.g. by writing things down, or by concentrating on the need to remember and constructing internal reminders. Hence, despite making more prospective memory errors than the young under laboratory conditions, in real life they may often make fewer errors.

For long a neglected topic, prospective memory is now a very active one, with studies based on observational and diary measures now supplemented with a range of laboratory-based methods. There is, I suspect, a danger that the more tractable laboratory tasks may come to dominate this area, suggesting the need for a continued attempt to check their validity outside the laboratory. My current suspicion is that prospective memory represents a type of task that we require our memory system to perform, rather than itself reflecting a single memory system or process. That does not, of course, make it any less important or interesting, but does suggest that we are unlikely to reach any simple unitary theoretical solution to the problems it raises.

One area in which the laboratory-based and everyday approaches to memory appear to work effectively together is in the assessment of memory deficits. Traditional measures of memory have tended to rely on classical laboratory techniques, such as paired associate learning and the recall of complex figures, with measures tailored to patient use and then standardized against normal control subjects. However, patients sometimes complain that their problem is not in learning to associate pairs of words or remember complicated figures, but rather in forgetting appointments and failing to remember people's names, or the way around the hospital. Sunderland et al. (1983) decided to check the validity of such standard laboratory-based memory tests against the incidence of memory errors reported by patients and their carers. They tested a group of head-injured patients and subsequently a group of normal elderly subjects (Sunderland et al., 1983, 1986). They found that head injury and age both led to a clear reduction in performance on the standardized tests, together with an increase in memory complaints. However, there was no reliable association between reports of memory errors by the patients or carers and performance on most of the objective tests, with the only task showing a significant correlation being the recall of a prose passage.

Concerned with this problem herself, Barbara Wilson devised a memory test that attempted to capture the range of problems reported most frequently by her patients, whose memory deficits typically resulted from some form of brain injury, most frequently resulting from head injury or cardiovascular accident. She developed the Rivermead Behavioural Memory Test (RMBT), which comprises 12 subcomponents, testing such features as the capacity to memorize and recall a new name, recognition of previously presented unfamiliar faces, and of pictures of objects, recalling a brief prose passage immediately and after a delay, and the immediate and delayed recall of a simple route. The test also involves measures of orientation in time and place, and some simple tests of prospective memory. The RMBT proved sensitive to memory deficits and, in contrast to more conventional methods, correlated well with frequency of memory lapses, as observed by therapists working with the patients over a period of many hours (Wilson et al., 1989). In a study following up a group of amnesic patients several years later, Wilson (1991) found that level of performance on the test accurately predicted capacity to cope independently, in contrast to more conventional measures, such as the Wechsler Memory Scale–Revised.

The strength of the RBMT and of other tests using a similar philosophy, such as the Behavioural Assessment of the Dysexecutive Syndrome Test (Wilson et al., 1996), typically stems from their attempting to provide sensitive objective measures that simulate the real-world problems typically confronting a patient. They are excellent for predicting how well a patient will cope, but should not be regarded as a substitute for tests that attempt to give a precise estimate of the various types of memory function. Such theoretically driven tests are likely to be crucial in understanding the nature of the patient's problems, and hence in providing advice and help (see Chapter 8 on assessment, this volume). It is typically the case, however, that patients feel more comfortable with material that appears to relate to their practical problems, and this has led to a development of a number of theoretically targeted tests that use naturalistic materials. The Doors and People Test of visual and verbal recall and recognition (Baddeley et al., 1994) and the Autobiographical Memory Inventory (Kopelman et al., 1990) are two examples.

CONCLUSION

The psychology of memory has developed enormously since the days when memory was regardèd as a single unitary faculty. The study of patients with memory deficits has played a major role in this development, and seems likely to continue to do so.

REFERENCES

Atkinson, R.C. & Shiffrin, R.M. (1968). Human memory: a proposed system and its control processes. In K.W. Spence (ed.), *The Psychology of Learning and Motivation: Advances in Research and Theory, Vol. 2* (pp. 89–195). New York: Academic Press.

Baddeley, A.D. (1986). *Working Memory*. Oxford: Clarendon Press.

Baddeley, A.D. (1996). Exploring the Central Executive. *Quarterly Journal of Experimental Psychology*, **49A**(1), 5–28.

Baddeley, A.D. (1997). *Human memory: Theory and Practice*, revised edn. Hove: Psychology Press.

Baddeley, A.D. (1999). *Essentials of Human Memory*. Hove: Psychology Press.

Baddeley, A.D. (2000). The episodic buffer: a new component of working memory? *Trends in Cognitive Sciences*, **4**(11), 417–423.

Baddeley, A.D., Aggleton, J.A. & Conway, M.A. (2002b). *Episodic Memory*. Oxford: Oxford University Press.

Baddeley, A.D., Emslie, H. & Nimmo-Smith, I. (1994). *Doors and People: A Test of Visual and Verbal Recall and Recognition*. Bury St. Edmunds: Thames Valley Test Company.

Baddeley, A.D., Gathercole, S.E. & Papagno, C. (1998). The phonological loop as a language learning device. *Psychological Review*, **105**(1), 158–173.

Baddeley, A.D. & Hitch, G.J. (1974). Working memory. In G.A. Bower (ed.), *Recent Advances in Learning and Motivation*, Vol. 8 (pp. 47–89). New York: Academic Press.

Baddeley, A.D., & Hitch, G. (1977). Recency re-examined. In S. Dornic (ed.), *Attention and Performance VI* (pp. 647–667). Hillsdale, NJ Erlbaum.

Baddeley, A.D. & Hitch, G.J. (1993). The recency effect: implicit learning with explicit retrieval? *Memory and Cognition*, **21**, 146–155.

Baddeley, A.D., Kopelman, M.D. & Wilson, B.A. (2002a). *The Handbook of Memory Disorders*, 2nd edn. Chichester: Wiley.

Baddeley, A.D., Vargha-Khadem, F. & Mishkin, M. (2001). Preserved recognition in a case of developmental amnesia: implications for the acquisition of semantic memory. *Journal of Cognitive Neuroscience*, **13**(3), 357–369.

Baddeley, A.D., & Wilson, B. (1988). Frontal amnesia and the dysexecutive syndrome. *Brain and Cognition*, **7**, 212–230.

Baddeley, A.D. & Wilson, B.A. (2002). Prose recall and amnesia: implications for the structure of working memory. *Neuropsychologia*, **40**, 1737–1743.

Banaji, M.R. & Crowder, R.G. (1989). The bankrupcy of everyday memory. *American Psychologist*, **44**, 1185–1193.

Bartlett, F.D. (1932). *Remembering*. Cambridge: Cambridge University Press.

Brooks, D.N. & Baddeley, A.D. (1976). What can amnesic patients learn? *Neuropsychologia*, **14**, 111–122.

Claperède, E. (1911). Recognition et moiité. *Archives de Psychologie*, **11**, 79–90.

Cohen, N.J. & Squire, L.R. (1980). Preserved learning and retention of pattern analyzing skill in amnesia: dissociation of knowing how and knowing what. *Science*, **210**, 207–210.

Corkin, S. (1968). Acquisition of motor skill after bilateral medial temporal lobe excision. *Neuropsychologia*, **6**, 255–265.

Craik, F.I.M. & Lockhart, R.S. (1972). Levels of processing: a framework for memory research. *Journal of Verbal Learning and Verbal Behavior*, **11**, 671–684.

da Costa Pinto, A. & Baddeley, A.D. (1991). Where did you park your car? Analysis of a naturalistic long-term recency effect. *European Journal of Cognitive Psychology*, **3**, 297–313.

Duncan, J. (1996). Attention, intelligence and the frontal lobes. In M. Gazzaniga (ed.), *The Cognitive Neurosciences* (pp. 721–733). Cambridge, MA: MIT Press.

Ebbinghaus, H. (1885). *Über das Gedächtnis*. Leipzig: Dunker.

Galton, F. (1883). *Inquiries into Human Faculty and Its Development* (Everyman edn). London: Dent.

Gardiner, J.M. & Java, R.J. (1993). Recognising and remembering. In A.F. Collins, S.E. Gathercole, M.A. Conway & P.E. Morris (eds), *Theories of Memory* (pp. 163–188). Hove: Erlbaum.

Glanzer, M. (1972). Storage mechanisms in recall. In G.H. Bower (ed.), *The Psychology of Learning and Motivation: Advances in Research and Theory*, Vol. 5. New York: Academic Press.

Greene J.D.W., Baddeley A.D. & Hodges J.R. (1996). Analysis of the episodic memory deficit in early Alzheimer's disease: evidence from the doors and people test. *Neuropsychologia*, **34**(6), 537–551.

Huppert, F.A. & Piercy, M. (1979). Normal and abnormal forgetting in amnesia: effect of locus of lesion. *Cortex*, **15**, 385–390.

Kapur, N., Millar, J. Colbourn, C. et al. (1997). Very long-term amnesia in association with temporal lobe epilepsy: evidence for multiple-stage consolidation processes. *Brain & Cognition*, **35**, 58–70.

Kolodny, J.A. (1994). Memory processes in classification learning—an investigation of amnesic performance in categorisation of dots, patterns and artistic styles. *Psychological Science*, **5**, 164–169.

Kopelman, M.D. (1985). Rates of forgetting in Alzheimer-type dementia and Korsakoff's syndrome. *Neuropsychologia*, **15**, 527–541.

Kopelman, M., Wilson, B.A. & Baddeley, A. (1990). The autobiographical memory interview. Bury St. Edmunds: Thames Valley Test Company.

Lockhart, R.S. (2000). Methods of memory research. In E. Tulving & F.I.M. Craik (eds), *The Oxford Handbook of Memory* (pp. 45–57). Oxford: Oxford University Press.

Miller, G.A. (1956). The magical number seven, plus or minus two: some limits on our capacity for processing information. *Psychological Review*, **63**, 81–97.

Milner, B. (1966). Amnesia following operation on the temporal lobes. In C.W.M. Whitty & O. L. Zangwill (eds), *Amnesia*. London: Butterworth.

Neisser, U. (1978). Memory: what are the important questions? In M.M. Gruneberg, P.E. Morris & R.N. Sykes (eds), *Practical Aspects of Memory*. London: Academic Press.

Norman, D.A. & Shallice, T. (1986). Attention to action: willed and automatic control of behaviour. In R.J. Davidson, G.E. Schwarts & D. Shapiro (eds), *Consciousness and Self-regulation. Advances in Research and Theory, Vol. 4* (pp. 1–18). New York: Plenum.

Parkin, A.J. & Leng, N.R.C. (1993). *Neuropsychology of the Amnesic Syndrome*. Hove: Erlbaum.

Roberts, A.C., Robbins, T.W. & Weiskrantz, L. (1998). *The Prefrontal Cortex: Executive and Cognitive Functions*. Oxford: Oxford University Press.

Rubin, D.C. (1995). *Memory in Oral Traditions: The Cognitive Psychology of Epic Ballads and Counting-out Rhymes*. New York: Oxford University Press.

Schacter, D.L. (1994). Priming and multiple memory systems: perceptual mechanisms of implicit memory. In D.L. Schacter & E. Tulving (eds), *Memory Systems*. Cambridge, MA: MIT Press.

Shallice, T. (1988). *From Neuropsychology to Mental Structure*. Cambridge: Cambridge University Press.

Shallice, T. & Burgess, P. (1996). The domain of supervisory processes and temporal organization of behaviour. *Philosophical Transactions of the Royal Society of London Series B—Biological Sciences*, **351**(1346), 1405–1411.

Shallice, T. & Warrington, E.K. (1970). Independent functioning of verbal memory stores: a neuropsychological study. *Quarterly Journal of Experimental Psychology*, **22**, 261–273.

Snowden, J. (2002). Disorders of semantic memory. In A.D. Baddeley, M.D. Kopelman & B.A. Wilson (eds), *The Handbook of Memory Disorders*, 2nd edn (pp. 293–314). Chichester: Wiley.

Squire, L.R. (1992). Declarative and non-declarative memory: multiple brain systems supporting learning and memory. *Journal of Cognitive Neuroscience*, **4**, 232–243.

Stuss, D. & Knight, R.T. (2002). *Principles of Frontal Lobe Function*. New York: Oxford University Press.

Sunderland, A., Harris, J.E. & Baddeley, A.D. (1983). Do laboratory tests predict everyday memory? *Journal of Verbal Learning and Verbal Behavior*, **22**, 341–357.

Sunderland, A., Watts, K., Harris, J.E. & Baddeley, A.D. (1986). Subjective memory assessment and test performance in the elderly. *Journal of Gerontology*, **41**, 376–385.

Tulving, E. (1962). Subjective organization in free recall of "unrelated" words. *Psychological Review*, **69**, 344–354.

Tulving, E. (1972). Episodic and semantic memory. In E. Tulving & W. Donaldson (eds), *Organization of Memory* (pp. 381–403). New York: Academic Press.

Tulving, E. (1989). Memory: performance, knowledge and experience. *European Journal of Cognitive Psychology*, **1**, 3–26.

Tulving, E. & Craik, F.I.M. (2000). *Handbook of Memory*. Oxford: Oxford University Press.

Tulving, E. & Patkau, J.E. (1962). Concurrent effects of contextual constraint and word frequency on immediate recall and learning of verbal material. *Canadian Journal of Psychology*, **16**, 83–95.

Vallar, G. & Baddeley, A.D. (1984). Fractionation of working memory. Neuropsychological evidence for a phonological short-term store. *Journal of Verbal Learning and Verbal Behaviour*, **23**, 151–161.

Vallar, G. & Papagno, C. (2002). Neuropsychological impairments of verbal short-term memory. In A.D. Baddeley, M.D. Kopelman & B.A. Wilson (eds), *The Handbook of Memory Disorders*, 2nd edn (pp. 249–270). Chichester: Wiley.

Vargha-Khadem, F., Gadian, D. & Mishkin, M. (2002). Dissociations in cognitive memory: the syndrome of developmental amnesia. In A. Baddeley, M. Conway & J. Aggleton (eds), *Episodic Memory* (pp. 153–163). Oxford: Oxford University Press.

Warrington, E.K. & Weiskrantz, L. (1968). New methods of testing long-term retention with special reference to amnesic patients. *Nature*, **217**, 972–974.

Wechsler, D. (1987). *Wechsler Memory Scale—Revised*. San Antonio, TX: The Psychological Corporation.

Wilson, B.A. (1991). Long-term prognosis of patients with severe memory disorders. *Neuropsychological Rehabilitation*, **1**, 117–134.

Wilson, B.A., Alderman, N., Burgess, P. et al. (1996). Behavioural assessment of the dysexecutive syndrome. Bury St Edmunds: Thames Valley Test Company.

Wilson, B., Cockburn, J., Baddeley, A. & Hiorns, R. (1989). The development and validation of a test battery for detecting and monitoring everyday memory problems. *Journal of Clinical and Experimental Neuropsychology*, **11**, 855–870.

CHAPTER 2

The Amnesic Syndrome: Overview and Subtypes

Margaret O'Connor

Beth Israel Deaconess Medical Center, Boston, MA, USA

and

Mieke Verfaellie

Memory Disorders Research Center, Boston, MA, USA

Global amnesia refers to a dense and circumscribed deficit in memory in the context of otherwise preserved intelligence. It encompasses the acquisition of events and facts encountered postmorbidly (anterograde amnesia), as well as the retrieval of information acquired premorbidly (retrograde amnesia). Patients with amnesia are capable of holding a limited amount of information in mind for a very brief period of time, but with increased retention interval or increased interference, their recall and recognition of the information inevitably fails. Anterograde amnesia is usually global, in that memory for all new information is affected—regardless of the nature of the information (i.e. verbal or nonverbal) or the modality in which it is presented (i.e. auditory or visual). In most patients, anterograde amnesia is associated with some degree of retrograde loss, although its extent is more variable. The reverse, however, is not necessarily the case, as some patients have been described who demonstrate relatively focal retrograde amnesia in the absence of anterograde memory loss (Kapur, 1993; Kopelman, 2000).

Although amnesia is characterized by a pervasive and devastating memory loss, it is important to note that some components of memory remain intact. Amnesic patients demonstrate normal performance on tasks of immediate memory and working memory (Cave & Squire, 1992; Parkin & Leng, 1993). This ability to hold and manipulate information "on-line" is critical for performance on a variety of cognitive tasks, ranging from language comprehension to simple arithmetic. Patients with amnesia are also able to retrieve overlearned semantic memories, as evidenced by the fact that their general world knowledge and knowledge of word meanings remains intact. Finally, even within the domain of new learning, some forms of memory are preserved. These include skill learning, classical conditioning and repetition priming, the bias or facilitation in processing a stimulus that results from prior exposure to that same or related stimulus (Squire et al., 1993). These forms of memory have in common the fact that knowledge can be expressed without a need for

The Essential Handbook of Memory Disorders for Clinicians. Edited by A.D. Baddeley, M.D. Kopelman and B.A. Wilson.
© 2004 John Wiley & Sons, Ltd. ISBN 0-470-09141-X.

conscious recollection, and without awareness of the episode in which learning took place. The dissociation between aware (declarative) and unaware (procedural) memory in patients with global amnesia has guided much research into the neural and functional organization of various components of memory (e.g. Gabrieli, 1999; Verfaellie & Keane, 2001).

The memory problem of the amnesic individual must be differentiated from more common forms of memory loss. In order for an individual to be diagnosed with amnesia, there must be evidence of a marked learning deficit and this problem must exist in relative isolation, so that other aspects of cognition remain intact. The severity of the learning deficit is the cardinal feature distinguishing amnesia from milder memory problems, such as those associated with age-related memory decline, depression or developmental learning difficulties. The preservation of attention, working memory and general reasoning abilities differentiate the amnesic patient from the patient who has memory problems in the context of global cognitive decline (e.g. dementia or delirium). It is noteworthy that some amnesics have superior cognitive abilities, a fact that underscores the relative independence of memory and intelligence (e.g. Cermak & O'Connor, 1983). Other amnesic patients show modest reductions on measures of verbal intelligence, but this decline can sometimes reflect decrements in semantic memory (e.g. Stefanacci et al., 2000).

Many clinical and theoretical insights into global amnesia find their origin in the study of patient H.M., a man who became amnesic following bilateral resection of the temporal lobes for treatment of refractory epilepsy (Scoville & Milner, 1957). Although H.M. still serves as a benchmark for characterizing amnesia, it has also become clear that the syndrome is functionally heterogeneous, comprising a number of different patterns of memory loss and associated processing deficits, which may be linked to distinct etiologies and associated patterns of neuroanatomical damage. In addition, it should be kept in mind that premorbid factors, such as baseline intelligence and personality style, can influence a patient's clinical presentation, as may associated neurocognitive problems.

Global amnesia occurs as a result of damage to the medial temporal lobes, the diencephalon and the basal forebrain. Such damage can be caused by a broad array of traumatic, vascular and infectious disease processes, the most common of which are anoxia, encephalitis, cerebrovascular accidents, Korsakoff syndrome and rupture and repair of anterior communicating artery aneurysms. In these conditions, amnesia is usually of a permanent nature. Transient forms of amnesia also occur secondary to seizure activity or temporary disruption of the vascular supply (see Goldenberg, 2002). In what follows, we first review the main etiologies leading to permanent amnesia and their associated neuropsychological profiles. We next consider to what extent each of the main brain regions implicated in amnesia causes a distinct pattern of processing deficits.

NEUROLOGICAL CONDITIONS ASSOCIATED WITH AMNESIA

ENCEPHALITIS

Herpes simplex encephalitis (HSE) occurs as a result of virus-induced hemorrhagic lesions in the brain. In the early stages of the infectious process, patients experience a "flu-like" illness that is often associated with fever, headaches and lethargy. Profound confusion and disorientation may follow and patients often develop other neurocognitive problems, including aphasia, agnosia and amnesia. For some patients these problems persist so that a broad array of cognitive abilities is compromised. For others, disorientation may be followed by complete recovery. A third group of patients presents with focal memory disturbances in the absence of other cognitive deficits. These are the patients who have been of particular interest to memory researchers, because they typically present with very dense amnesic syndromes, quite similar to that of patient H.M. (e.g. Cermak, 1976; Damasio et al., 1985a; Stefanacci et al., 2000).

Like the clinical presentation, the neuroanatomical damage associated with encephalitis is heterogeneous, but typically centers on limbic regions in the temporal lobe, including the hippocampus and adjacent entorhinal, perirhinal and parahippocampal cortices, the amygdala and polar limbic cortices. Damage frequently also extends laterally, resulting in varying degrees of damage to the anterolateral and inferior aspects of the temporal neocortex. Extension of the lesion anteriorly can result in damage to ventromedial areas, such as the insular cortex and basal forebrain (Damasio & Van Hoesen, 1985).

S.S., a patient we have followed for many years, experienced dense memory loss as a result of HSE (Cermak, 1976; Cermak & O'Connor, 1983). S.S.'s initial presentation was noteworthy for lethargy and headaches followed by a 1 month coma. In the acute stage of his illness, S.S. was aphasic and hemiparetic, but these problems resolved and he was left with a dense amnesia associated with bilateral lesions in anterolateral and medial portions of the temporal lobes, the insula and the putamen. S.S.'s anterograde amnesia is profound. He has not been able to form any new declarative memories for the last three decades. He has not retained any episodic information regarding important family matters and is totally unaware of recent public facts or events. He has also failed to acquire any new semantic knowledge. Strikingly, he has not learned any novel vocabulary introduced into the English language since the onset of his illness, even though he has been exposed to these words repeatedly through television programs and newspapers (Verfaellie et al., 1995a). S.S. also has a very extensive retrograde memory loss for autobiographical as well as personal semantic information that encompasses most of his adult life. Despite this dense amnesia, S.S. is of superior intelligence. Even at age 70, 30 years after the onset of his amnesia, he has a Full Scale IQ of 130. He continues to perform in the superior range on tasks of working memory, frontal/executive abilities, language and deductive reasoning skills. Like other amnesic patients who have suffered encephalitis, S.S. has insight into his memory loss, a fact that is likely due to the relative preservation of frontal brain regions.

As with all amnesic etiologies, there are variations in the severity of memory loss. While some patients may be totally unable to benefit from repeated exposure to new material or to benefit from extended study time, others are able gradually to acquire a limited amount of information (e.g. Haslam et al., 1997). This likely reflects the extent of medial temporal damage (Stefanacci et al., 2000). Lesions may be asymmetrical and, as expected, the laterality of lesion affects the nature of the neurobehavioral presentation. Greater damage to right temporal regions has a more pronounced effect on nonverbal/visual memory, such as memory for faces and spatial aspects of stimuli (Eslinger et al., 1993), while disproportionate damage to left temporal regions has a more pronounced effect on verbal memory (Tranel et al., 2000).

The distribution of the encephalitis-induced lesion also affects the nature and severity of the remote memory loss. Patients with extensive retrograde amnesia typically have lesions extending into lateral temporal regions (Damasio et al., 1985a; O'Connor et al., 1992; Stefanacci et al., 2000). Damasio and colleagues attribute the profound loss of remote memories in these patients to the destruction of convergence zones in anterior temporal areas (Tranel et al., 2000). Asymmetrical patterns of damage can result in distinct patterns of remote memory loss. Several case studies have indicated that damage to right anterior temporal regions severely interferes with retrieval of autobiographical memories (O'Connor et al., 1992; Ogden, 1993). Patient L.D., who has been studied extensively by our group, demonstrated a dramatic loss of personal episodic memories, whereas her knowledge of semantic aspects of past memories was preserved. This dissociation took place in the context of pervasive damage to her right temporal lobe vs. much more restricted damage to her left temporal lobe. L.D.'s remote memory was evaluated using various tests of autobiographical memory and public events. Her recollection of personal experiences from childhood years was devastated: she was unable to produce any episodic memories of personal events in response to verbal cues or upon directed questioning. Interestingly, L.D. demonstrated better recall of factually based information (e.g. the name of her first grade teacher, the fact that she owned a poodle). However, she was unable to elaborate upon these facts with experiential information. L.D.'s nonverbal memory and visual imaging problems were examined in relation to her pronounced episodic memory impairment. It was hypothesized that L.D.'s nonverbal memory and imaging deficits augmented her autobiographical memory impairment because visual images provide an organizational framework for retrieval of experiential information.

The reverse pattern, a disproportionate loss of semantic knowledge, occurs in the context of mainly left temporal cortex damage. An illustrative case is that of patient L.P., described by De Renzi and colleagues (1987a). Following an episode of encephalitis, L.P. demonstrated greatly impoverished knowledge of the meaning and attributes of words and pictures. She was severely anomic and unable to define or classify either verbal concepts or their pictorial referents, while non-semantic aspects of language and perception were preserved. Her lesion was centered in the anterior inferotemporal cortex. While L.P. demonstrated semantic difficulties for all types of information, other patients have been described with category-specific deficits. Although such category-specific impairments are rare, a number of cases have been described with differential impairments for concrete vs. abstract concepts, and for animate vs. inanimate concepts (for review, see McKenna & Warrington, 2000).

Anoxia

Anoxic brain injury occurs as a result of reduced oxygen to the brain, due to decreased vascular perfusion or reduced oxygen content in the blood. This may be caused by a variety of conditions, such as cardiac arrest or respiratory distress, which in turn may be a result of severe allergic reactions, strangulation or near-drowning episodes. When the brain is deprived of oxygen, excitatory neurotransmitters are released which are accompanied by increased sodium, cell swelling and neuronal damage. Persistent oxygen deprivation leads to neuronal excitation, which results in increased calcium, and to increased free radicals—events that cause significant cell damage (Caine & Watson, 2000). Specific brain areas are vulnerable to anoxic injury, in part due to their physical location and in part due to their biochemical make-up. Peripheral blood vessels are particularly sensitive to reductions in oxygenation (Brierley & Graham, 1984). Also sensitive to damage are areas with high metabolic demands (Moody et al., 1990). In addition, the neurochemical properties of particular areas render them more vulnerable than others to changes in oxygen content. For instance, the hippocampus is vulnerable to oxygen deprivation due to the neurotoxic effects of excessive release of glutamate and aspartate (Caine & Watson, 2000). It is of interest that anoxic damage affects different parts of the brain over different time courses. While the basal ganglia and cerebral cortex are affected shortly after the anoxic event, hippocampal damage may not occur until days after the initial insult (Kuroiwa & Okeda, 1994; Levine & Grek, 1984).

Studies have shown that initial markers of anoxic insult, such as mental status examination, length of coma and laboratory tests, do not necessarily correlate with long-term indices of behavioral outcome and neuropathological change. Hopkins and colleagues (1995) studied three patients who were severely impaired during the early stage of recovery from anoxia but who presented with very different clinical outcomes. A recent review of 58 studies of cerebral anoxia (Caine & Watson, 2000) discussed the range of neuropathological and neuropsychological outcomes associated with this etiology. This review indicated that the watershed zone of the cerebral cortex and basal ganglia structures are the most common sites of damage. Damage to hippocampal structures was also common, although isolated damage to the hippocampus was seen in only 18% of the cases.

One well-documented example of amnesia following anoxia-induced hippocampal damage is that of patient R.B. (Zola-Morgan et al., 1986). R.B.'s clinical presentation was noteworthy for moderate-level learning difficulties alongside mild remote memory loss covering just a few years preceding the anoxic event. Neuropathological studies revealed that R.B. sustained bilateral damage limited to the CA1 area of the hippocampus. Several other cases of amnesia secondary to anoxia have come to autopsy since then (Rempel-Clower et al., 1996). More extensive lesions beyond CA1, but still limited to the hippocampal formation, appear to produce more severe anterograde memory impairment as well as extensive retrograde amnesia covering up to 15 years or more.

Recently, Vargha-Khadem and colleagues (Gadian et al., 2000; Vargha-Khadem et al., 1997) have drawn attention to the fact that anoxic episodes shortly after birth can lead to a relatively selective form of developmental amnesia. Their most recent report concerned a group of five young patients with amnesia, none of whom demonstrated other signs of neurological dysfunction. Detailed imaging studies confirmed selective bilateral hippocampal atrophy in all cases. Neuropsychological test findings revealed that all of the children performed deficiently on tasks of episodic memory, whereas attention, reasoning abilities and visuospatial skills were intact. Strikingly, these children were able to acquire a considerable amount of new semantic knowledge, as indicated by the fact that they were successfully able to attend mainstream schools. Vargha-Khadem et al. (1997) argued that semantic learning was mediated by preserved subhippocampal cortical areas, including entorhinal and perirhinal cortex. We have recently observed a similar, albeit less striking, dissociation between semantic and episodic learning in P.S., a patient with adult-onset amnesia secondary to anoxic injury (Verfaellie et al., 2000). In line with Vargha-Khadem et al., we ascribed this pattern to relative preservation of subhippocampal cortices.

Although there is clear evidence that anoxia-induced amnesia can result from hippocampal damage (e.g. patient R.B.), it is important to note that damage is not always selective and that lesions often extend beyond the hippocampus to involve other brain areas. Markowitsch et al. (1997) studied a patient with anoxia secondary to a heart attack, in whom PET imaging revealed widespread regions of hypoactivity that could not be predicted from the structural neuroimaging findings. In another study, Reed and colleagues (1999) described thalamic hypometabolism in addition to hippocampal atrophy in a group of four hypoxic patients.

As the review by Caine & Watson (2000) indicates, the neuropathology associated with anoxia is often more widespread, involving the basal ganglia, the thalamus, white matter projections and diffuse cortical areas. Accordingly, many patients present with more generalized cognitive deficits. A number of studies have shown that anoxia is associated with significant changes in frontal/executive abilities, so that the individual's capacities for complex attention (i.e. mental tracking and cognitive flexibility), planning and abstract thinking are compromised (Bengtsson et al., 1969; Volpe & Hirst, 1983). Some patients with extensive posterior neocortical damage have shown visual recognition problems, including prosopagnosia and visual object agnosia (Parkin et al., 1987). Although most anoxic patients present with normal language abilities, there are reports of patients who present with name retrieval difficulties (Bengtsson et al., 1969; Parkin et al., 1987). Tranel and colleagues (2000) have described a patient with diminished lexical and semantic knowledge of concrete items. Other possible sequelae of anoxic brain injury are marked changes in personality, with increased emotional lability and irritability (McNeill et al., 1965), reduced capacity for empathy (Reich et al., 1983) or apathy (Parkin et al., 1987).

Wernicke–Korsakoff Syndrome

Patients with Wernicke–Korsakoff Syndrome (WKS) develop amnesia as a result of the convergent effects of chronic alcohol abuse and malnutrition (Victor et al., 1989). The onset of WKS is usually marked by an acute phase in which the patient is disoriented, confused and apathetic, and unable to maintain a coherent conversation. This confusional state is often accompanied by occulomotor problems and ataxia. Traditionally, this triad of neurological signs was a prerequisite for a diagnosis of Wernicke's encephalopathy, but it is now clear that these problems do not necessarily co-occur in a single patient (Harper et al., 1986). More recently, it has been suggested that the diagnosis of Wernicke's encephalopathy should be based on at least two of the following criteria: (a) dietary deficiencies; (b) occulomotor abnormalities; (c) cerebellar dysfunction; and (d) altered mental status (Caine et al., 1997).

Once the acute confusion clears, the patient is typically left with an enduring dense amnesia, characteristic of the Korsakoff stage of the disorder. Although some patients have been described to recover to a premorbid level of functioning, this is a rare occurrence. Because of considerable variability in its presentation, Wernicke's encephalopathy may at times go unrecognized until autopsy (Harper et al., 1986). Indeed, some patients may evolve to the Korsakoff stage of the disorder without clinical evidence of an antecedent Wernicke encephalopathy.

Neuroanatomical studies of WKS patients have highlighted damage in thalamic nuclei, the mammillary bodies and frontal network systems (Mair et al., 1979; Victor et al., 1989). For many years there was a great deal of controversy regarding the relative contributions of damage to specific thalamic nuclei vs. damage to the mammillary bodies in the etiology of amnesia in this patient group. Many studies were confounded by the poor operational criteria for diagnosis of Korsakoff's syndrome and also by use of inadequate control groups. Chronic alcoholism and Wernicke's encephalopathy cause damage to the entire brain (Kril et al., 1997) and may result in neurodegeneration in specific regions, including the basal forebrain, prefrontal cortex, mammillary nuclei and mediodorsal thalamic nuclei (Cullen et al., 1997; Harding et al., 2000). Hence, inclusion of nonamnesic alcoholics and patients with Wernicke's encephalopathy is necessary in order to examine the neural substrates necessary and sufficient to cause amnesia in the Korsakoff group. A recent comparison (Harding et al., 2000) of Korsakoff patients, patients with Wernicke's encephalopathy and nonamnesic alcoholic controls revealed shared pathology in the hypothalamic mammillary nuclei and in the mediodorsal thalamic nuclei. However, neuronal loss in the anterior thalamic nuclei was found only in the Korsakoff group. The authors therefore concluded that damage to the anterior nucleus of the thalamus is necessary for the amnesic disorder in WKS. Although less emphasis has been placed on the role of hippocampal damage in WKS, several studies have documented hippocampal pathology as well (Jernigan et al., 1991; Sullivan, 2001). However, this is not an invariant finding and other investigators have found that WKS patients do not have reduced medial temporal lobe volume (Colchester et al., 2001). In fact, the latter study documented a double dissociation between WKS and HSE patients: WKS patients demonstrated reduced volume in thalamic structures but no significant atrophy in medial temporal lobe structures, whereas HSE patients showed the reverse pattern.

Patients with WKS amnesia have profound and global learning difficulties that have been viewed as a consequence of increased sensitivity to interference. Patients are able to repeat information in the absence of any delay, but given distracting activity for as little as 9 s, performance can be markedly impaired. Some information may be learned on an initial learning trial, but on subsequent trials marked deficits occur because of interference from information that was presented earlier. Historically, several explanations were proposed for this sensitivity to interference. Butters & Cermak (1980) emphasized the role of superficial and deficient encoding strategies. When left to their own devices, WKS patients process the phonemic and structural aspects of incoming information, rather than more meaningful semantic attributes (Biber et al., 1981; Cermak & Reale, 1978). Others pointed to patients' inability to inhibit competition from irrelevant material at the time of retrieval (Warrington & Weiskrantz, 1970, 1973). More recently, a consensus has emerged that considers the interaction between encoding and retrieval processes as being critical for a full understanding of WKS patients' learning deficit (Verfaellie & Cermak, 1991).

In addition to anterograde amnesia, WKS patients present with a severe retrograde amnesia that is "temporally graded", in that memories from the more recent decades (leading up to the onset of WKS) are more severely affected than very remote memories. There has been controversy regarding the cause of this temporally graded retrograde amnesia. Some investigators conjectured that social deprivation and deficient learning of information in the decades leading up to the onset of WKS contributed to the pattern of impairment (Albert et al., 1981; Cohen & Squire, 1981). However, this interpretation was called into question by the study of P.Z. (Butters & Cermak, 1986), an eminent scientist who had just completed his autobiography prior to the onset of WKS. P.Z.'s writings and his daily log provided comprehensive records regarding his experiences and his knowledge of events that occurred a short while before the onset of his amnesia. P.Z. demonstrated a temporally graded loss for material mentioned in his autobiography. Likewise, he showed a temporally graded loss for knowledge of scientific information that he clearly knew before the onset of amnesia, as indicated by his publications and lecture notes. Thus, it was certain that P.Z.'s temporally graded retrograde amnesia was not due to progressive anterograde memory loss secondary to alcohol abuse. Instead, it was suggested that this pattern might be due to the fact that information from different time periods taps qualitatively different forms of memory. Information from the recent past, which is still anchored in time and space, may tap primarily episodic memory, whereas remote information, which has been rehearsed more frequently, may tap primarily semantic memory. According to this view, a temporally graded pattern would suggest that episodic memories are more vulnerable to disruption in WKS than are semantic memories. Recent evidence, however, suggests that memory for semantic information acquired prior to the onset of amnesia is also impaired in WKS and shows a similar temporal gradient (Verfaellie et al., 1995b). It appears, therefore, that more recent memories, regardless of their episodic or semantic nature, are more vulnerable to disruption than are more remote memories.

We have followed a group of over 20 WKS patients over the last two decades. All of them had significant anterograde amnesia that undermined their management of daily affairs. All demonstrated greatly impaired performance on standard tasks of delayed recall and recognition. However, we have observed variability among patients with regard to how quickly information is lost from memory. Most patients showed deficits on tasks of working memory, such as the Brown–Peterson paradigm (i.e. recall of three items over 0–18 s distractor intervals), whereas several WKS patients demonstrated superior perfor-mance on this task. Even though recall has been invariably deficient in our WKS group, in some patients recognition has benefited considerably from extended exposure. Patients have also varied with respect to other aspects of their neuropsychological profiles, such as confab-ulation, perseveration and executive dysfunction. These latter tendencies are likely linked to frontal brain damage. Whether these tendencies are central features of the WKS syndrome or whether they represent additive neurotoxic effects of alcohol is not certain. Our group of WKS patients vary markedly in their social and psychological dispositions. Many are prone to apathy and low motivation, problems that compound their memory deficits. In addition, there is a great deal of heterogeneity with respect to general intellectual abilities—many, but not all, WKS patients are from educationally deprived backgrounds. Limited academic exposure may confound assessment of baseline intelligence.

Cerebrovascular Accidents

Bilateral posterior cerebral artery (PCA) infarction is a well-recognized cause of amnesia. Because the left and right PCA's originate from a common source, strokes in the posterior circulation system often affect the temporal lobes bilaterally (including the posterior aspect of the hippocampal complex) and may result in severe memory deficits (Benson et al., 1974). Neuroanatomical studies of patients who have suffered PCA infarctions have underscored lesions in the posterior parahippocampus or collateral isthmus (a pathway connecting the posterior parahippocampus to association cortex) as critical in the memory disturbance (Von Cramon et al., 1988). When the lesion extends posteriorly to include occipitotemporal cortices, deficits beyond amnesia are often seen.

As far back as 1900 a patient was described who exhibited severe memory loss in asso-ciation with bilateral infarction of the PCA (Bechterew, 1900). Since then numerous case reports have documented significant memory disturbances in patients who have suffered similar damage (Benson et al., 1974; Victor et al., 1961). In the early phase of recovery from PCA infarction, patients present with global confusion. This may subsequently resolve into an isolated amnesic syndrome or may be associated with other neuropsychological deficits, such as visual field defects, alexia, color agnosia and anomia (Benson et al., 1974). The memory disturbance of these patients adheres to the classic amnesic profile of consolidation deficits in the context of normal working memory and normal intelligence. Some PCA patients have retrograde memory problems but this is not an invariant feature of the syndrome. Some patients who have suffered PCA infarctions have presented with unusual memory problems. Ross (1980) described the neuropsychological profiles of two patients who sustained bilateral PCA strokes, both of whom had isolated deficits in the domain of visual memory. Their memory for tactile, verbal and nonverbal auditory information remained intact. Imaging studies revealed that both patients had sustained bilateral occipital lobe infarctions and bilateral lesions involving deep white matter in occipital and temporal lobes. Neither patient had lesions in medial temporal areas. The patients' sensory-specific amnesic syndromes were viewed as a consequence of a disconnection between striate cortices involved in visual processing and temporal brain regions involved in learning and memory.

While the majority of cases of amnesia secondary to infarction have involved bilateral hippocampal damage, memory problems have also been described in association with unilateral (primarily left) PCA infarction (Geschwind & Fusillo, 1966; Mohr et al., 1971; Ott & Saver, 1993; Von Cramon et al., 1988). In some of the unilateral PCA patients, the memory deficit has been transient (Geschwind & Fusillo, 1966), whereas permanent memory loss has been present in others (Mohr et al., 1971). Though many of these patients have been labeled "amnesic", there is scant documentation of the extent and nature of their memory problems. Many investigations of patients who sustained unilateral PCA infarction have failed to assess both verbal and nonverbal memory and have not included tests sensitive to rate of forgetting. Consequently, it has been difficult to determine whether the memory deficits of unilateral PCA patients are qualitatively and quantitatively similar to those of other amnesic patients.

One of the more comprehensive studies of patients with left PCA infarction was conducted by De Renzi and colleagues (1987b), who described the neuropsychological profile of 16 PCA patients with damage to left occipitotemporal brain areas. These patients presented with pure alexia, visual naming problems and verbal amnesia. The reading and naming problems were attributed to a disconnection of posterior (occipital) regions from left hemisphere language zones. The most common problem encountered by these patients was verbal amnesia, presumably related to damage in left medial temporal areas. The mnestic abilities of right PCA patients have not been well studied. Von Cramon and colleagues (1988) noted that verbal memory remained intact in 10 right PCA patients, whereas the visual processing abilities of these patients were impaired. Tests of visual memory were not administered as part of the study. Likewise, Goldenberg & Artner (1991) reported that unilateral right PCA infarction may be associated with perceptual discrimination problems but the memory abilities of the patients were not examined.

Thalamic strokes have also been associated with amnesia, although the severity of the memory deficit varies in relation to the site of damage within the thalamus (Graff-Radford et al., 1990; Von Cramon et al., 1985). The small size and close proximity of thalamic nuclei (Jones, 1985) limits analyses based on lesion location. Nonetheless, some conditions, such as lacunar infarctions, result in more spatially restricted lesions in the thalamus, and therefore provide valuable information regarding the differential contributions of specific thalamic nuclei in memory processes.

A recent review (Van der Werf et al., 2000) of 60 patients who sustained damage to the thalamus as a result of infarctions revealed that damage to the mammillo–thalamic tract (MTT) was necessary and sufficient for anterograde amnesia. Since this tract contains fibers bound for the anterior thalamic nucleus, it is to be expected that infarctions that directly affect the anterior nucleus can produce similar deficits.

Others have focused on the role of the medial dorsal nucleus in the memory disturbance of patients who have suffered thalamic strokes. Several patients have been described who demonstrated amnesia following discrete medial dorsal lesions (Isaac et al., 2000; Speedie & Heilman, 1982, 1983), but in other cases of medial dorsal damage, no evidence of a memory impairment was apparent (Kritchevsky et al., 1987; Von Cramon et al., 1985). Based on their review, Van der Werf et al. (2000) concluded that medial dorsal lesions may lead to mild memory disturbances, but that severe amnesia is typically associated with lesions that extend beyond the medial dorsal nucleus to include the MTT or anterior nucleus.

As is to be expected, thalamic amnesia shares many characteristics with the amnesia associated with Korsakoff's syndrome. Patients demonstrate a severe anterograde memory deficit, characterized by increased sensitivity to interference. Impairments in executive functioning frequently accompany the mnestic disturbance (Isaac et al., 2000; Pepin & Auray-Pepin, 1993; Speedie & Heilman, 1982). Deficits in retrograde amnesia also occur in conjunction with thalamic amnesia, but studies have shown that there is variability with respect to the persistence and extent of remote memory loss. In some thalamic patients, retrograde amnesia was seen during the early phases of recovery, but this subsequently resolved (Kapur et al., 1996; Winocur et al., 1984). In other patients, more severe, persistent retrograde deficits were observed (Hodges & McCarthy, 1993; Stuss et al., 1988). Material-specific memory deficits have also been described in association with unilateral thalamic stroke: left-sided damage results in memory deficits on tasks of verbal learning (Sandson et al., 1991; Speedie & Heilman, 1982), whereas right-sided thalamic damage results in nonverbal/visual memory difficulties (Speedie & Heilman, 1983).

Aneurysm Rupture of the Anterior Communicating Artery (ACoA)

Intracranial aneurysms throughout the circle of Willis can result in severe memory problems (Richardson, 1989) but most of the neuropsychological studies over the past few decades have focused on patients who develop amnesia secondary to anterior communicating artery (AcoA) aneuryms. The ACoA and its branches perfuse the basal forebrain, the anterior cingulate, the anterior hypothalamus, the anterior columns of the fornix, the anterior commissure and the genu of the corpus callosum. The behavioral deficits observed following ACoA aneurysm may be a result of infarction, either directly or secondary to subarachnoid hemorrhage, vasospasm and hematoma formation (Alexander & Freedman, 1984; Damasio et al., 1985b).

Because of the various neuropathological sequelae, the cognitive disorders resulting from rupture of ACoA aneurysms are more variable than those seen following diencephalic or medial temporal damage and may be more global in nature (for review, see DeLuca & Diamond, 1995). Nonetheless, memory deficits are often the primary presenting symptom and may range from relatively mild impairments to significant amnesia. Here, we focus on the moderate to severe end of the spectrum of memory disorders to facilitate comparison with other subtypes of amnesia.

In the acute phase of the disorder, patients typically present with a severe confusional state and gross attentional disturbances. When the confusional state clears, significant deficits in new learning become apparent. Patients may be disoriented to time, and there is often a severe retrograde amnesia that appears temporally graded. Confabulation and lack of insight may also occur, especially in patients with additional frontal lobe lesions (D'Esposito et al., 1996; DeLuca, 1993). D'Esposito et al. (1996) observed that executive dysfunction in the early stages of illness was much greater in patients whose lesion extended into the medial frontal lobes than in those whose lesion was restricted to the basal forebrain. Additionally, patients with frontal lesions had more severe retrograde amnesia. Their executive dysfunction and remote memory loss improved significantly by 3 months post-onset, but remained worse than that seen in patients with focal basal forebrain lesions. Anterograde memory loss, however, persisted in both groups and was of equal severity.

During the chronic phase, most patients show preserved immediate memory, as measured by Digit Span Forwards (e.g. Delbecq-Derouesne et al., 1990; DeLuca, 1992; Parkin et al., 1988), but working memory deficits are not uncommon. Several studies have documented impaired performance on the Brown–Peterson distractor paradigm (Corkin et al., 1985; Delbecq-Derouesne et al., 1990; DeLuca, 1992; Parkin et al., 1988; Talland et al., 1967). This impairment may be due to a susceptibility to interference that affects both working memory and long-term memory performance.

The anterograde memory performance of ACoA patients is characterized by severe deficits in recall, especially following a delay, while performance on recognition tasks is often much better preserved. Volpe & Hirst (1983) first drew attention to this pattern, and it has been confirmed in several subsequent studies (Beeckmans et al., 1998; Hanley et al., 1994; Parkin et al., 1988). The disproportionate impairment in recall reflects a disruption of strategic search processes that enable access to information stored in memory.

Not all ACoA patients, however, show a sparing of recognition memory. Particularly striking is the report by Derousne-Delbecque et al. (1990) of a patient whose recognition memory was more severely impaired than his recall. This pattern arose because of the patient's high tendency to produce false alarms in recognition tests. Since then, a number of other patients have been described who show pathological levels of false recognition (Beeckmans et al., 1998; Parkin et al., 1990; Rapscak et al., 1998). This problem is thought to reflect a disruption in the processes that evaluate the outcome of a memory search.

Strategic memory processes are not only important for memory retrieval; they also support adequate encoding of information. In light of the "executive" nature of the memory impairment seen in ACoA patients, it is not surprising to see evidence of inefficient encoding as well. In at least some cases, however, patients' encoding can be supported by the use of strategies. For instance, Parkin et al. (1988) described a patient who performed very poorly when asked to learn paired associates by rote, but whose performance was dramatically improved when given instructions to use imagery to aid encoding. Along the same lines, Diamond et al. (1997) found that in a subgroup of ACoA patients, recall of the Rey Complex Figure could be greatly enhanced by providing an organizational strategy for encoding details of the figure.

ACoA patients also exhibit striking contextual memory deficits. Several studies have demonstrated disproportionate deficits in spatial memory (Mayes et al., 1991; Shoqeirat & Mayes, 1991) and in memory for source (Parkin et al., 1988). Deficits in temporal tagging have also been emphasized (Damasio et al, 1985b; Ptak & Schnider, 1999). Whether these deficits are part of a core basal forebrain amnesia or result from associated frontal deficits remains unclear at present.

It has been difficult to isolate the minimal lesion necessary to cause amnesia in ACoA patients, in part because of clip artifact during scanning. Irle and colleagues (1992) suggested that lesions extending beyond the basal forebrain to include the striatum or frontal regions were necessary to cause amnesia. A number of studies, however, have documented severe amnesia in patients with circumscribed basal forebrain lesions. In several cases lesions have been centered in the septal nuclei (Alexander & Freedman, 1984; Von Cramon et al., 1993) but the nucleus accumbens has also been implicated (Goldenberg et al., 1999). Because several basal forebrain nuclei contain a large number of cholinergic neurons that innervate the hippocampus as well as large sectors of neocortex, the amnesia of ACoA patients may be due, at least in some cases, to disruption of hippocampal functioning caused by basal forebrain damage (Volpe et al., 1984).

SUBTYPES OF AMNESIA

Amnesic patients present with a variety of medical and psychosocial conditions. One approach to dealing with this variability has been to search for specific patterns of memory loss in relation to etiology of amnesia or location of neural damage. A number of investigators have compared the amnesic profiles of patients classified according to site of neural damage (Butters et al., 1984; Huppert & Piercy, 1979; Lhermitte & Signoret, 1972). These early studies suggested that distinct profiles of amnesia were associated with damage in diencephalic and medial temporal brain areas. Patients with diencephalic amnesia were described as having tendencies toward superficial and inefficient encoding, confabulation, diminished insight, sensitivity to interference, and temporally graded retrograde amnesia. Patients with medial temporal amnesia were described as having consolidation deficits, intact insight, lack of confabulation, and limited retrograde amnesia. Studies of patients with basal forebrain amnesia revealed that they displayed many of the same characteristics as the diencephalic group, including limited insight, confabulation, sensitivity to interference, and remote memory problems (DeLuca, 1992; O'Connor & LaFleche, in press).

Despite initial acceptance of amnesia subtypes, questions arose as to whether there were consistent differences in the pattern of memory loss associated with various etiological subgroups (Weiskrantz, 1985). Within the domain of working memory, several studies compared the performance of patients with medial temporal lesions to that of diencephalic patients on the Brown–Peterson task. Leng & Parkin (1988, 1989) found that patients with diencephalic lesions showed disproportionate deficits on this task, but their poor performance was linked to frontal involvement. On the other hand, Kopelman & Stanhope (1997) found no differences on the Brown–Peterson test in their comparison of diencephalic, medial temporal and frontal patients. Hence, differences in the ability to maintain information within working memory did not appear to represent a core distinction between amnesic subtypes.

Within the domain of long-term memory, one area in which differences between groups were initially observed concerns rate of forgetting. Several studies demonstrated that medial temporal patients forget at a faster rate than diencephalic patients (Huppert & Piercy, 1979; Squire, 1981). However, these findings have not stood up to scrutiny (Freed et al., 1987; Kopelman & Stanhope, 1997; McKee & Squire, 1992) and it is now generally accepted that forgetting from long-term memory does not differentiate medial temporal and diencephalic amnesics.

Profiles of retrograde amnesia have also been examined in relation to etiological distinctions. Early studies suggested that diencephalic and medial temporal amnesics differed substantially on tasks of remote memory. Diencephalic patients were described as having extensive "temporally-graded" retrograde amnesia, characterized by relative preservation of early memories (Albert et al., & Levin, 1979; Kopelman, 1989), whereas the retrograde amnesia of the medial temporal group was described as limited (Milner, 1966; Zola-Morgan et al., 1986). More recent studies have indicated significant variability within diencephalic and medial temporal subgroups with respect to the severity and nature of remote memory loss (Kopelman et al., 1999). Patients with focal damage to diencephalic structures secondary to tumors, vascular causes and irradiation have only brief (i.e. less than three years) or no remote memory loss, in contrast to WKS patients, who have extensive retrograde amnesia. Within the medial temporal group, some patients have been described who have brief retrograde loss in the context of circumscribed damage to medial temporal structures (Zola-Morgan et al., 1986), whereas more extensive retrograde amnesia has been associated with widespread pathology in bitemporal brain regions (Rempel-Clower et al., 1996).

A number of issues confound comparisons across etiological groups. One of these concerns the fact that some patients have concomitant damage to brain structures that, although not part of the core neural system mediating memory, may nonetheless affect performance on memory tasks. For instance, in patients with WKS, the extensive retrograde amnesia has been attributed to additional frontal pathology, which may contribute to generalized deficits in memory retrieval (Kopelman, 1991; Kopelman et al., 1999). Likewise, frontal damage may explain some of the qualitative differences in performance on new learning tasks in WKS or basal forebrain amnesics compared to medial temporal amnesics. Two studies from our group serve to illustrate this phenomenon. In one study, we (Kixmiller et al., 1995) compared the occurrence of intrusion errors on the Visual Reproduction subtest of the WMS-R among medial temporal amnesics, Korsakoff patients and ACoA patients. Korsakoff patients showed much higher intrusion rates than medial temporal patients. Further, high intrusion rates were also seen in ACoA patients, but only when patients were tested after a delay, when their memory became more clearly depressed. We concluded that the occurrence of intrusions is linked to a combination of severe memory deficits and frontal dysfunction; neither deficit in isolation is sufficient to cause high rates of intrusion errors.

In a second study, Kixmiller et al., (2000) compared the performance of the same three subgroups on the Rey Osterrieth Complex Figure. Even though the Korsakoff patients and medial temporal amnesics were matched in terms of overall severity of amnesia, Korsakoff patients' delayed recall was strikingly worse than that of the medial temporal group. This was ascribed, at least in part, to visual-perceptual and organizational deficits exhibited by the Korsakoff group—deficits that compounded their severe amnesia.

The above studies indicate that nonobligatory frontal deficits in some amnesic patients may account for observed disparities in the memory profile of different etiological groups. Another issue that complicates subtype comparisons concerns selection criteria influencing referral to a memory clinic. In some cases, etiology of amnesia (e.g. a diagnosis of WKS) precipitates such a referral; in other cases, behavioral evidence of significant memory loss may be the reason for referral. Differences in selection factors may influence the nature and severity of the memory deficit exhibited by each etiological group. In addition, it is often the case that subtype comparisons are flawed by between-group differences in level of intelligence. It is well known that intelligence influences performance on a broad array of neuropsychological measures; baseline intellectual abilities may distort the profile of strengths and deficits exhibited by each group.

Table 2.1 Summary of neuropscholgical characteristics of amnesic patients with medial-temporal (n = 10), diencephalic (n = 10), and basal forebrain (n = 10) damage

Group	WAIS-R[1] VIQ	PIQ	WMS-R[2] Logical Memory I	Logical Memory II	RMT[3] Words	Faces	BNT[4]	WCST[5] Categories (n)	Pers. errors (%)
Medial-temporal	103	107	19	3	33	33	52	5	20
Diencephalic	99	100	17	1	34	33	53	5	19
Basal Forebrain	102	103	16	2	37	35	56	4	29

[1] Wechsler Adult Intelligence Scale—Revised.
[2] Wechsler Memory Scale—Revised.
[3] Recognition Memory Test.
[4] Boston Naming Test.
[5] Wisconsin Card Sorting Test.

To examine the memory profiles of different groups of patients while controlling for level of intelligence, we recently reviewed clinical data from 30 patients, selected on the basis of IQ, from a larger group of amnesics at the Memory Disorders Research Center (Table 2.1). Using a traditional lesion-based approach, we compared medial temporal amnesics (i.e. patients with diverse etiologies, such as encephalitis, stroke and anoxia), diencephalic amnesics (i.e. Korsakoff patients) and basal forebrain amnesics (i.e. patients with ACoA aneurysms). All patients underwent comprehensive neuropsychological evaluations and all performed normally on tests of language skills and general reasoning abilities. As we expected, when groups were matched for IQ, their performance on many clinical tests of memory was similar. All three groups demonstrated equivalent forgetting of information from working memory (e.g. recall of items on the Brown–Peterson paradigm) and from long-term memory (e.g. delayed recall and recognition of prose stories, word lists, etc.). Analysis of performance on tests of retrograde amnesia (e.g. the Famous Faces Test and the Transient Events Test) also revealed striking similarities across groups. All three groups demonstrated sparse recall and recognition of events from the last three decades and all demonstrated evidence of mild temporal gradients. Because diencephalic and basal forebrain groups often have frontal involvement, we expected that these groups might demonstrate heightened tendencies towards false-positive errors on tests of recognition memory, but this did not turn out to be the case. All groups demonstrated similar rates of false alarms.

Our comparison of amnesic groups suggests that the pattern of performance is largely similar among patients who are matched for baseline intelligence when tests are used that focus on quantitative aspects of performance (i.e. amount of information retained) rather than specific processing strategies. Aside from these clinical comparisons, several studies have compared the performance of medial temporal and diencephalic amnesics on experimental paradigms in an attempt to identify information processing domains in which these subgroups may differ. Most prominently, Parkin and colleagues have suggested that medial temporal and diencephalic amnesics differ in their memory for the temporal context in which target information is presented. In one study (Parkin et al., 1990) they found that diencephalic amnesics performed worse than medial temporal patients on a recognition task that required the encoding of distinctive temporal context to distinguish which stimuli were targets or distractors on any given trial. In another study (Hunkin et al., 1994) they found that diencephalic patients performed worse on a list discrimination task than medial temporal patients, even though their recognition memory was similarly impaired. Although in several studies, memory for temporal context has been linked to frontal dysfunction (Shimamura et al., 1990; Squire, 1982), in neither of the studies by Parkin and colleagues did performance on the temporal memory tasks correlate with performance on frontal tasks. Furthermore, similar impairments in temporal memory were observed in two patients with diencephalic lesions who showed no evidence of impairment on tasks of executive functioning (Parkin et al., 1994; Parkin & Hunkin, 1993). Based on these findings, Parkin and colleagues suggested that amnesics with diencephalic damage present with a qualitatively distinct memory deficit from that seen in amnesics with medial temporal lobe damage. According to their view, structures within the diencephalon, possibly through connections with dorsolateral frontal cortex, may be critically involved in the encoding of temporal information. In the face of diencephalic lesions, contextual input to the hippocampal system is greatly (and selectively) impoverished. In contrast, lesions of the hippocampal system are thought to interfere with consolidation of all types of information, contextual as well as item-related.

More recently, Kopelman et al. (1997) have directly compared memory for temporal and spatial context in patients with medial temporal and diencephalic lesions. Their findings for temporal context were generally consistent with those of Parkin, in that diencephalic patients performed worse than medial temporal patients. The inverse pattern was observed with respect to spatial (position) memory, where the medial temporal group performed worse than the diencephalic group. The latter finding was seen as support for the idea that the hippocampus plays a pivotal role in spatial memory (see also Chalfonte et al., 1996).

Despite reports of some differences between diencephalic and medial temporal amnesic patients, the similarities in the cognitive presentation of these patient groups are striking. Some researchers have argued that these commonalities are to be expected because the medial temporal and diencephalic structures are part of the same functional system required for the encoding of episodic information (Delay & Brion, 1969). Recently, Aggleton & Brown (1999) have argued that the core structures within this system are the hippocampus, fornix, mammillary bodies, anterior thalamus and possibly, more diffusely, the cingulum bundle and prefrontal cortex. According to their model, lesions anywhere in this system can cause deficits in episodic memory. More specifically, these deficits arise because of this system's role in linking target information to the spatial and temporal context that give an event its uniquely episodic character. Aggleton & Brown also postulate the existence of a second memory system, consisting of the perirhinal cortex and its connections to the medial dorsal thalamus. This system is thought to be involved in the detection of stimulus familiarity, a process that can support performance on recognition tasks, but not on recall tasks.

The notion that there are two medial temporal–diencephalic memory circuits that make qualitatively distinct contributions to memory leads to the prediction that patients with lesions restricted to the hippocampal circuit should have normal or near-normal item recognition memory. Aggleton & Shaw (1996) provided evidence in support of this view in a meta-analysis of studies in which the Recognition Memory Test (Warrington, 1984) was given to amnesic patients. They found that patients with lesions restricted to the hippocampus, fornix or mammillary bodies performed at a normal level, even though their recall was as severely impaired as was that of patients with more extensive medial temporal lesions.

A number of other reports of preserved recognition memory in patients with lesions to the hippocampal circuit provide further support for this view. These include several studies of patients with selective fornix lesions (Hodges & Carpenter, 1991; McMakin et al., 1995), a report of three young children who suffered relatively selective hippocampal damage due to anoxic injury early in life (Vargha-Khadem et al., 1997), and the study of a patient with adult-onset selective bilateral hippocampal injury (Mayes et al., 2002). Findings in the latter case are especially striking, as the patient was tested on a very extensive battery of recognition tests that varied the nature of to-be-remembered information, list length, retention interval and task difficulty.

Despite this evidence, the notion that different memory circuits subserve qualitatively distinct memory processes remains highly controversial. An alternative view, articulated most forcefully by Squire and colleagues (Squire & Zola, 1998; Zola & Squire, 2000), is that the hippocampus is important not only for recall but also for recognition. By this view, differences between patients with selective hippocampal lesions and more extensive medial temporal lobe lesions are only a matter of severity. Supporting this notion are findings from three patients with selective hippocampal lesions (Reed & Squire, 1997), who showed moderate levels of impairment not only in recall but also in recognition.

In an attempt to reconcile the report by Reed & Squire of impaired recognition following selective hippocampal damage with their own findings of preserved recognition, Mayes and colleagues (2002) have pointed to the possibility of hidden extra-hippocampal damage in Reed & Squire's patients. Further, they raise the possibility that partial damage to the hippocampus may disrupt the functioning of connected structures (such as the perirhinal cortex) more than complete damage. Another possibility, until now not considered, is that the location of lesion within the hippocampus affects the pattern of deficit. Clearly, a resolution of this debate will require convergent evidence from animal and human studies. In this context, careful analysis of patients with selective lesions to the hippocampal circuit, using state-of-the-art measures of structural integrity as well as indices of metabolic activity, will be of great importance.

CONCLUSION

Over the past four decades we have learned a great deal about the diversity of etiologies that may result in amnesia. Initial attempts to classify patients according to site of neuropathology in medial temporal, diencephalic and basal forebrain regions seemed promising, but subsequent investigations revealed that much of the variability between patients was due to extraneous factors rather than core features of the memory disorder. Recent clinical comparisons have emphasized similarities in the neuropsychological profiles of amnesic subgroups. Experimental studies focused on isolated aspects of information processing have revealed only subtle differences between these groups. Against this background, the current emphasis on differentiating the role of specific regions within the medial temporal lobe and its afferents may lead to a more useful framework for patient classification. Regardless of whether this framework turns out to be correct, detailed description of the anatomical and cognitive characteristics of amnesic patients remains an important endeavor. Such studies may lead to better clinical diagnosis and treatment of patients with memory disorders and may contribute a unique source of information to the cognitive neuroscience of memory.

ACKNOWLEDGEMENTS

Preparation of this chapter was supported by Program Project Grant NS 26985 from the National Institute of Neurological Disorders and Stroke and by the Medical Research Service of the U.S. Department of Veterans Affairs.

REFERENCES

Aggleton, J.P. & Brown, M.W. (1999). Episodic memory, amnesia, and the hippocampal–anterior thalamic axis. *Behavioral and Brain Sciences*, **22**, 425–489.

Aggleton, J.P. & Shaw, C. (1996). Amnesia and recognition memory: a re-analysis of psychometric data. *Neuropsychologia*, **34**, 51–62.

Albert, M., Butters, N. & Brandt, J. (1981). Patterns of remote memory in amnesic and demented patients. *Archives of Neurology*, **38**, 495–500.

Albert, M., Butters, N. & Levin, J. (1979). Temporal gradients in the retrograde amnesia of patients with alcoholic Korsakoff's disease. *Archives of Neurology*, **36**, 211–216.

Alexander, M.P. & Freedman, M. (1984). Amnesia after anterior communicating artery rupture. *Neurology*, **34**, 752–759.

Bechterew, W. (1900). Demonstration eines Gehirnes mit Zerstorung der vorderen und inneren Theile der Hirnrinde beider Schlafenlappen. *Neurologisches Zentralblatt*, **19**, 990–991.

Beeckmans, K., Vancoillie, P. & Michiels, K. (1998). Neuropsychological deficits in patients with an anterior communicating artery syndrome: a multiple case study. *Acta Neurologica Belgica*, **98**, 266–278.

Bengtsson, M., Holmberg, S. & Jansson, B. (1969). A psychiatric–psychological investigation of patients who had survived circulatory arrest. *Acta Scandinavica Psychiatrica*, **45**, 327–346.

Benson, D., Marsden, C. & Meadows, J. (1974). The amnesic syndrome of posterior cerebral artery occlusion. *Acta Neurologica Scandinavia*, **50**, 133–145.

Biber, C., Butters, N., Rosen, J. et al. (1981). Encoding strategies and recognition of faces by alcoholic Korsakoff and other brain damaged patients. *Journal of Clinical Neuropsychology*, **3**, 315–330.

Brierley, J.B. & Graham, D.I. (1984). Hypoxia and vascular disorders of the central nervous system. In W. Blackwood & J. A. N. Corsellis (eds), *Greenfield's Neuropathology* (pp. 125–207). London: Edward Arnold.

Butters, N. & Cermak, L.S. (1980). *Alcoholic Korsakoff's Syndrome: An Information Processing Approach*. New York: Academic Press.

Butters, N. & Cermak, L.S. (1986). A case study of the forgetting of autobiographical knowledge: implications for the study of retrograde amnesia. In D. Rubin (ed.), *Autobiographical Memory* (pp. 253–272). New York: Cambridge University Press.

Butters, N., Miliotis, P., Albert, M. & Sax, D. (1984). Memory assessment: evidence of the heterogeneity of amnesic symptoms. *Advances in Clinical Neuropsychology*, **1**, 127–159.

Caine, D., Halliday, G., Kril, J. & Harper, C. (1997). Operational criteria for the classification of chronic alcoholics: identification of Wernicke's encephalopathy. *Journal of Neurology, Neurosurgery and Psychiatry*, **62**, 51–60.

Caine, D. & Watson, D.G. (2000). Neuropsychological and neuropathological sequelae of cerebral anoxia: a critical review. *Journal of the International Neuropsychological Society*, **6**, 86–99.

Cave, C. & Squire, L. (1992). Intact and long-lasting repetition priming in amnesia. *Journal of Experimental Psychology: Learning, Memory and Cognition*, **1992**, 509–520.

Cermak, L.S. (1976). The encoding capacity of a patient with amnesia due to encephalitis. *Neuropsychologia*, **14**, 311–326.

Cermak, L.S. & Reale, L. (1978). Depth of processing and retention of words by alcoholic Korsakoff patients. *Journal of Experimental Psychology: Human Learning and Memory*, **4**, 165–174.

Cermak, L.S. & O'Connor, M.G. (1983). The anterograde and retrograde retrieval ability of a patient with amnesia due to encephalitis. *Neuropsychologia*, **21**, 213–234.

Chalfonte, B.L., Verfaellie, M., Johnson, M.K. & Reiss, L. (1996). Spatial location memory in amnesia: binding item and location information under incidental and intentional encoding conditions. *Memory*, **4**, 591–614.

Cohen, N. & Squire, L. (1981). Retrograde amnesia and remote memory impairment. *Neuropsychologia*, **19**, 337–356.

Colchester, A., Kingsley, D., Lasserson, B. et al. (2001). Structural MRI volumetric analysis in patients with organic amnesia, 1: methods and comparative findings across diagnostic groups. *Journal of Neurology, Neurosurgery and Psychiatry*, **71**, 13–22.

Corkin, S., Cohen, N.J., Sullivan, E.V. et al. (1985). Analyses of global memory impairments of different etiologies. *Annals of the New York Academy of Sciences*, **444**, 10–40.

Cullen, K.M., Halliday, G.M., Caine, D. & Kril, J.J. (1997). The nucleus basalis (Ch4) in the alcoholic Wernicke–Korsakoff syndrome: reduced cell number in both amnesic and non-amnesic patients. *Journal of Neurology, Neurosurgery and Psychiatry*, **63**, 315–320.

D'Esposito, M., Alexander, M.P., Fisher, R. et al. (1996). Recovery of memory and executive function following anterior communicating artery aneurysm rupture. *Journal of the International Neuropsychological Society*, **2**, 565–570.

Damasio, A.R., Eslinger, P.J., Damasio, H. et al. (1985a). Multi-modal amnesic syndrome following bilateral temporal and frontal damage: the case of patient D.R.B. *Archives of Neurology*, **42**, 252–259.

Damasio, A.R., Graff-Radford, N.R., Eslinger, P.J. et al. (1985b). Amnesia following basal forebrain lesions. *Archives of Neurology*, **42**, 263–271.

Damasio, A.R. & Van Hoesen, G.W. (1985). The limbic system and the localisation of herpes simplex encephalitis. *Journal of Neurology, Neurosurgery and Psychiatry*, **48**, 297–301.

De Renzi, E., Liotti, M. & Nichelli, P. (1987a). Semantic amnesia with preservation of autobiographical memory: a case report. *Cortex*, **23**, 575–597.

De Renzi, E., Zambolin, A. & Crisi, G. (1987b). The pattern of neuropsychological impairment associated with left posterior cerebral artery infarcts. *Brain*, **110**, 1099–1116.

Delay, J. & Brion, S. (1969). *Le Syndrome de Korsakoff*. Paris: Masson.

Delbecq-Derouesne, J., Beauvois, M.F. & Shallice, T. (1990). Preserved recall versus impaired recognition. *Brain*, **113**, 1045–1074.

DeLuca, J. (1992). Cognitive dysfunction after aneurysm of the anterior communicating artery. *Journal of Clinical and Experimental Neuropsychology*, **14**, 924–934.

DeLuca, J. (1993). Predicting neurobehavioral patterns following anterior communicating artery aneurysm. *Cortex*, **29**, 639–647.

DeLuca, J. & Diamond, B.J. (1995). Aneurysm of the anterior communicating artery: a review of neuroanatomical and neuropsychological sequelae. *Journal of Clinical and Experimental Neuropsychology*, **17**, 100–121.

Diamond, B.J., DeLuca, J. & Kelley, S.M. (1997). Memory and executive functions in amnesic and non-amnesic patients with aneurysms of the anterior communicating artery. *Brain*, **120**, 1015–1025.

Eslinger, P.J., Damasio, H., Damasio, A.R. & Butters, N. (1993). Nonverbal amnesia and asymmetric cerebral lesions following encephalitis. *Brain and Cognition*, **21**, 140–152.

Freed, D.M., Corkin, S. & Cohen, N.J. (1987). Forgetting in HM: a second look. *Neuropsychologia*, **25**, 461–471.

Gabrieli, J.D.E. (1999). The architecture of human memory. In J. K. Foster & M. Jelicic (eds), *Memory: Systems, Process or Function?* (pp. 205–231). Oxford: Oxford University Press.

Gadian, D., Aicari, J., Watkins, K. et al. (2000). Developmental amnesia associated with early hypoxic–ischemic injury. *Brain*, **123**, 499–507.

Geschwind, N. & Fusillo, M. (1966). Color naming defects in association with alexia. *Archives of Neurology*, **15**, 137–146.

Goldenberg, G. (2002). Transient global amnesia. In A.D. Baddeley, M.D. Kopelman. & B.A. Wilson (eds), *The Handbook of Memory Disorders*, 2nd edn (pp. 209–232). Chichester: Wiley.

Goldenberg, G. & Artner, C. (1991). Visual imagery and knowledge about the visual appearance of objects in patients with posterior cerebral lesions. *Brain and Cognition*, **15**, 160–186.

Goldenberg, G., Schuri, U., Gromminger, O. & Arnold, U. (1999). Basal forebrain amnesia: does the nucleus accumbens contribute to human memory? *Journal of Neurology, Neurosurgery and Psychiatry*, **67**, 163–168.

Graff-Radford, N.R., Tranel, D., Van Hoesen, G.V. & Brandt, J. (1990). Diencephalic amnesia. *Brain*, **113**, 1–25.

Hanley, J., Davies, A., Downes, J. & Mayes, A. (1994). Impaired recall of verbal material following rupture and repair of an anterior communicating artery aneurysm. *Cognitive Neuropsychology*, **11**, 543–578.

Harding, A., Halliday, G., Caine, D. & Kril, J. (2000). Degeneration of anterior thalamic nuclei differentiates alcoholics with amnesia. *Brain*, **123**, 141–154.

Harper, C., Giles, M. & Finlay-Jones, R. (1986). Clinical signs in the Wernicke–Korsakoff complex: a retrospective analysis of 131 cases diagnosed at necropsy. *Journal of Neurology, Neurosurgery and Psychiatry*, **49**, 341–345.

Haslam, C., Coltheart, M. & Cook, M.L. (1997). Preserved category learning in amnesia. *Neurocase*, **3**, 337–347.

Hodges, J.R. & Carpenter, K. (1991). Anterograde amnesia with fornix damage following removal of IIIrd ventricle colloid cyst. *Journal of Neurology, Neurosurgery and Psychiatry*, **54**, 633–638.

Hodges, J.R. & McCarthy, R.A. (1993). Autobiographical amnesia resulting from bilateral paramedian thalamic infarction: a case study in cognitive neurobiology. *Brain*, **116**, 921–940.

Hopkins, R., Gale, S., Johnson, S. et al. (1995). Severe anoxia with and without concomitant brain damage. *Journal of the International Neuropsychological Society*, **1**, 501–509.

Hunkin, N.M., Parkin, A.J. & Longmore, B.E. (1994). Aetiological variation in the amnesic syndrome: comparisons using the list discrimination task. *Neuropsychologia*, **32**, 819–825.

Huppert, F.A. & Piercy, M. (1979). Normal and abnormal forgetting in organic amnesia: effects of locus of lesion. *Cortex*, **15**, 385–390.

Irle, E., Wowra, B., Kunert, H.J. et al. (1992). Memory disturbance following anterior communicating artery rupture. *Annals of Neurology*, **31**, 473–480.

Isaac, C., Holdstock, J., Cezayirli, E. et al. (2000). Amnesia in a patient with lesions to the dorsomedial thalamic nucleus. *Neurocase*, **4**, 497–508.

Jernigan, T.L., Shafer, K., Butters, N. & Cermak, L.S. (1991). Magnetic resonance imaging of alcoholic Korsakoff patients. *Neuropsychopharmacology*, **4**, 175–186.

Jones, E. (1985). *The Thalamus*. New York: Plenum.

Kapur, N. (1993). Focal retrograde amnesia in neurological disease: a critical review. *Cortex*, **29**, 217–234.

Kapur, N., Thompson, S., Cook, P. et al. (1996). Anterograde but not retrograde memory loss following combined mammillary body and medial thalamic lesions. *Neuropsychologia*, **43**, 1–8.

Kixmiller, J.S., Verfaellie, M., Chase, K.A. & Cermak, L.S. (1995). Comparison of figural intrusion errors in three amnesic subgroups. *Journal of the International Neuropsychological Society*, **1**, 561–567.

Kixmiller, J.S., Verfaellie, M., Mather, M.M. & Cermak, L.S. (2000). Role of perceptual and organizational factors in amnesics' recall of the Rey–Osterrieth complex figure: a comparison of three amnesic groups. *Journal of Clinical and Experimental Neuropsychology*, **22**, 198–207.

Kopelman, M.D. (1989). Remote and autobiographical memory, temporal context memory and frontal atrophy in Korsakoff and Alzheimer patients. *Neuropsychologia*, **27**, 437–460.

Kopelman, M.D. (1991). Frontal dysfunction and memory deficits in the alcoholic Korsakoff syndrome and Alzheimer-type dementia. *Brain*, **114**, 117–137.

Kopelman, M.D. (2000). Focal retrograde amnesia and the attribution of causality: an exceptionally critical review. *Cognitive Neuropsychology*, **17**, 585–621.

Kopelman, M.D. & Stanhope, N. (1997). Rates of forgetting in organic amnesia following temporal lobe, diencephalic, or frontal lobe lesions. *Neuropsychology*, **11**, 343–356.

Kopelman, M.D., Stanhope, N. & Kingsley, D. (1997). Temporal and spatial context memory in patients with focal frontal, temporal lobe and diencephalic lesions. *Neuropsychologia*, **35**(12), 1533–1545.

Kopelman, M.D., Stanhope, N. & Kingsley, D. (1999). Retrograde amnesia in patients with diencephalic, temporal lobe or frontal lesions. *Neuropsychologia*, **37**, 939–958.

Kril, J.J., Halliday, G.M., Svoboda, M.D. & Cartwright, H. (1997). The cerebral cortex is damaged in chronic alcoholics. *Neuroscience*, **79**, 983–998.

Kritchevsky, M., Graff-Radford, N. & Damasio, A. (1987). Normal memory after damage to the medial thalamus. *Archives of Neurology*, **44**, 959–962.

Kuroiwa, T. & Okeda, R. (1994). Neuropathology of cerebral ischemia and hypoxia: Recent advances in experimental studies on its pathogenesis. *Pathology International*, **44**, 171–181.

Leng, N.R.C. & Parkin, A.J. (1988). Double dissociation of frontal dysfunction in organic amnesia. *British Journal of Clinical Psychology*, **27**, 359–362.

Leng, N.R.C. & Parkin, A.J. (1989). Aetiological variation in the amnesic syndrome: comparisons using the Brown Peterson task. *Cortex*, **25**, 251–259.

Levine, D. & Grek, A. (1984). The anatomic basis of delusions after right cerebral infarction. *Neurology*, **34**, 577–582.

Lhermitte, F. & Signoret, J.L. (1972). Analyse neuropsychologique et differentiation des syndromes amnesiques. *Revue Neurologique*, **126**, 161–178.

Mair, W., Warrington, E. & Weiskrantz, L. (1979). Memory disorder in Korsakoff's psychosis: a neuropathological and neuropsychological investigation of two cases. *Brain*, **102**, 749–783.

Markowitsch, H.J., Weber-Luxemburger, G., Ewald, K. et al. (1997). Patients with heart attacks are not valid models for medial temporal lobe amnesia. A neuropsychological and FDG–PET study with consequences for memory research. *European Journal of Neurology*, **4**, 178–184.

Mayes, A.R., Holdstock, J.S., Isaac, C.L. et al. (2002). Relative sparing of item recognition memory in a patient with adult-onset damage limited to the hippocampus. *Hippocampus*, **12**, 325–340.

Mayes, A.R., Meudell, P.R. & MacDonald, C. (1991). Disproportionate intentional spatial-memory impairments in amnesia. *Neuropsychologia*, **29**, 771–784.

McKee, R.D. & Squire, L.R. (1992). Equivalent forgetting rates in long-term memory in diencephalic and medial temporal lobe amnesia. *Journal of Neuroscience*, **12**, 3765–3772.

McKenna, P. & Warrington, E. (2000). The neuropsychology of semantic memory. In L.S. Cermak (ed.), *Memory and Its Disorders*, 2nd edn, Vol. 2 (pp. 355–382). Amsterdam: Elsevier.

McMakin, D., Cockburn, J., Anslow, P. & Gaffan, D. (1995). Correlation of fornix damage with memory impairment in six cases of colloid cyst removal. *Acta Neurochirurgica*, **135**, 12–18.

McNeill, D.L., Tidmarsh, D. & Rastall, M.L. (1965). A case of dysmnesic syndrome following cardiac arrest. *British Journal of Psychiatry*, **111**, 697–699.

Milner, B. (1966). Amnesia following operation on the temporal lobes. In C.W.M. Whitty & O.L. Zangwill (eds), *Amnesia* (pp. 109–133). London: Butterworths.

Mohr, J., Leicester, J., Stoddard, T. & Sidman, M. (1971). Right hemianopia with memory and color deficits in circumscribed left posterior cerebral artery territory infarction. *Neurology*, **21**, 1104–1113.

Moody, D.M., Bell, M.A. & Challa, R. (1990). Features of the cerebral vascular pattern that predict vulnerability to perfusion or oxygenation deficiency: an anatomic study. *American Journal of Neuroradiology*, **11**, 431–439.

O'Connor, M.G., Butters, N., Miliotis, P. et al. (1992). The dissociation of anterograde and retrograde amnesia in a patient with herpes encephalitis. *Journal of Clinical and Experimental Neuropsychology*, **14**, 159–178.

O'Connor, M.G. & LaFleche, J. (in press). The retrograde memory profile of patients with amnesia secondary to rupture and surgical repair of anterior communicating artery aneurysms. *Journal of the International Neuropsychological Society*.

Ogden, J.A. (1993). Visual object agnosia, prosopagnosia, achromatopsia, loss of visual imagery, and autobiographical amnesia following recovery from cortical blindness: case M.H. *Neuropsychologia*, **31**, 571–589.

Ott, B.R. & Saver, J.L. (1993). Unilateral amnesic stroke: six new cases and a review of the literature. *Stroke*, **24**, 1033–1042.

Parkin, A.J. & Hunkin, N.M. (1993). Impaired temporal context memory on anterograde but not retrograde tests in the absence of frontal pathology. *Cortex*, **29**, 267–280.

Parkin, A.J., Leng, N.R.C. & Hunkin, N. (1990). Differential sensitivity to context in diencephalic and temporal lobe amnesia. *Cortex*, **26**, 373–380.

Parkin, A.J., Leng, N.R.C., Stanhope, N. & Smith, A.P. (1988). Memory impairment following ruptured aneurysm of the anterior communicating artery. *Brain and Cognition*, **7**, 231–243.

Parkin, A.J. & Leng, R.C. (1993). *Neuropsychology of the Amnesic Syndrome*. Hillsdale, NJ: Erlbaum.

Parkin, A.J., Miller, J. & Vincent, R. (1987). Multiple neuropsychological deficits due to anoxic encephalopathy: a case study. *Cortex*, **23**, 655–665.

Parkin, A.J., Rees, J., Hunkin, N. & Rose, P. (1994). Impairment of memory following discrete thalamic infarction. *Neuropsychologia*, **32**, 39–51.

Pepin, E. & Auray-Pepin, L. (1993). Selective dorsolateral frontal lobe dysfunction associated with diencephalic amnesia. *Neurology*, **43**, 733–741.

Ptak, R. & Schnider, A. (1999). Spontaneous confabulations after orbito-frontal damage: the role of temporal context confusion and self-monitoring. *Neurocase*, **5**, 243–250.

Rapscak, S.Z., Kaszniak, A.W., Reminger, S.L. et al. (1998). Dissociation between verbal and autonomic measures of memory following frontal lobe damage. *Neurology*, **50**, 1259–1265.

Reed, J.M. & Squire, L.R. (1997). Impaired recognition memory in patients with lesions limited to the hippocampal formation. *Behavioral Neuroscience*, **111**, 1163–1170.

Reed, L.J., Lasserson, D., Marsden, P. et al. (1999). FDG–PET analysis and findings in amnesia resulting from hypoxia. *Memory*, **7**, 599–612.

Reich, P., Regstein, Q.R., Murawski, B.J. et al. (1983). Unrecognized organic mental disorders in survivors of cardiac arrest. *American Journal of Psychiatry*, **140**, 1194–1197.

Rempel-Clower, N.L., Zola, S.M., Squire, L.R. & Amaral, D.G. (1996). Three cases of enduring memory impairment after bilateral damage limited to the hippocampal formation. *Journal of Neuroscience*, **16**, 5233–5255.

Richardson, J.T. (1989). Performance in free recall following rupture and repair of intracranial aneurysm. *Brain and Cognition*, **9**, 210–226.

Ross, E.D. (1980). Sensory-specific and fractional disorders of recent memory in man: I. Isolated loss of visual recent memory. *Archives of Neurology*, **37**, 193–200.

Sandson, T., Daffner, K., Carvalho, P. & Mesulam, M. (1991). Frontal lobe dysfunction following infarction of the left-sided medial thalamus. *Archives of Neurology*, **48**, 1300–1303.

Scoville, W.B. & Milner, B. (1957). Loss of recent memory after bilateral hippocampal lesions. *Journal of Neurology, Neurosurgery and Psychiatry*, **20**, 11–12.

Shimamura, A.P., Janowski, J.S. & Squire, L.R. (1990). Memory for the temporal order of events in patients with frontal lobe lesions and amnesic patients. *Neuropsychologia*, **28**, 803–813.

Shoqeirat, M. & Mayes, A.R. (1991). Disproportionate incidental spatial-memory and recall deficits in amnesia. *Neuropsychologia*, **29**, 749–769.

Speedie, L.J. & Heilman, K.M. (1982). Amnestic disturbance following infarction of the left dorsomedial nucleus of the thalamus. *Neuropsychologia*, **20**, 597–604.

Speedie, L.J. & Heilman, K.M. (1983). Anterograde memory deficits for visuospatial material after infarction of the right thalamus. *Archives of Neurology*, **40**, 183–186.

Squire, L.R. (1981). Two forms of human amnesia: an analysis of forgetting. *Journal of Neuroscience*, **6**, 635–640.

Squire, L.R. (1982). Comparisons between forms of amnesia: some deficits are unique to Korsakoff's syndrome. *Journal of Experimental Psychology: Learning, Memory and Cognition*, **8**, 560–571.

Squire, L.R., Knowlton, B. & Musen, G. (1993). The structure and organization of memory. *Annual Review of Psychology*, **44**, 453–495.

Squire, L.R. & Zola, S.M. (1998). Episodic memory, semantic memory and amnesia. *Hippocampus*, **8**, 205–211.

Stefanacci, L., Buffalo, E.A., Schmolck, H. & Squire, L.R. (2000). Profound amnesia after damage to the medial temporal lobe: a neuroanatomical and neuropsychological profile of patient E.P. *Journal of Neuroscience*, **20**, 7024–7036.

Stuss, D.T., Guberman, A., Nelson, R. & Larochelle, S. (1988). The neuropsychology of paramedian thalamic infarction. *Brain and Cognition*, **8**, 348–378.

Sullivan, E. (2001). *Equivalent hippocampal volume loss in Korsakoff's syndrome and Alzheimer's disease*. Paper presented at the International Neuropsychological Society, Chicago.

Talland, G.A., Sweet, W.H. & Ballantine, H.T. (1967). Amnesic syndrome with anterior communicating artery aneurysm. *Journal of Nervous and Mental Diseases*, **145**, 179–192.

Tranel, D., Damasio, H. & Damasio, A. (2000). Amnesia caused by herpes simplex encephalitis, infarctions in basal forebrain, and anoxia/ischemia. In L.S. Cermak (ed.), *Handbook of Neuropsychology*, 2nd edn, Vol. 2 (pp. 85–110). Oxford: Elsevier.

Van der Werf, Y., Witter, M., Uylings, H. & Jolles, J. (2000). Neuropsychology of infarctions in the thalamus: a review. *Neuropsychologia*, **38**, 613–627.

Vargha-Khadem, F., Gadian, D.G., Watkins, K.E. et al. (1997). Differential effects of early hippocampal pathology on episodic and semantic memory. *Science*, **277**, 376–380.

Verfaellie, M. & Cermak, L.S. (1991). Neuropsychological Issues in Amnesia. In J. L. Martinez & R. P. Kersner (eds), *Learning and Memory: A Biological View* (pp. 467–497). San Diego, CA: Academic Press.

Verfaellie, M. Croce, P. & Milberg, W.P. (1995a). The role of episodic memory in semnatic learning: an examination of vocabulary acquisition in a patient with amnesia due to encephalitis. *Neurocase*, **1**, 291–304.

Verfaellie, M. & Keane, M.M. (2001). Scope and limits of implicit memory in amnesia. In B. De Gelder, E. De Haan & C. Heywood (eds), *Unconscious Minds* (pp. 151–162). Oxford: Oxford University Press.

Verfaellie, M., Koseff, P. & Alexander, M.P. (2000). Acquisition of novel semantic information in amnesia: effects of lesion location. *Neuropsychologia*, **38**, 484–492.

Verfaellie, M., Reiss, L. & Roth, H. (1995b). Knowledge of new English vocabulary in amnesia: an examination of premorbidly acquired semantic memory. *Journal of the International Neuropsychological Society*, **1**, 443–453.

Victor, M., Adams, R.D. & Collins, G.H. (1989). *The Wernicke–Korsakoff Syndrome and Related Neurologic Disorders due to Alcoholism and Malnutrition*, 2nd edn. Philadelphia, PA: Davis.

Victor, M., Angevine, J., Mancall, E. & Fischer, M. (1961). Memory loss with lesions of hippocampal formation. *Archives of Neurology*, **5**, 244–263.

Volpe, B. T., Herscovitch, P. & Raichle, M. E. (1984). Positron emission tomography defines metabolic abnormality in mesial temporal lobes of two patients with amnesia after rupture and repair of anterior communicating artery aneurysm. *Neurology*, **34**, 188.

Volpe, B.T. & Hirst, W. (1983). Amnesia following the rupture and repair of an anterior communicating artery aneurysm. *Journal of Neurology, Neurosurgery and Psychiatry*, **46**, 704–709.

Von Cramon, D., Hebel, N. & Schuri, U. (1985). A contribution to the anatomical basis of thalamic amnesia. *Brain*, **108**, 993–1008.

Von Cramon, D., Hebel, N. & Schuri, U. (1988). Verbal memory and learning in unilateral posterior cerebral infarction. *Brain*, **111**, 1061–1077.

Von Cramon, D.Y., Markowitsch, H.J. & Shuri, U. (1993). The possible contribution of the septal region to memory. *Neuropsychologia*, **31**, 1159–1180.

Warrington, E.K. (1984). *Recognition Memory Test*. Western Psychological Services.

Warrington, E.K. & Weiskrantz, L. (1970). Amnesic syndrome: consolidation or retrieval? *Nature*, **228**, 628–630.

Warrington, E.K. & Weiskrantz, L. (1973). An analysis of short-term and long-term memory deficits in man. In J.A. Deutsch (ed.), *The Physiological Basis of Memory* (pp. 365–396). New York: Academic Press.

Weiskrantz, L. (1985). On issues and theories of the human amnesic syndrome. In N. Weinberger, J. McGaugh & G. Lynch (eds), *Memory Systems of the Brain* (pp. 380–415). New York: Guilford.

Winocur, G., Oxbury, S., Roberts, R. et al. C. (1984). Amnesia in a patient with bilateral lesions to the thalamus. *Neuropsychologia*, **22**, 123–143.

Zola, S.M. & Squire, L.R. (2000). The medial temporal lobe and the hippocampus. In E. Tulving & F. I. M. Craik (eds), *The Oxford Handbook of Memory* (pp. 485–500). Oxford: Oxford University Press.

Zola-Morgan, S., Squire, L. & Amaral, D. (1986). Human amnesia and the medial temporal region: enduring memory impairment following a bilateral lesion limited to field CA1 of the hippocampus. *Journal of Neuroscience*, **6**, 2950–2967.

CHAPTER 3

Posttraumatic Amnesia and Residual Memory Deficit after Closed Head Injury

Harvey S. Levin

and

Gerri Hanten

Department of Physical Medicine and Rehabilitation,
Baylor College of Medicine, Houston, TX, USA

Early concepts of amnesia following closed-head injury (CHI) can be traced to ancient descriptions (for review see Levin et al., 1983). However, detailed serial observations of resolving anterograde and posttraumatic amnesia following CHI were first widely disseminated in the nineteenth century reports (Brodie, 1854), which influenced the theoretical writings by Ribot (1882) on dissolution of memory. In this review of research on memory disorder after CHI, we will use studies from our laboratory and other centers to illustrate recent advances in understanding the consequences of CHI on different aspects of memory performance.

PATHOPHYSIOLOGIC FEATURES CONTRIBUTING TO MEMORY DEFICIT

Brain damage associated with CHI can be classified as primary or secondary (Graham et al., 2000). Primary brain damage, which occurs or is initiated at the time of injury, includes focal brain lesions, diffuse axonal injury (DAI) and intracranial hemorrhage.

Focal brain lesions, including contusions and intracranial hematomas, primarily occur in the frontal and temporal lobes in association with a wide spectrum of CHI severity (Adams et al., 1980; Eisenberg et al., 1990; Levin et al., 1987). Temporal lobe hematomas and contusions have been implicated in residual memory disturbance after CHI (Jennett, 1969; Levin et al. 1982), which is consistent with amnesic disorder arising from other etiologies of mesial temporal lobe damage (Scoville & Milner, 1957). During the past 20 years, studies of patients with focal brain lesions arising from various etiologies have elucidated the role

The Essential *Handbook of Memory Disorders for Clinicians.* Edited by A.D. Baddeley, M.D. Kopelman and B.A. Wilson.
© 2004 John Wiley & Sons, Ltd. ISBN 0-470-09141-X.

of the prefrontal cortex in declarative memory. Patients with frontal lesions have been shown to exhibit impaired knowledge and deployment of memory strategies (Shimamura et al., 1991). Consistent with frontal lobe involvement in declarative memory, prefrontal activation on positron emission tomography (PET) occurs with memory retrieval in neurologically intact adults (Lepage et al., 2000). In agreement with the focal lesion and functional brain imaging literatures, a recent volumetric magnetic resonance imaging (MRI) study showed that frontal lesion volume (but not extrafrontal lesion volume) was predictive of recall of categorized words by children and adolescents who had sustained CHI that ranged from mild to severe in acute severity (DiStefano et al., 2000). Distefano et al. found that the volume of frontal lesion was related to total recall across five recall trials of the California Verbal Learning Test—Children's Version (CVLT-C; Delis et al., 1994), using a regression analysis that first adjusted for the effects of overall CHI severity and the patient's age (Figure 3.1).

In addition to focal lesions involving the frontal and temporal lobes, the hippocampus is especially vulnerable to the effects of ischemia (Adams et al., 1980). Neuropathological studies have documented hippocampal damage in more than 90% of fatal cases of CHI (Kotapka et al., 1994).

Frontotemporal connections, which are postulated to mediate strategic aspects of declarative memory, such as rehearsal and selective processing of rewarded items (Miller, 2000), can presumably be disrupted by DAI even in the absence of focal lesions. However, the relationship between structural brain imaging findings and memory functioning has been inconsistent across studies (Wilson et al., 1988; Levin et al., 1992), suggesting that areas of cerebral dysfunction can be larger than the lesions detected by conventional CT and MRI. This interpretation has been supported by metabolic imaging, in which abnormalities in neurotransmitters (N-aspartate, choline), detected in lesion-free brain regions such as the frontal white matter by MRI, corresponded to neuropsychological outcome in chronic survivors of CHI (Friedman et al., 1998; Garnett et al., 2000). Regional cerebral glucose metabolism, as measured by PET in adult CHI patients without cortical contusions on MRI, were studied between 2 and 12 months postinjury (Fontaine et al., 1999). Fontaine et al. found that verbal memory was correlated with glucose metabolism primarily in the left mesial prefrontal region, the left dorsolateral prefrontal area and the left posterior cingulate gyrus. In addition, less robust correlations with verbal memory were found with glucose metabolism in the left anterior cingulate gyrus, the orbitofrontal cortex and the right mesial prefrontal cortex. Preliminary findings using functional MRI (fMRI) to study working memory after mild CHI (McAllister et al., 1999) suggest that altered patterns of brain activation might elucidate the mechanisms mediating memory disorder in more severe injuries.

Secondary brain insult, including hypoxia and hypotension, also complicate efforts to isolate the effects of focal brain lesions on memory. Secondary brain damage, which also arises during the first few hours after CHI from a cascade of excitotoxic neurotransmitters such as glutamate, can lead to cellular injury or death, even in patients without evidence of structural brain lesions on CT (Bullock et al., 1998). Programmed cell death, or apoptosis, also contributes to diffuse brain damage (Graham et al., 2000; Kochanek et al., 2000). Other forms of secondary brain injury associated with CHI include increased intracranial pressure, swelling, ischemia and infection. Secondary brain injury occurs more frequently with moderate to severe CHI, but delayed brain swelling and/or hematomas can develop occasionally in patients who initially have mild impairment of consciousness. Although the distinctive

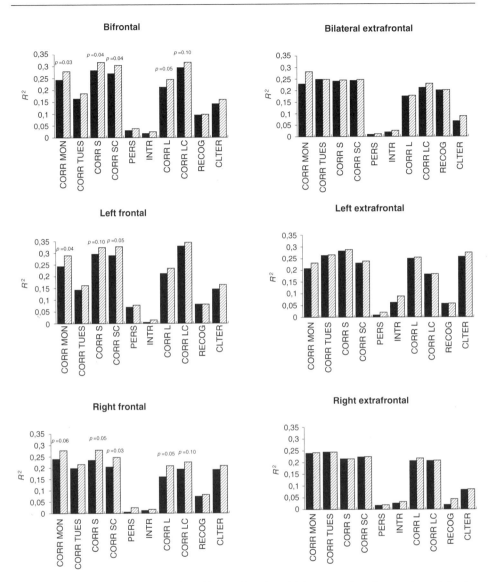

Figure 3.1 Summary of the results of hierarchical multiple regression that evaluated the incremental contributions of bilateral frontal (top left), bilateral extrafrontal (top right), left frontal (middle left), left extrafrontal (middle right), right frontal (bottom left) and right extrafrontal (bottom right) lesions to predicting the verbal learning and memory test scores after entering the severity of injury and age at testing alone. Closed bars indicate R^2 when entering GCS score and age at testing into the regression equation; hatched bars indicate incremental R^2 when additionally entering lesion size into regression equation. CORR MON, correct words on Monday list; CORR TUES, correct words on Tuesday list; CORR S, correct words on short delay free recall; CORR SC, correct words on short delay cued recall; PERS, perseverations on Monday list recall; INTR, intrusions on Monday list recall; CORR L, correct word on long delay free recall; CORR LC, correct word on long delay cued recall; RECOG, correct recognitions; CLTER, clusters on Monday list recall. Reproduced from DiStefano et al. (2000). © 2000, BMJ Publishing Group

contribution of specific pathophysiologic features to residual memory disturbance is difficult to isolate because of the heterogeneity of injury in patient samples and the confounding by co-morbidities such as alcohol abuse in some studies, several pathophysiologic features of CHI have been implicated in producing memory deficit.

In addition to the primary vs. secondary distinction, brain damage produced by CHI includes focal brain lesions and diffuse brain insult. Investigating the relationship between localization of traumatic focal lesions and memory disorder is complicated by variation across patients in type and size of lesion, in addition to concomitant diffuse and multifocal neuropathology in many cases. Further, the weak correlation between structural damage detected by imaging and performance on neuropsychological tests (Wilson et al., 1988; Levin et al., 1992) suggests that areas of cerebral dysfunction are more extensive than the abnormalities detected by conventional imaging procedures. This interpretation has been supported by evidence from metabolic imaging, in which abnormalities detected with MRI corresponded to neuropsychological outcome in chronic survivors of traumatic brain injury (Langfitt et al., 1986; Friedman et al., 1998; Garnett et al., 2000).

POSTTRAUMATIC AMNESIA

Measurement of Posttraumatic Amnesia

Posttraumatic amnesia (PTA), an early stage of recovery during which the patient fails to retain information about ongoing events, is a characteristic feature of CHI which can occur even in mild injuries which produce no coma (Ommaya & Gennarelli, 1974; Russell, 1932). Apart from anterograde amnesia, PTA also involves a variable constellation of behavioral disturbances, including defective attention, agitation, lethargy, inappropriate and disinhibited behavior and speech. Early reports of PTA duration (Russell, 1971; Russell & Nathan, 1946; Russell & Smith, 1961) were based on the patient's retrospective estimate due to circumstances of assessing injured servicemen evacuated after the acute injury phase to the Oxford Hospital for Head Injury. However, subsequent research has shown that objective, serial assessment of mild CHI patients, beginning in the emergency room, yields durations of PTA which are discrepant from later subjective estimates by the patients (Gronwall & Wrightson, 1980). In contrast to Russell's inclusion of the comatose period in estimating PTA duration, widespread use of the Glasgow Coma Scale (GCS) of Teasdale & Jennett (1974) has facilitated separate assessment of the acute amnesic period after the patient begins to follow commands consistently.

In response to the aforementioned problem in retrospective estimates of PTA (see Schacter & Crovitz, 1977), Levin et al. (1979) developed the Galveston Orientation and Amnesia Test (GOAT), a brief bedside evaluation of orientation and retention of ongoing events. The test includes items from a temporal orientation questionnaire (Benton et al., 1964), recall of the first postinjury event and the last event that occurred prior to the injury. Error points are awarded for each item and deducted from 100, yielding a total score that we found to range from 75 to 100 in patients who had recovered from a mild CHI. Duration of PTA, which was operationally defined by the interval from injury to the point of reaching a stable score within the normal range on this brief test, was related to both the severity of initial injury and the outcome of head injury 6 months later (Levin et al., 1979). Ellenberg

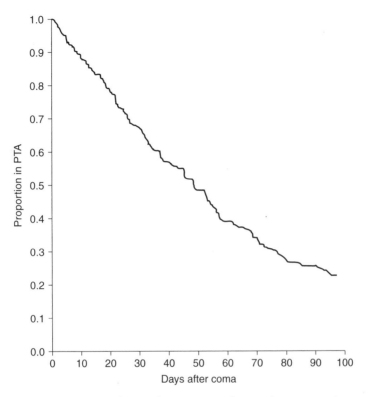

Figure 3.2 Kaplan–Meier survival curve for time to resolution of posttraumatic amnesia (PTA) as defined by achieving a Galveston Orientation and Amnesia Test score of 75 or more after termination of coma. At 30 days, approximately 65% of the cohort remained in PTA. At 65 days after awakening from coma, approximately 35% were still in PTA. Reproduced from Ellenberg et al. (1996). © 2000, American Medical Association

et al. (1996) accessed the National Institutes of Health Traumatic Coma Data Bank to plot a survival curve for the proportion of severe CHI patients remaining in PTA with a GOAT score of 75 or higher as the criterion for recovery. Ellenberg et al. found that half of the patients were still in PTA at 50 days after recovery of consciousness and that PTA duration was predictive of 6 months outcome after taking into account the duration of coma. Initial postresuscitation GCS score, pupillary reactivity, coma duration and use of phenytoin were all predictive of PTA duration, as measured by serial administration of the GOAT (Figure 3.2).

A second method of directly assessing PTA was developed by Artiola et al. (1980) of the Neuropsychology Unit at Oxford. This method defined resolution of PTA according to recall of three pictures, the examiner's name and the examiner's face on the day after the previous assessment. If recall was not perfect, recognition memory was tested. The Westmead Test, a variant of the Oxford procedure, has also been published (Shores et al., 1986). The Oxford and Westmead procedures offer the advantage of more specific testing of declarative memory, exclusive of orientation, as compared to the GOAT. As described

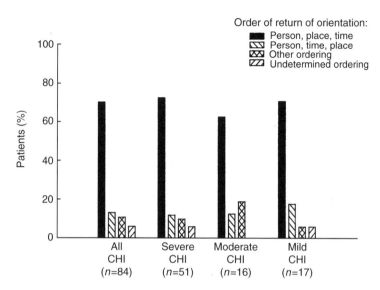

Figure 3.3   Order of return of orientation shown for the closed head-injured patients, combined and separately, according to severity of injury as assessed by the Glasgow Coma Scale. Reproduced from High et al. (1990). © 1990, Swets Zeitlinger

below, the decision regarding measurement method should be based on the specific clinical or research application and practical issues.

Features of Posttraumatic Amnesia

Sequence of Recovery

Recovery of orientation during PTA was studied by High et al. (1990) in a series of 84 survivors of CHI of varying severity who were serially tested during their acute hospitalization. As shown in Figure 3.3, orientation recovered in the sequence of person, place and time in the majority (70%) of patients. Estimates of the date were displaced backward in time (up to 5 years for severe injuries), and the discrepancies between the estimate and the actual date diminished as orientation improved. This receding of retrograde amnesia was observed for moderate and severe but not mild head injuries. Accordingly, the investigators postulated that backward displacement of time may shrink in parallel with the resolution of loss of information for events preceding the injury. This pattern of recovery of orientation was corroborated in a study of 31 severely injured patients which also compared the results of the GOAT with the Westmead and Oxford procedures (Tate et al., 2000).

In contrast to the finding that orientation recovered before recognition memory of items presented on the preceding day to patients recovering from mild CHI (Gronwall & Wrightson, 1980), Tate et al. (2000) found that recognition of three line drawings of concrete items presented on the preceding day improved to a normal level before temporal disorientation resolved in adults following severe CHI. Orientation to place recovered before free recall of the three items and the examiner's name, but there was no significant difference between the duration of PTA, as measured by the GOAT, and time to recover free recall. The inconsistency in findings obtained in these studies might reflect the patient samples with a mild CHI group studied by Gronwall & Wrightson, as compared to severe CHI patients assessed by Tate et al.

Attentional Disturbance or Memory Deficit?

Descriptions of recovery of CHI patients initially after they began comprehending commands and opening their eyes have implicated attentional disturbance concomitant with memory and learning problems (Russell, 1971; Russell & Nathan, 1946; Russell & Smith, 1961). Experimental support for the role of attentional disturbance in PTA was obtained by Stuss et al. (1999), who serially administered attention tests of varying complexity, the GOAT, and recognition memory to patients during the early stage of recovery from mild, moderate or severe CHI. Stuss and colleagues found that performance on attention control tasks, such as reciting overlearned sequences (counting forward, months of year), typically recovered concurrent with improvement in scores to within the normal range on the GOAT, whereas recovery on these simple attention tasks preceded resolution of PTA as defined by the GOAT in severely injured patients. Parallel investigation of recognition and recall memory generally showed a pattern of earlier recovery on less effortful tasks, followed by improved memory performance on more difficult measures (Stuss et al., 1999). Analysis of the sequence of recovery of attention, memory and performance on the GOAT generally reflected a closer correspondence between changes on the GOAT and the attentional measures with later improvement on the memory tests.

To summarize, there is general agreement that resolution of PTA as measured by the GOAT is paralleled by improvement in performance on simple attentional and memory tests. Although the findings reported by Tate et al. indicate that the GOAT might be sufficient to measure PTA duration, it is apparent from Stuss et al.'s findings that recovery measured by more challenging tests of recall will be delayed after patients attain a normal score on the GOAT. From a cognitive perspective it is appropriate to differentiate PTA from residual memory disorder. For clinical applications, it is important to determine the complexity of bedside testing that is relevant to monitoring recovery and planning rehabilitation in relation to the time required for assessment and the effort asked of the patient.

Frequency, Specificity and Impact of Residual Memory Disorder

Russell (1971) reported that residual memory disturbance (i.e. persisting after resolution of PTA) was present in 23% of the 1000 servicemen he examined while they were convalescing from a CHI. This figure rose to 50% of the severely injured patients. Interviews with survivors of severe CHI and their families have corroborated the results of Russell's clinical examinations, indicating a high frequency of residual memory impairment observed in performance of daily activities. Oddy et al. (1985) found that 53% of patients and 79% of their families reported that memory deficit was still present 7 years after injury. This was the most common problem mentioned by the patients and their relatives. Other studies have found that survivors of CHI frequently underestimate the severity of their memory deficit, as measured by experimental tests (Baddeley et al., 1987b; Sunderland et al., 1983). More recently, Brooks et al. (1987) identified verbal memory deficit as one of the two neurobehavioral sequelae (the other being slowed information-processing rate) which were most strongly related to unemployment 7 years after severe head injury.

Whether memory deficit can persist as a relatively specific sequel of CHI or is invariably a manifestation of global cognitive impairment was addressed by Gronwall & Wrightson (1980), who were able to show that verbal memory deficit was dissociable from information-processing rate on a test of paced auditory addition. To further address the specificity of memory impairment after head injury, we analyzed the findings of 87 young adults and adolescents who had sustained moderate or severe CHI and who participated in a prospective outcome study (Levin et al., 1988a). Memory was assessed for two postinjury intervals (5–15 months, 16–42 months) using the Verbal Selective Reminding Test (Buschke & Fuld, 1974) and the Continuous Memory Test (Hannay et al., 1979), which involved recognition of recurring line drawings of familiar living things. To evaluate the presence of a dissociation between intellectual function and memory, the analysis was confined to patients (about two-thirds of the series) whose Wechsler Verbal and Performance IQs were at least 85 at the time of the follow-up examination. The number of words consistently recalled across trials (CLTR) and d', an index of memory sensitivity, were the dependent measures for selective reminding and recognition memory tests, respectively. To facilitate within-subjects comparison of intellectual and memory functioning, the raw scores of the memory tests were transformed into standard scores (i.e. a mean of 100 and a standard deviation of 15) based on normative data obtained from a sample of 50 young adults.

Figures 3.4A and 3.4B are box-plots showing the distribution of IQ and transformed memory scores for controls, moderate and severe head-injured patients. It is seen that intellectual functioning in these groups did not significantly differ, whereas severely injured patients exhibited impaired verbal memory (Selective Reminding Test) relative to the moderate CHI and control groups who did not differ from each other. A similar pattern emerged for visual recognition memory, but the group differences did not reach statistical significance. To evaluate the presence of a relatively specific impairment of memory, a disparity of at least 15 standard score points was used to compare verbal memory with verbal intelligence quotient (VIQ) and visual recognition memory with performance intelligence quotient (PIQ).

Disproportionate memory impairment, defined by standard scores on both memory tests that were below 85 and at least 15 points less than the corresponding VIQ or PIQ score (VIQ > CLTR, PIQ > d'), was present in about 15% of the moderate and 30% of the severe head-injured patients whose intellectual level had recovered to within the normal range. The feature of verbal memory that most consistently distinguished the memory-impaired patients from the other head-injured patients with normal intellectual function (who comprised about one-half of the total sample at each interval) was their difficulty in recalling the test words after a 30 minute delay. About one-third of the total series had global cognitive impairment (i.e. IQ below 85, associated with poor memory). These patients had more severe injuries than the patients with IQ 85 and above, as reflected by the degree and duration of impaired consciousness and their frequency of nonreactive pupils during the acute stage of injury. In contrast, the indices of CHI severity of the patients with a relatively specific memory deficit did not significantly differ from the patients who recovered to the normal range of both intellectual and memory functions.

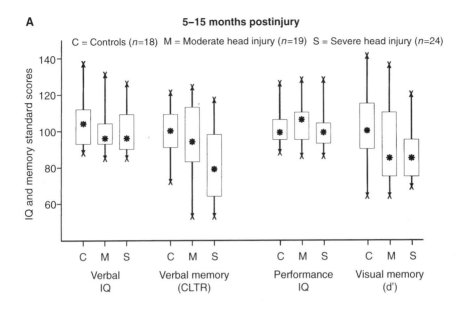

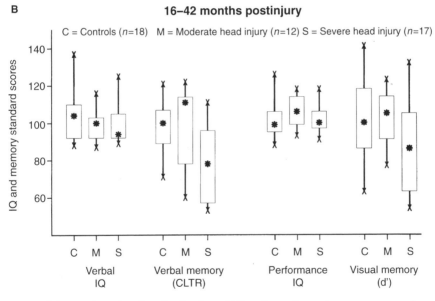

Figure 3.4 (A) Box-plots showing distribution of IQ and transformed memory scores for controls, moderate and severe head-injured patients who obtained IQ scores within the normal range (<85) at 5–15 months after injury. (B) IQ and transformed memory test data obtained at 16–42 months postinjury. Each asterisk signifies the median, upper and lower horizontal lines of each bar indicate the 75th and 25th centile scores, respectively, and the maximum and minimum scores are depicted by the letter "X". Reproduced from Levin et al. (1988b). © 1988, BMJ Publishing Group

PATTERNS OF MEMORY DEFICIT AFTER CLOSED HEAD INJURY

In recent years memory theorists have come to substantial agreement that human memory is not a unitary construct, but rather is made up of dissociable components sensitive to differing stimulus characteristics and demands (see Baddeley, 1998). Much of the progress in this area has resulted from cognitive neuropsychological studies of individuals who have demonstrated differential patterns of performance on tests of memory subsequent to brain injury. The precise nature of the components has yet to be completely specified, and discussion of the various theories relating to memory components and systems, although beyond the scope of this chapter, are addressed in other chapters in this volume. However, in reporting research concerning the effects of traumatic brain injury on memory, we will make certain assumptions based on widely reported functional dissociations in memory performance; for example, there is ample evidence from both the neuropsychological and the normal cognitive literature to support a functional distinction between short-term memory and long-term memory, regardless of theoretical approach. In addition to discussing aspects of short- and long-term memory performance, we will also report recent findings on the effect of CHI on some "hybrid" memorial abilities, specifically prospective memory and metacognition, illustrated by descriptions of studies from our laboratory and others where appropriate.

Impairments of Working Memory

The term "working memory" as used here refers to a limited capacity system for the temporary storage of information held for further manipulation (Baddeley, 1986). Working memory is central to performance in many cognitive domains, including learning, planning and problem solving, as well as language acquisition, comprehension and production. The effect of traumatic brain injury on task performance has been investigated for various forms of memory, including verbal and nonverbal memory, spatial memory, and phonological and semantic components of working memory.

Auditory–Verbal Memory Deficits

Probably the most well-characterized area of cognitive impairment after traumatic brain injury is auditory–verbal memory. Many studies have directly or indirectly investigated the characteristics of auditory–verbal memory after CHI using recall, cued recall or recognition tests. The tests employed have frequently been standardized list-learning tests using the repeated presentation and recall of a single supraspan list of related words, such as the California Verbal Learning Test (Delis et al., 1986, 1991, 1994) or the Auditory–Verbal Learning Test (Rey, 1964), although other types of tests, such as the Selective Reminding Test (Buschke & Fuld, 1974) and the Continuous Recognition Memory Test (Hannay et al., 1979), have also been used.

The general finding is that both adults and children who have had severe CHI and are in the postacute stages of injury show deficits in immediate and delayed recall (e.g. Baddeley et al., 1987a; Brooks, 1975; Crosson et al., 1988; Hanten & Martin, 2000; Jaffe et al.,

1992; Levin, 1989; Levin et al., 1979, 1982, 1988a, 2000; Reid & Kelly, 1993; Roman et al., 1998; Wiegner & Donders, 1999; Yeates et al., 1995). Tests of recognition memory and cued recall also generally show that persons with severe CHI are impaired relative to uninjured controls (Baddeley et al., 1987; Dennis & Barnes, 1990; Levin et al., 1988a; Roman et al., 1998). In some studies persons with severe CHI have been found to show increased errors in recall, including intrusions and perseverations, and impairment in the ability to utilize semantic information to aid recall (Hanten & Martin, 2000; Levin et al., 1996, 2000; Levin & Goldstein, 1986). This will be discussed in more detail later.

Specific Components of STM

Essential to the eventual development of effective intervention techniques is the elucidation of the specific underlying causes of impairment. Although various studies have used cluster analyses in order to determine factors that contribute to the impairments in verbal learning exhibited by CHI patients (Wiegner & Donders, 1999; Gardner & Vrbancic, 1998; Millis, 1995; Wilde & Boake, 1994), the factors used in such analyses tend to be general. As clinical research tools, verbal learning tests, such as the CVLT, have proved useful in identifying general verbal learning impairment in various populations, including CHI. However, one of the disadvantages of such tests is that they do not provide measures of specific memory processes in isolation. The variables are usually complex, and therefore difficult to dissociate into discrete components. Experimental neuropsychological studies of individuals who have short-term memory deficits have been more successful in isolating specific components of short-term memory (Baddeley & Wilson, 1993; Hulme et al., 1993; Jarrold et al., 1999; Martin et al., 1994; Saffran & Martin, 1990). Using this approach, studies of adult patients with brain injury have revealed individuals with severely reduced memory span whose impairments appear to arise from a phonological short-term memory deficit (see Shallice & Vallar, 1990). Other recent studies have elucidated that there are separable components of phonological and semantic short-term memory, and that brain damage can selectively affect these components (Hanten & Martin, 2000, 2001; Martin & Romani, 1994; Saffran & Martin, 1990; Shelton et al., 1992). One recent study (Hanten & Martin, 2000), investigating the short-term memory and sentence-processing abilities of two children who had sustained severe CHI, found a dissociation in performance, such that one child appeared to have a relatively pure phonological STM deficit, whereas the other child showed a pattern of performance, consistent with a deficit in semantic STM coupled with a milder impairment of phonological STM. Such studies may provide a clearer understanding of the specific functional impairment underlying memory deficits and may be important in terms of remediation efforts.

Non-verbal/Visual Memory Deficits

A number of group studies have investigated memory deficits after head injury using visual, non-verbal stimuli. Many studies have found that individuals with severe CHI are impaired on recognition tests of nonverbal memory, using abstract, nonverbalizable stimuli (Brooks, 1974, 1976; Reid & Kelly, 1993; Shum et al., 2000), drawings of nameable objects (Hannay et al., 1979; Levin et al., 1988b) and unfamiliar faces (Millis & Dijkers,

1993). In studies that have looked at individual performance, dissociations in patterns of impairment have been found with recognition or matching of faces dissociated from facial expression recognition (Parry et al., 1991). In studies requiring recall of an unnameable object, as in the Rey Complex figure (Rey, 1964), some group studies have shown no persistent impairment (Hellawell et al., 1999), although other studies have revealed impairments (Donders, 1993). A study done by Spikeman et al. (1995) may shed some light on the conditions under which recognition memory may be preserved or impaired. They found that 22 adults with severe CHI demonstrated preserved recognition memory for complex pictorial scenes but impaired recognition memory for unfamiliar faces. The authors of the study noted that the two sets of visual stimuli varied in at least one notable way. The pictures of faces used in the task comprised a set of common features that varied from face to face; thus, recognition had to be based on subtle differences among common features. On the other hand, the complex pictures had different and distinct features from picture to picture, and thus had more unique information to support recognition. The difference in recognition performance in the two conditions suggests that the patients may have utilized the distinctive features in the complex pictures as an aid in recognition, but in the absence of such supporting features showed impairment in face recognition performance. A recent study in our laboratory using non-verbal stimulus items is consistent with this interpretation. We investigated the ability of adults with severe CHI to perform an ongoing task that required the subject to select each member of a full set of abstract stimulus items during a series of trials in a sequence of their choice without pointing to the same alternative twice (adapted from Petrides & Milner, 1982). The number of designs that had to be kept in mind increased with each successful trial, thus increasing the working memory load. The task was untimed, and responses were made by pointing to the items, thus eliminating speed of cognitive processing and language as contributing factors to impaired performance. Importantly, in this study, the stimulus items, although easily discriminable, shared many features, and the stimulus items themselves were randomly rearranged between trials; thus, neither unique features nor spatial context could contribute to performance. The results of the study indicated that adults with severe CHI made significantly more errors (Figure 3.5)

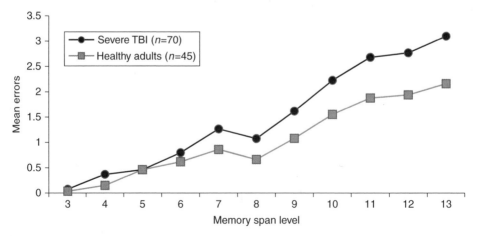

Figure 3.5 Average errors per trial by memory load in persons with severe TBI and age-matched uninjured controls. From Stallings et al. (submitted)

and achieved a lower memory span than did age- and education-matched uninjured control subjects.

This and other studies showing impaired recognition in the absence of context but spared recognition under conditions of rich contextual support (Mangels et al., 2000; Tsukiura et al., 2000) suggests that persons with CHI may be able to use contextual support as an aid in memory performance.

In summary, most studies of auditory–verbal memory and working memory in persons with CHI indicate that memory impairment is a likely consequence of severe head injury. In addition, the magnitude of the impairment has been found to be related to the severity of the injury, as determined by the GCS (Levin et al., 1988a). Studies of components of working memory have indicated that it may be possible to isolate impairments of specific components of working memory.

Impairment of Long-term and Remote Memory

Various aspects of long-term memory after traumatic brain injury have been investigated, including varieties of knowledge (semantic, declarative, procedural), autobiographical and remote memory, and memory for names of familiar objects or faces. Within the semantic/declarative knowledge domain, studies have tended to look at either the ability to acquire knowledge or the selective loss or preservation of (presumably) already existing knowledge. In the procedural knowledge domain, most studies have focused only the ability to acquire knowledge, rather than on the selective loss or preservation of specific areas of procedural knowledge.

Semantic/Declarative Knowledge

Selective impairments of semantic knowledge have been reported in patients with acquired brain damage arising from various etiologies; however, such deficits have not been commonly reported in studies of CHI. However, many studies of memory deficits after CHI employ group study designs, which may occlude relatively rare semantic deficits. In studies that have reported deficits on tasks that assess semantic knowledge, the impairments tend to be revealed in tasks that require the spoken output of a lexical item. In a study comparing the nature of semantic deficits exhibited by nonprogressive brain injury (CHI) as compared to progressive brain injury, Wilson (1997) described two CHI patients who appeared to have semantic knowledge deficits. The deficits were similar to those reported for patients with dementia but appeared to be limited to tasks in which spoken output of the actual lexical item was required. The patients were very impaired on a verbal fluency test, in which they produced exemplars from specific categories, and on naming to pictures and descriptions of exemplars. However, they performed normally on picture sorting for both superordinate and subordinate categories and on picture–word matching for nonliving categories, and were only mildly impaired on picture–word matching for living categories. This pattern of impaired verbal production of exemplars with spared semantic knowledge is consistent with other studies investigating semantic impairments after CHI (Haut et al., 1991; Hough et al., 1997; Lohman et al., 1989; Levin et al., 1996; Levin & Goldstein, 1986). It should be noted that when generating words beginning with a specified letter, CHI subjects have been found to produce significantly fewer items than normal controls (Adamovich & Henderson, 1984; Crowe, 1992; Levin et al., 1981; Sarno, 1984), suggesting that at least a portion of the reported impairments may be accounted for by lexical factors unrelated to semantic organization.

Although patients with CHI may display relatively spared semantic knowledge, there is evidence that the mechanism of access is not only slowed or very effortful, but may be qualitatively different than in uninjured persons (Goldstein et al., 1990; Haut et al., 1991). Several investigators have reported that CHI patients at varying levels of functioning and time postinjury produce excessive intrusions on tests of verbal recall (Hough et al., 1997; Levin, 1989; Richardson, 1984). Further, the ability to either benefit from or use semantic information to facilitate recall has been shown to be impaired in children (Hanten & Martin, 2000; Levin et al., 1996) and adults with CHI (Gruen et al., 1990; Levin & Goldstein, 1986). A further issue to be addressed is the ability of persons with CHI to acquire categorical knowledge, separate from the ability to make use of preserved categorical knowledge. Although we are not aware of any studies specifically investigating this aspect of memory after CHI, the ability of persons with amnesia from various etiologies to acquire categorical knowledge has been studied. Knowlton & Squire (1993) found that after training on sets of dot patterns to learn "categories", amnesic patients and control subjects performed similarly when asked to decide if novel patterns belonged to the same category as the set of training patterns. In contrast, the amnesic subjects were impaired relative to the controls at recognizing which dot patterns had been presented for training, thus demonstrating preserved category acquisition in the presence of impaired recognition. Other studies have investigated category knowledge acquisition with more life-like stimulus items with similar results (Reed et al., 1999). These results are suggestive of categorical knowledge acquisition relying on preserved implicit learning in amnesic patients. It remains to be determined whether a similar pattern is present for patients with CHI.

Episodic/Remote/Autobiographical Memory

One variety of long-term memory is that for personally experienced events. Falling under the general rubric of episodic memory, i.e. memory for events (Tulving, 1983), it has sometimes been called "remote" memory for events having to do with historical events, and "autobiographical" memory when the memory episodes are personal in nature. As mentioned above, temporary retrograde amnesia occurs as an immediate consequence of brain trauma, and usually gradually resolves until the patient can remember all but the very immediate moments prior to the trauma. Less common is more persistent retrograde amnesia, in which loss of memory from events in the past may be experienced for much longer duration, up to years or even permanently. Deficits of remote and autobiographical memory have been described in which patients with brain injury from various etiologies (including CHI) show selective loss of memory for specific time periods (Albert et al., 1979; Barr et al., 1990; Ellis et al., 1989; Evans et al., 1993; Markowitsch et al., 1993; McCarthy & Warrington, 1992; Squire, 1974). Memory loss has been reported to occur in a temporal gradient, with memory for more remote events better than memory for recent events (e.g. Albert et al., 1979). This phenomenon has been explained as a disruption by trauma of the "consolidation" of immediate memory (Squire, 1992; Squire & Zola-Morgan, 1988). However, methodological issues somewhat cloud this area of research. Primarily, in the absence of a measure of the premorbid state of

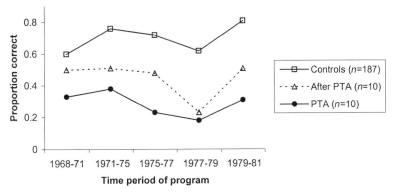

Figure 3.6 Mean proportion of correct recognition of titles of television programs, plotted across the time period of broadcast for oriented (after PTA) and amnesic (PTA) head-injured patients and control subjects. Reproduced from Levin et al. (1985b). © 1985, BMJ Publication Group

remembering of an individual for a specific event, it is difficult to determine how memorial abilities or knowledge has been changed as a consequence of trauma. This is compounded for events that are autobiographical in nature, as the events themselves are difficult to verify. A second problem relating to the measurement of temporal gradients in remote memory is the difficulty in equating the salience of memory items across chronological intervals. As has been pointed out by McCarthy & Warrington (1992), items that are remembered from the remote past might be of higher salience than those from the recent past. Methodological issues aside, impairments for remote/autobiographical memory do appear to accompany brain injury, although only a few studies have focused on the consequences of traumatic brain injury. Studies done by Levin et al. (1977, 1984, 1985a) investigated the remote memory of oriented (After) and amnesic (PTA) head-injured patients by testing their memory on a questionnaire for television programs that had been shown for only one season, thus equating the difficulty of the items to be remembered (Squire & Slater, 1975). The amnesic CHI patients showed a clear impairment in recognition memory, but no evidence for a temporal gradient (Figure 3.6).

Similarly, Leplow et al. (1997) investigated remote memory for patients with CHI and two other patient groups, as well as a large control group of 214 persons. To control for the increased salience effect, the authors tested memory for events across six decades that had been on the front page of the newspapers for 3 days. Further, the study was confined to people who had not left the geographical area for more than 6 months throughout their lifetime. The results of the recall and recognition tests for events and people indicated that the patients with CHI were very impaired in remote memory, especially in recall, when compared to the controls. However, as in the studies by Levin, there was no indication of a memory gradient for more impairment for more recent events, and in fact, performance was slightly better for recent as compared to more remote events.

Levin et al. (1985a) also investigated recall of autobiographic events in survivors of moderate to severe CHI undergoing inpatient rehabilitation. In contrast to the lack of a temporal gradient for salience-matched remote memory on the questionnaire of television programs (Figure 3.6), Levin et al. (1985a) found relative preservation of recall for autobiographical events from the primary school years, as compared to later development periods, in these

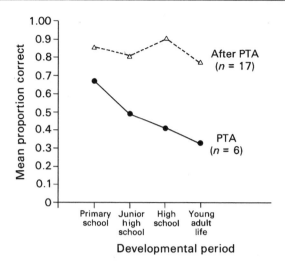

Figure 3.7 Mean proportion of correct recall of autobiographical events, compiled for developmental periods of the head-injured patients during and after PTA. Reproduced from Levin et al. (1985b). © 1985, BMJ Publication Group

young adult patients (Figure 3.7). The temporal gradient obtained for autobiographical events is similar to the sparing of memory for faces of famous persons and retention of public events from the remote past, which has been reported in amnesics with alcoholic Korsakoff syndrome (Albert et al., 1979).

Methodological issues notwithstanding, the studies described above suggest that loss of memory for remote and for autobiographical memory is associated with CHI. However, the findings of a temporal gradient for preserved distant memory with loss for recent memory, although theoretically plausible, is yet not consistent and requires further investigation.

Naming

There have been a number of studies that have found impaired naming of people and objects after CHI. Specific naming impairments have been described in the presence of the ability to produce accurate and specific semantic knowledge of the people that could not be named (Brooks et al., 1984; Carney & Temple, 1993; Fery et al., 1995; Hittmaier-Delazer et al., 1994; Lucchelli & de Renzi, 1992; Parry et al., 1991; Sunderland et al., 1983). Impaired naming of familiar objects following closed head injury has also been found to be relatively frequent in adults with CHI; for example, Levin et al. (1977) found impaired object naming in 40% of the 50 patients they studied in whom PTA had resolved. Similar findings have been reported in other studies of adults with CHI (Hellawell et al., 1999; Kerr, 1995; Mattson et al., 2000); for example, Mattson et al. (2000) reported a case of prosopagnosia following moderate CHI with left hemisphere focal lesion. Color vision was intact on screening, although shape detection was borderline. Impairments in higher order visual perception were evident to varying degrees on nonfacial tasks. Matching of unfamiliar faces was very slow but accurate, and identification of characteristics of faces (gender, age) and identification and matching of facial expressions were relatively intact. However, the patient showed a marked impairment in the ability to recognize familiar faces and learn new face–name associations relative to healthy control subjects.

In summary, research on the long-term memory consequences has demonstrated that deficits in declarative knowledge can be a consequence of traumatic brain injury, especially under conditions that require naming of an item. Although semantic category information is generally reported to be intact, there is some evidence that the acquisition of new categorical knowledge may be impaired.

PRODEDURAL KNOWLEDGE

Within the procedural memory domain, most studies have focused only on the acquisition of knowledge, rather than systematically testing loss or preservation of knowledge. Studies of the ability to acquire procedural knowledge (i.e. learning "how to" do something) after CHI have generally shown intact procedural learning, even in the presence of impaired verbal learning; for example, Ewert et al. (1989) investigated the acquisition of procedural knowledge as compared to declarative knowledge in adults with severe CHI. They reported that individuals with CHI were impaired on declarative learning tasks relative to a group of matched uninjured adults but they showed learning across sessions on all procedural memory tasks. Timmerman & Brouwer (1999) used reaction time tasks to evaluate the effect of task difficulty on performance in acquiring declarative and procedural knowledge. They found that patients with CHI were generally slower than controls on both declarative and procedural tasks, but task difficulty affected performance only on the declarative tasks. Further, analysis of errors indicated that only on the declarative tasks did the CHI patients make more errors than the controls. However, it should be noted that both of the declarative knowledge tasks were machine-paced. One of the procedural tasks was self-paced and the other task, although machine paced, had a presentation time substantially longer than for the declarative tasks. Because no distinction was made between omission of responses and incorrect responses, it is possible that some of the differences observed may be accounted for by slowed processing. Nonetheless, the finding that task difficulty affected only declarative knowledge supports the general results of other studies that the ability to acquire procedural knowledge is less susceptible to disruption by traumatic brain injury than is declarative knowledge.

IMPLICIT MEMORY

Implicit memory occurs when the response to a stimulus is influenced by previous experience in the absence of intentional, conscious recollection of that experience (Roediger, 1990; Schacter, 1987). The findings that implicit memory was spared in persons with dense amnesia (Warrington & Weiskrantz, 1968) incited a riot of recent research on the dissociation between explicit and implicit memory in both normal and patient populations (e.g. Bassili et al., 1989; Challis & Brodbeck, 1992; Craik et al., 1994; Gabrieli et al., 1995; Graf & Masson, 1993; Graf et al., 1985; Jacoby & Dallas, 1981; Rajaram & Roediger, 1993; Roediger & Blaxton, 1987; Roediger et al., 1992; Schacter, 1987; Schacter & Church, 1992). In the studies investigating memory deficits, the general finding is that patients who show impairment on explicit tests of memory perform normally on implicit tests of memory. This pattern has been shown for a wide variety of stimulus materials, including verbal, nonverbal, procedural and even memory for context (McAndrews et al., 1987; Vakil et al., 1998). Studies with memory-impaired patients in various populations have indicated that priming for words (used to measure implicit learning) in word-stem completion tasks is spared in patients with frontal lesions (Shimamura et al., 1992), and supports previous neuropsychological and PET findings, which indicate that word priming depends critically on posterior cortical areas (e.g. Dhond et al., 2001). Although studies directly comparing implicit and explicit tests of memory in CHI patients are relatively sparse, such studies that have been done suggest that implicit memory is more resistant to impairment after CHI than is explicit memory in both adults (Ewert et al., 1989; Glisky, 1993; Shum et al., 1996; Watt et al., 1999) and children (Shum et al., 1999a); for example, Shum et al. (1999a) investigated the abilities of 12 children with severe CHI and 12 matched uninjured children on a picture fragment completion task under explicit or implicit instructions. In the study phase of both conditions the children were shown complete pictures in a naming task, after which there was a filled delay. Under implicit instructions, the children were shown fragments of the pictures that had been presented in the study phase intermixed with non-studied picture fragments. Without reference to the previous study stage, the children were asked to identify pictures from the fragments. Under explicit instructions, the children were shown fragments and were asked to identify pictures from the fragments, but were told that they had seen the pictures earlier in the testing session. The authors found that the children with CHI performed similarly to the uninjured control children in the implicit task, but were significantly impaired on the explicit task.

IMPAIRMENTS OF METACOGNITION

The term "metacognition" has been applied to different processes. Some theorists (Flavell, 1981; Flavell et al., 1970; Metcalfe & Shimamura, 1996) have used the word to mean conscious awareness of one's cognitive abilities, in other words, what we know about what we know. A different use of the term metacognition is a product of the information-processing approach to theoretical models of cognition, which assume a system whose activities and resources are monitored by a central executive. In these models, metacognition refers to the self-regulatory activities of the cognitive system (Brown, 1978; Brown & Deloache, 1978). This aspect might be conceptualized as what we *do* about what we know. As has been alluded to above, successful memorial performance involves more than the passive registration and retrieval of information. It can also involve strategic manipulation of information, assessment of ongoing processes, monitoring of performance or appraisal of feedback. There is a rich tradition of metacognitive research—mostly metamemory—in normal adults and children (e.g. Flavell, 1981; Flavell et al., 1970; Hart, 1967), which has been extended to neuropsychological research (e.g. Mazzoni & Nelson, 1998; Metcalfe & Shimamura, 1996). Studies of individuals with CHI have revealed that in performance of memory tasks they may fail to apply the appropriate metacognitive processes; for example, studies of verbal learning using the CVLT-C have shown that children with head injury show increased numbers of intrusions and perseverations in list recall (Levin et al., 1996) and in procedural learning (Beldarrain et al., 1999), suggesting a failure of metacognitive monitoring and control processes. Adults with CHI have also demonstrated a passive learning strategy with semantically related lists, leading to poorer recall (Levin & Goldstein, 1986). In studies that have directly investigated metacognition, previous research in adults with acquired brain damage has shown that feeling-of-knowing judgments (the ability to judge whether one can recognize a previously unrecallable target item) are impaired in individuals with frontal lobe damage (Janowsky et al., 1989; Shimamura et al., 1991; Shimamura & Squire, 1986). These impairments in metacognitive abilities were evident even when item recall level was matched across groups. Thus, the impairment in metacognitive processing in these patients was apparently not related to any general memory impairment, but rather to an impairment of executive level monitoring processes. In studies that have directly addressed metacognitive processing in persons with CHI, deficits have been reported in "feeling-of-knowing" judgments in adults and children (Hanten et al., 2000; Jurado et al., 1998). In our laboratory we have investigated metacognitive control within the memory domain in children with CHI and in uninjured children using a modification of a selective learning task for adults (Watkins & Hanten, unpublished manuscript). In this task we tested children's ability to selectively learn high-value items over low-value items in list recall (Hanten et al., 2001).

We studied 13 children with chronic severe CHI, ages 9–15, and 24 normally developing uninjured children matched for age and parental education. The children were presented lists of 16 words, of which eight words are designated as "high-value" words, and eight words are "low-value" words, with value indicated by category membership. The subjects were to make as high a score as possible by learning the words in the list. The measure of metacognitive control was the *selective efficiency* demonstrated in learning the words of differing value, independent of the number of words recalled. Children with CHI appeared to recall slightly fewer words than did control children (Figure 3.8A), although the difference was not significant. In contrast, the children with CHI were impaired relative to the control children on the measure of selective efficiency (Figure 3.8B). The different pattern of performance demonstrated for memory span and the measure of selective learning may be interpreted as a dissociation in memory capacity and metacognitive control in children with CHI.

Although research investigating the relationship between metacognition and memory performance after CHI is in the early stages, such results as have been reported suggest that impairments in metacognitive monitoring and control are a possible consequence of CHI and may interact with memory processes. Such interactions may have implications for outcome after CHI.

PROSPECTIVE MEMORY

Prospective memory, the recall of future intentions or actions to be performed, is a hybrid or multicomponent form of memory. Prospective memory has a "declarative" component (the *what* element to be recalled, which in this case is an action or intention), and also has a temporal–contextual element (the *when* and sometimes *where* the intention or action is to be executed). Relatively little research has been conducted on prospective memory after CHI. Self-reports on a questionnaire of memory failures indicate that adult CHI patients report significantly impaired prospective memory compared to uninjured adults (Mateer et al., 1987). In studies utilizing experimental tasks to investigate prospective memory in adults after CHI, impairments have been reported after short delay (Shum et al., 1999b) but not long delay (Hannon et al., 1995; Kinsella et al., 1996). In our laboratory, we studied the prospective memory performance of children with severe CHI and normally developing children (McCauley & Levin, 2000). Children were tested on several versions of event-based

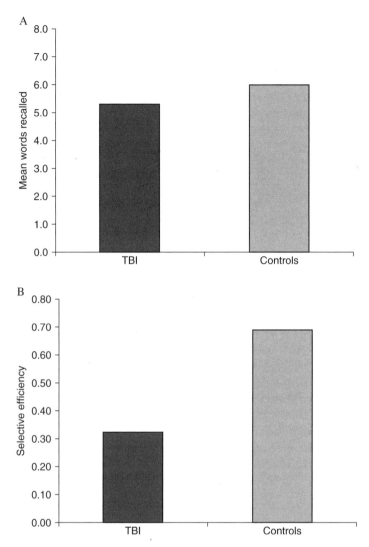

Figure 3.8 Memory span (A) and selective learning efficiency (B) of children with TBI and uninjured control children. From Hanten et al. (2001)

(EB) and activity-based (AB) prospective memory tasks. The tasks were designed to be ecologically valid and included such tasks as requiring the child to place his/her hands in his/her lap as quickly as possible (in spite of any ongoing activity) at the sound of a bell, or to pick up an envelope and give it to his/her parent at the conclusion of the testing session. We found that children with CHI were impaired relative to the control children on both EB and AB prospective memory tasks (Figure 3.9). These results support the hypothesis that severe CHI in children can result in prospective memory deficits across a variety of ecologically valid prospective memory tasks.

To summarize, neuropsychological findings in consecutive admissions for moderate to severe CHI support the impression that memory disturbance is a frequent and perhaps the

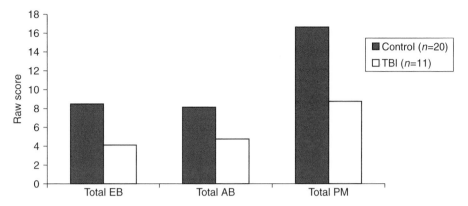

Figure 3.9 Raw score for tests of prospective memory in children with severe TBI and age-matched control children. In these tasks, a higher score indicates better performance. From McCauley & Levin (2000)

most prominent residual cognitive deficit after CHI. These results are also consonant with reports by patients and their families indicating that memory deficit is a common, persisting complaint (Oddy et al., 1985).

SEVERITY AND CHRONICITY OF HEAD INJURY

Numerous studies have documented the relationship between severity of acute CHI and the degree and persistence of the resulting memory deficit (Brooks, 1974, 1975; Dikmen et al., 1987; Levin et al., 1987, 1988a). The influence of chronicity of injury is particularly apparent in recovery from an initial memory deficit in patients examined within the first week after sustaining a mild head injury (Levin et al., 1987). In a three-center study, Levin et al. (1987) found that an initial impairment of verbal learning and memory resolved between 1 and 3 months after a mild head injury characterized at the time of hospital admission by brief loss of consciousness, normal neurologic findings and confusion, with preserved eye opening and ability to follow commands. This recovery pattern is depicted by the box plots shown in Figure 3.10. Support for our conclusion was provided by Dikmen et al. (1987), who found evidence of residual memory deficit in patients tested a year after sustaining a severe, but not a mild, injury. Findings from the Traumatic Coma Data Bank have documented remarkable individual variation in memory recovery curves among a cohort of severe CHI patients studied serially over 2 years (Levin et al., 1990; Ruff et al., 1991). These investigators found subgroups that exhibited recovery of verbal memory to within the normal range, as opposed to relatively flat functions showing minimal or no improvement over time, and a subgroup that showed evidence of deterioration in performance.

Analysis of the one year neurobehavioral follow-up data collected in the Traumatic Coma Data Bank has provided an opportunity to investigate the relationship between acute neurologic indices of severe CHI and later memory functioning (Levin et al., 1990). The lowest postresuscitation GCS score was predictive of verbal memory (Selective Reminding Test) one year later in patients who also had nonreactive pupils during their initial hospitalization. In contrast, the GCS score was unrelated to memory performance in

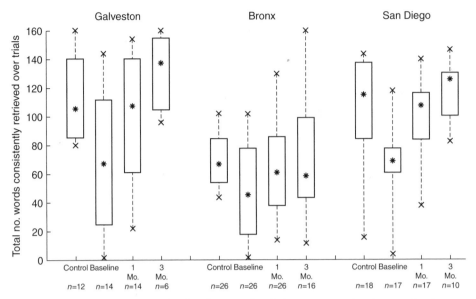

Figure 3.10 Box-plot showing the distribution of verbal memory retrieval scores by the controls and mild head-injured group studied in Galveston, the Bronx and San Diego. The distributions of scores are given for the head-injured groups at baseline (within 1 week postinjury) and at 1 and 3 months (Mo.) after injury; n = number of patients. See Figure 3.4A for explanation of symbols. Reproduced from Levin et al. (1987). © 1987 *Journal of Neurosurgery*

patients who had normal pupillary reactivity in the emergency room and throughout their initial hospitalization. Levin and colleagues interpreted this interaction as evidence for long-term consequences of severely impaired consciousness on memory, provided that it is accompanied by other signs of neurologic deterioration, as reflected by abnormal pupillary reactivity. In contrast, recovery of verbal memory within one year after a severe CHI appears to be unrelated to the lowest GCS score, provided that there is no other evidence of neurologic deterioration. Further analysis of the interrelationships among indices of acute brain injury could potentially elucidate the wide variation in recovery of memory observed among survivors of severe CHI.

IMPLICATIONS FOR REHABILITATION

Memory theorists and clinical neuropsychologists have published case reports and studies of small groups of CHI patients that lend support to various remedial techniques for memory disorder (Crosson & Buenning, 1984; Crovitz et al., 1979; Glasgow et al., 1977; Glisky & Schacter, 1988; Glisky et al., 1986; Harris & Sunderland, 1981; Richardson, 1979; Wilson & Moffat, 1984). Although visual imagery and semantic elaboration techniques have received preliminary support (Glasgow et al., 1977; Kovner et al., 1983), evidence from controlled clinical trials is limited to a single study that evaluated the efficacy of a total program, rather than a specific technique (Prigatano et al., 1984). Apart from the modest empirical support for remediation of memory deficit, practical issues include the compliance of severely brain-injured patients with unfamiliar techniques, such as bizarre imagery. Other limitations include the lack of generalization across situations and erosion of gains after termination of training (Crosson & Buenning, 1984, Crovitz et al., 1979).

A primary objection to attempts to "retrain" memory through role experience is that repeatedly tested amnesics, such as patient H.M., have exhibited no improvement despite exhaustive practice and exposure to various mnemonic techniques (Milner et al., 1968). Similarly, we have reported that survivors of severe CHI frequently exhibit persistent impairment of memory, despite intensive rehabilitation (Levin et al., 1985a).

In recent years a broader spectrum of rehabilitation techniques has been explored, in part as a consequence of expanding knowledge of physiology and neurochemistry of the brain, as well as advances in understanding of the mechanisms underlying basic cognitive processes. Traditional psychological approaches to rehabilitation have employed compensatory strategies, such as utilization of internal or external memory cues or memory aid devices, with variable results (for review, see Sohlberg & Mateer, 1989). More recently, researchers have taken the approach of devising strategies that build on preserved cognitive components, such as procedural and/or implicit memory (e.g. Evans et al., 2000; Glisky, 1993; Glisky & Schacter, 1988; Thoene & Glisky,1995; Wilson & Evans, 1996). As with more traditional approaches, the results of these types of strategies are inconclusive. More research is needed to specify the conditions under which such interventions are effective. Several more biological approaches to rehabilitation have shown promise when implemented in animal models, including methods to stimulate regeneration or reorganization of brain structure (e.g. Kolb et al., 1997; McEwen & Wooley, 1994), and intracerebral transplantation (see Dickinson-Anson et al., 1999). In humans, pharmacological agents have been used to mitigate the effects of brain trauma (e.g. Arnsten & Smith, 1999; McIntosh, 1993; McIntosh et al., 1996; Stein et al., 1999; Zhu et al., 2000) with some success, although experimental evidence for the efficacy of such treatments is at present equivocal.

ACKNOWLEDGEMENT

Research presented in this chapter was supported by grants NS21889, H133B990014, and H133A980073. The authors are indebted to Angela D. Williams for word processing and editorial assistance.

REFERENCES

Adamovich, B. & Henderson, J. (1984). Can we learn more from word fluency measures with aphasic, right brain-injured, and closed head trauma patients? In R. Brookshire (ed.), *Clinical Aphasiology Conference Proceedings* (pp. 124–131). Minneapolis, MN: BRK.

Adams, J.H., Graham, D., Scott, G. et al. (1980). Brain damage in fatal non-missile head injury. *Journal of Clinical Pathology*, **33**, 1132–1145.

Albert, M.S., Butters, N. & Levin, J. (1979). Temporal gradients in the retrograde amnesia of patients with alcoholic Korsakoff's disease. *Archives of Neurology*, **36**, 211–216.

Arnsten, A.F.T. & Smith, D.H. (1999). Pharmacological strategies for neuroprotection and rehabilitation. In D.T. Stuss, G. Winocur & I.H. Robertson (eds), *Cognitive Neurorehabilitation* (pp. 113–135). Cambridge: Cambridge University Press.

Artiola, L., Fortuny, I., Briggs, M. et al. (1980). Measuring the duration of post-traumatic amnesia. *Journal of Neurology, Neurosurgery, and Psychiatry*, **43**, 377–379.

Baddeley, A. (1986). *Working Memory*. Oxford: Clarendon/Oxford University Press.

Baddeley, A. (1998). Recent developments in working memory. *Current Opinion in Neurobiology*, **8**(2), 234–238.

Baddeley, A., Harris, J., Sunderland, A. et al. (1987). Closed head injury and memory. In H.S. Levin, J. Grafman & H.M. Eisenberg (eds), *Neurobehavioral Recovery from Head Injury* (pp. 295–316). Oxford: Oxford University Press.

Baddeley, A. & Wilson, B.A. (1993). A developmental deficit in short-term phonological memory: implications for language and reading. *Memory*, **1**, 65–78.

Barr, W.B., Goldberg, E., Wasserstein, J. & Novelly, R.A. (1990). Retrograde amnesia following unilateral temporal lobectomy. *Neuropsychologia*, **28**, 243–255.

Bassili, J.N., Smith, M.C. & MacLeod, C.M. (1989). Auditory and visual word-stem completion: separating data-driven and conceptually driven processes. *Quarterly Journal of Experimental Psychology, A Human Experimental Psychology*, **41**, 439–453.

Beldarrain, M., Grafman, J., Pascual-Leone, A. & Garcia-Monco, J.C. (1999). Procedural learning is impaired in patients with prefrontal lesions. *Neurology*, **52**, 1853–1860.

Benton, A.L., Van Allen, M.W. & Fogel, M.L. (1964). Temporal orientation in cerebral disease. *Journal of Nervous and Mental Disorders*, **139**, 110–119.

Brodie, B. (1854). *Psychological Enquiries*. London: Longman.

Brooks, D.N. (1974). Recognition memory and head injury. *Journal of Neurology, Neurosurgery, and Psychiatry*, **37**, 224–230.

Brooks, D.N. (1975). Long- and short-term memory in head injured patients. *Cortex*, **11**, 329–340.

Brooks, D.N. (1976). Recognition memory after head injury: a signal detection analysis. *Cortex*, **10**, 224–230.

Brooks, D.N., Deelman, B.G., van Zomeren, A.H. et al. (1984). Problems in measuring cognitive recovery after acute brain injury. *Journal of Clinical Neuropsychology*, **6**(1), 71–85.

Brooks, N., McKinlay, W., Simington, C., Beattie, A. & Campsie, L. (1987). Return to work within the first seven years of severe head injury. *Brain Injury*, **1**, 5–19.

Brown, A.L. (1978). Knowing when, where, and how to remember: a problem of metacognition. In R. Glaser (ed), *Advances in Instructional Psychology* (pp. 367–406). Hillsdale, NJ: Erlbaum.

Brown, A.L. & DeLoache, J.S. (1978). Skills, plans, and self-regulation. In R. Siegler (ed.), *Children's Thinking: What Develops?* Hillsdale, NJ: Erlbaum.

Bullock R., Zauner A., Woodward, J.J. et al. (1998). Factors affecting excitatory amino acid release following severe human head injury. *Journal of Neurosurgery*, **89** (4), 507–518.

Buschke, H. & Fuld, P.A. (1974). Evaluating storage, retention, and retrieval in disordered memory and learning. *Neurology*, **14**, 1019–1025.

Carney, R. & Temple, C.M. (1993). Prosopagnosia: a possible category specific anomia for faces. *Cognitive Neuropsychology*, **10**, 185–195.

Challis, B.H. & Brodbeck, D.R. (1992). Level of processing affects priming in word fragment completion. *Journal of Experimental Psychology: Learning, Memory, and Cognition*, **18**, 595–607.

Craik, F.I.M., Moscovitch, M. & McDowd, J.M. (1994). Contribution of surface and conceptual information to performance on implicit and explicit memory tasks. *Journal of Experimental Psychology: Learning, Memory, and Cognition*, **20**, 864–875.

Crosson, B. & Buenning, W. (1984). An individualized memory retraining program after closed head injury: a single-case study. *Journal of Clinical Neuropsychology*, **6**, 287–301.

Crosson, B., Novack, T.A., Trenerry, M.R. & Craig, P.L. (1988). California Verbal Learning (CVLT) performance in severely head-injured and neurologically normal adult males. *Journal of Clinical and Experimental Neuropsychology*, **10**, 754–768.

Crovitz, H.F., Harvey, M.T. & Horn, R.W. (1979). Problems in the acquisition of imagery mnemonics: three brain-damaged cases. *Cortex*, **15**, 225–234.

Crowe, S.F. (1992.) Dissociation of two frontal lobe syndromes by a test of verbal fluency. *Journal of Clinical and Experimental Neuropsychology*, **14**, 327–339.

Delis, D.C., Kramer, J.H., Kaplan, E. et al. (1986). *The California Verbal Learning Test, research edition*. New York, NY: Psychological Corporation.

Delis, D.C., Kramer, J.H., Kaplan, E. & Ober, B.A. (1994). *The California Verbal Learning Test, Children's Version Manual*. San Antonio, TX: Psychological Corporation.

Delis, D.C., Massman, P.J., Butters, N. et al. (1991). Profiles of demented and amnesic patients on the California Verbal Learning Test: implications for the assessment of memory disorders. *Psychological Assessment*, **3**, 19–26.

Dennis, M. & Barnes, M.A. (1990). Knowing the meaning, getting the point, bridging the gap, and carrying the message: aspects of discourse following closed head injury in childhood and adolescence. *Brain and Language*, **39**, 428–446.

Dhond, R.P., Buckner, R.L., Dale., A.M. et al. (2001). Spatiotemporal maps of brain activity underlying word generation and their modification during repetition priming. *Journal of Neuroscience*, **21**, 3564–3571.

Dickinson-Anson, H., Aubert, I. & Gage, F.H. (1999). Intracerebral transplantation and regeneration: practical implications. In D.T Stuss & G. Winocur (eds), *Cognitive Neurorehabilitation* (pp. 26–46). New York: Cambridge University Press.

Dikmen S., Temkin, N., McLean, A. et al. (1987). Memory and head injury severity. *Journal of Neurology, Neurosurgery and Psychiatry*, **50**, 1613–1618.

DiStefano, G., Bachevalier, J., Levin, H.S. et al. (2000). Volume of focal brain lesions and hippocampal formation in relation to memory function after closed head injury in children. *Journal of Neurology, Neurosurgery, and Psychiatry*, **69**, 210–216.

Donders J. (1993). Memory functioning after traumatic brain injury in children. *Brain Injury*, **7**, 431–437.

Eisenberg, H.M., Gary, H.E. Jr, Aldrich, E.F. et al. (1990). Initial CT findings in 753 patients with severe head injury: a report from the NIH Traumatic Coma Data Bank. *Journal of Neurosurgery*, **73**, 688–698.

Ellenberg, J.H., Levin, H.S. & Saydjari, C. (1996). Posttraumatic amnesia as a predictor of outcome after severe closed head injury: prospective assessment. *Archives of Neurology*, **53**, 782–786.

Ellis, A.W., Young, A.W. & Critchley, M.R. (1989). Loss of memory for people following temporal lobe damage. *Brain*, **112**, 1469–1483.

Evans, J.J., Wilson, B.A., Schuri, U. et al. (2000). A comparison of "errorless" and "trial-and-error" learning methods for teaching individuals with acquired memory deficits. *Neuropsychological Rehabilitation*, **10**, 67–101.

Evans, J., Wilson, B., Wright, E. & Hodges, J.R. (1993). Neuropsychological and SPECT scan findings during and after transient global amnesia: evidence for the differential impairment of remote episodic memory. *Journal of Neurology, Neurosurgery, and Psychiatry*, **56**, 1227–1230.

Ewert, J., Levin, H.S., Watson, M.G. & Kalisky, Z. (1989). Procedural memory during posttraumatic amnesia in survivors of closed head injury: implications for rehabilitation. *Archives of Neurology*, **46**, 911–916.

Fery, P., Vincent, E. & Brédart, S. (1995). Personal name anomia: a single case study. *Cortex*, **31**, 191–198.

Flavell, J.H. (1981). Cognitive monitoring. In W.P. Dickson (ed.), *Children's Oral Communication Skill*. New York: Academic Press.

Flavell, J.H., Friedrichs, A. & Hoyt, J. (1970). Developmental changes in memorization processes. *Cognitive Psychology*, **1**, 324–340.

Fontaine, A., Azouvi, P., Remy, P. et al. (1999). Functional anatomy of neuropsychological deficits after sever traumatic brain injury. *American Academy of Neurology*, **53**, 1963–1968.

Friedman, S.D., Brooks, W.M., Jung, R.E. et al. (1998). Proton MR spectroscopic findings correspond to neuropsychological function in traumatic brain injury. *American Journal of Neuroradiology*, **19**, 1879–1885.

Gabrieli, J.D.E., Fleischman, D.A., Keane, M.M. et al. (1995). Double dissociation between memory systems underlying explicit and implicit memory in the human brain. *Psychological Science*, **6**, 76–82.

Gardner, S.D. & Vrbancic, M.I. (1998). Which California Verbal Learning Test factors discriminate moderate and severe head injury from normals? *Brain and Cognition*, **37**, 10–13.

Garnett, M.R., Blamire, A.M., Rajagopalan B. et al. (2000.). Evidence for cellular damage in normal-appearing white matter correlates with injury severity in patients following traumatic brain injury. A magnetic resonance spectroscopy study. *Brain*, **123**, 1403–1409.

Glasgow, R.E., Zeiss, R. A., Barreara, M. Jr & Lewinsohn, P.M. (1977). Case studies on remediating memory, deficits in brain-damaged individuals. *Journal of Clinical Psychology*, **33**, 1049–1054.

Glisky, E. (1993). Computer-assisted instructions for patients with traumatic brain injury: teaching of domain-specific knowledge. *Journal of Head Trauma Rehabilitation*, **7**, 1–12.

Glisky, E.L. & Schacter, D.L. (1988). Long-term retention of computer learning by patients with memory disorders. *Neuropsychologia*, **26**, 173–178.

Glisky, E.L., Schacter, D.L. & Tulving, E. (1986.) Computer learning by memory-impaired patients: acquisition and retention of complex knowledge. *Neuropsychologia*, **24**, 313–328.

Goldstein, F.C., Levin, H.S., Boake, C., Lohrey, J.H. (1990). Facilitation of memory performance through induced semantic processing in survivors of closed head injury. *Journal of Clinical and Experimental Neuropsychology*, **12**, 286–300.

Graf, P. & Masson, E. (eds) (1993). *Implicit Memory: New Directions in Cognition, Development, and Neuropsychology*. Hillsdale, NJ: Erlbaum.

Graf, P., Shimamura, A.P. & Squire, L.R. (1985). Priming across modalities and priming across category levels: extending the domain of preserved function in amnesia. *Journal of Experimental Psychology: Learning, Memory, & Cognition*, **11**, 386–396.

Graham, D.I., McIntosh, T.K., Maxwell, W.L. & Nicoll, J.A.R. (2000). Recent advances in neurotrauma. *Journal of Neuropathology and Experimental Neurology*, **59**, 641–651.

Gronwall, D. & Wrightson, P. (1980). Duration of post-traumatic amnesia after mild head injury. *Journal of Clinical Neuropsychology*, **2**, 51–60.

Gruen, A.K., Frankle, B.C. & Schwartz, R. (1990). Word fluency generation skills of head-injured patients in an acute trauma center. *Journal of Communication Disorders*, **23**, 163–170.

Hannay, H.J., Levin, H.S. & Grossman, R.G. (1979). Impaired recognition memory after head injury. *Cortex*, **15**, 269–283.

Hannon, R., Adams, P., Harrington, S. et al. (1995). Effects of brain injury and age on prospective memory self-rating and performance. *Rehabilitation Psychology*, **40**, 289–298.

Hanten, G., Bartha, M. & Levin, H.S. (2000). Metamemory following pediatric traumatic brain injury: a preliminary study. *Developmental Neuropsychology*, **18**, 383–390.

Hanten, G., Dennis, M. & Levin, H.S. (2001). Knowing about knowing: metacognition after childhood closed head injury. In M. Dennis (Chair), *Neurobehavioral Outcome of Traumatic Brain Injury in Children*. Symposium conducted at the 29th Annual Meeting of the International Neuropsychological Society, Chicago, IL, February.

Hanten, G. & Martin, R. C. (2000). Contributions of phonological and semantic short-term memory to sentence processing: evidence from two cases of closed head injury in children. *Journal of Learning and Memory*, **43**, 335–361.

Hanten, G. & Martin, R.C. (2001). A developmental phonological short-term memory deficit: a case study. *Brain and Cognition*, **45**, 164–188.

Harris, J.E. & Sunderland, A. (1981). A brief survey of the management of memory disorders in rehabilitation units in Britain. *International Journal of Rehabilitation Medicine*, **3**, 206–209.

Hart, J.T. (1967). Memory and the memory-monitoring process. *Journal of Verbal Learning and Verbal Behavior*, **6**, 685–691.

Haut, M.W., Petros, T.V., Frank, R.G. & Haut, J.S. (1991). Speed of processing within semantic memory following severe closed head injury. *Brain and Cognition*, **17**, 31–41.

Hellawell, D.J., Taylor, R.T. & Pentland, B. (1999). Cognitive and psychosocial outcome following moderate or severe traumatic brain injury. *Brain Injury*, **13**, 489–504.

High, W.M. Jr, Levin, H.S. & Gary, H.E. Jr. (1990). Recovery of orientation and memory following closed-head injury. *Journal of Clinical and Experimental Neuropsychology*, **12**, 703–714.

Hittmaier-Delazer, M., Denes, G., Semenza, C. & Mantovan, M.C. (1994). Anomia for proper names. *Neuropsychologia*, **32**, 465–476.

Hough, M.S. (1993). Categorization in aphasia: access and organization of goal-derived and common categories. *Aphasiology*, **7**, 335–357.

Hough, M, S., Pierce, R.S, Difilippo, M. & Pabst, MJ. (1997). Access and organization of goal-derived categories after traumatic brain injury. *Brain Injury*, **11**, 801–814.

Hulme, C., Lee, G., Brown, G.D. (1993). Short-term memory impairments in Alzheimer-type dementia: evidence for separable impairments of articulatory rehearsal and long-term memory. *Neuropsychologia*, **31**(2), 161–172.

Jacoby, L.L. & Dallas, M. (1981). On the relationship between autobiographical memory and perceptual learning. *Journal of Experimental Psychology: General*, **110**, 306–340.

Jaffe, K.M., Fay, G.C., Polissar, N.L. et al. (1992). Severity of pediatric traumatic brain injury and early neurobehavioral outcome: a cohort study. *Archives of Physical Medicine and Rehabilitation*, **73**, 540–547.

Janowsky, J.S., Shimamura, A.P. & Squire, L.R. (1989). Memory and metamemory: comparisons between patients with frontal lobe lesions and amnesic patients. *Psychobiology*, **17**, 56–61.

Jarrold, C., Baddeley, A.D. & Hewes, A.K. (1999). Genetically dissociated components of working memory: evidence from Down's and Williams' syndrome. *Neuropsychologia*, **37**, 637–651.

Jennett, W.B. (1969). Head injuries and the temporal lobe. R.N. Herrington (ed). *Current Problems in Neuropsychiatry. British Journal of Psychiatry*, special publication No. 4. Ashford, Kent, UK: Headly Brothers, Ltd.

Jurado, M.A., Junque, C., Vendrell, P. et al. (1998). Overestimation and unreliability in "feeling-of-doing" judgments about temporal ordering performance: impaired self-awareness following frontal lobe damage. *Journal of Clinical and Experimental Neuropsychology*, **20**, 353–364.

Kerr, C. (1995). Dysnomia following traumatic brain injury: an information-processing approach to assessment. *Brain Injury*, **9**, 777–796.

Kinsella, G., Murtagh, D., Landry, A. et al. (1996). Everyday memory following traumatic brain injury. *Brain Injury*, **10**, 499–507

Knowlton B.J. & Squire L.R. (1993). The learning of categories: parallel brain systems for item memory and category knowledge. *Science*, **10**, 1747–1749.

Kochanek, P.M., Clark, R.S.B., Ruppel, R.A. et al. (2000). Biochemical, cellular and molecular mechanisms in the evolution of secondary damage after severe traumatic brain injury in infants and children: lessons learned from the bedside. *Pediatric Critical Care Medicine*, **1**, 4–19.

Kolb, B., Cote, S., Ribeiro-da-Silva, A. & Cuello, A.C. (1997). NGF stimulates recovery of function and dendritic growth after unilateral motor cortex lesion in rats. *Neuroscience*, **76**, 1139–1151.

Kotapka, M.J., Graham, D.I., Adams, J.H. et al. (1994). Hippocampal pathology in fatal human head injury without high intracranial pressure. *Journal of Neurotrauma*, **11**, 317–324.

Kovner, R., Mattis, S., Goldmeier. E. (1983). A technique for promoting robust free recall in chronic organic amnesia. *Journal of Clinical Neuropsychology*, **5**(1), 65–71.

Langfitt, T.W., Obrist, W.D., Alavi, A. et al. (1986). Computerized tomography, magnetic resonance imaging and positron emission tomography in the study of brain trauma: preliminary observations. *Journal of Neurosurgery*, **64**, 760–767.

Lepage, M., Ghaffar, O., Nyberg, L. & Tulving, E. (2000). Prefrontal cortex and episodic memory retrieval mode. *Proceedings of the National Academy of Sciences*, **97**(1), 506–511.

Leplow, B., Dierks, C.H., Lehnung, M. et al. (1997). Remote memory in ptients with acute brain injuries. *Neuropsychologia*, **35**, 881–892.

Levin, H.S. (1989). Memory deficit after closed head injury. *Journal of Clinical and Experimental Neuropsychology*, **12**, 129–153.

Levin, H.S., Benton, A.L. & Grossman, R.G. (1982). *Neurobehavioral Consequences of Closed Head Injury*. New York: Oxford University Press.

Levin, H.S., Fletcher, J.M., Kusnerik, L. et al. (1996). Semantic memory following pediatric head injury: relationship to age, severity of injury, and MRI. *Cortex*, **32**, 461–478.

Levin H.S., Gary, H.E., Eisenberg, H.M. et al. (1990). Traumatic Coma Data Bank Research Group. Neurobehavioral outcome 1 year after severe head injury: experience of the Traumatic Coma Data Bank. *Journal of Neurosurgery*, **73**, 699–709.

Levin, H.S. & Goldstein, F.C. (1986). Organization of verbal memory after severe closed head injury. *Journal of Clinical and Experimental Neuropsychology*, **8** (6), 643–656.

Levin, H.S., Goldstein, F.C., High, W.M. Jr & Eisenberg, H.M. (1988a). Automatic and effortful processing after severe closed head injury. *Brain and Cognition*, **7**, 283–297.

Levin, H.S., Goldstein, F.C., High, W.M. Jr & Eisenberg, H.M. (1988b). Disproportionately severe memory deficit in relation to normal intellectual functioning after closed head injury. *Journal of Neurology, Neurosurgery, and Psychiatry*, **51**, 1294–1301.

Levin, H.S., Grossman, R.G. & Kelly, P.J.(1977). Aphasic disorder in patients with closed head injury. *Journal of Neurology, Neurosurgery, and Psychiatry*, **39**,1062–1070.

Levin, H.S., Grossman, R., Sarwar, M. et al. (1981). Linguistic recovery after closed head injury. *Brain and Language*, **12**, 360–374.

Levin, H.S., Handel, S.F., Goldman, A.M. et al. (1985a). Magnetic resonance imaging after "diffuse" nonmissile head injury. *Archives of Neurology*, **42**, 963–968.

Levin, H.S., High, W.M. Jr, Meyers, C.A. et al. (1985b). Impairment of remote memory after closed head injury. *Journal of Neurology, Neurosurgery and Psychiatry*, **45**, 556–563.

Levin, H.S., High, W.M., Ewing-Cobbs, L. et al. (1988c). Memory functioning during the first year after closed head injury in children and adolescents. *Neurosurgery*, **22**, 1043–1052.

Levin, H.S., Mattis, S., Ruff, R.M. et al. (1987). Neurobehavioral outcome following minor head injury: a three-center study. *Journal of Neurosurgery*, **66**, 234–243.

Levin, H.S., O'Donnell, V.M. & Grossman, R.G. (1979). The Galveston Orientation and Amnesia Test: a practical scale to assess cognition after head injury. *Journal of Nervous and Mental Disease*, **167**, 675–684.

Levin, H.S., Papanicolaou, A.C. & Eisenberg, H.M. (1984). Observations of amnesia after nonmissile head injury. In: L.R. Squire and N. Butters (eds), *Neuropsychology of Memory* (pp. 247–257). New York: Guilford.

Levin, H.S., Peters, B.H. & Hulkonen, D.A. (1983). Early concepts of anterograde and retrograde amnesia. *Cortex*, **19**, 427–440.

Levin, H.S., Song, J., Scheibel, R.S. et al. (2000) Dissociation of frequency and recency processing from list recall after severe closed head injury in children and adolescents. *Journal of Clinical and Experimental Neuropsychology*, **22**, 1–15.

Levin H.S., Williams, D.H., Eisenberg, H.M. et al.(1992). Serial MRI and neurobehavioral findings after mild to moderate closed head injury. *Journal of Neurology, Neurosurgery, Psychiatry*, **55**, 255–262.

Lohman, T., Ziggas, D. & Pierce, R.S. (1989). Word fluency performance on common categories by subjects with closed head injuries. *Aphasiology*, **3**, 685–693.

Lucchelli, F. & de Renzi, E. (1992). Proper name anomia. *Cortex*, **28**, 221–230.

Mangels, J., Craik, F., Levine, B. et al. (2000). Chronic deficits in item and context memory following traumatic brain injury: a function of attention and injury severity. *Brain and Cognition*, **44**, 98–112.

Markowitsch, H.J., Calabrese, P, Liess, J. et al. (1993). Retrograde amnesia after traumatic brain injury of the frontal temporal cortex. *Neurology, Neurosurgery, and Psychiatry*, **56**, 988–992.

Martin, R.C. & Romani, C. (1994). Verbal working memory and sentence comprehension: a multiple components view. *Neuropsychology*, **8**, 506–523.

Martin, R.C., Shelton, J.R. & Yaffee, L.S. (1994). Language processing and working memory: neuropsychological evidence for separate phonological and semantic capacities. *Journal of Memory and Language*, **33**, 83–111.

Mateer, C.A., Sohlberg, M.M. & Crinean, J. (1987). Focus on clinical research: perceptions of memory function in individuals with closed-head injury. *Journal of Head Trauma Rehabilitation*, **2**, 74–84.

Mattson, A.J., Levin, H.S. & Grafman J. (2000). A case of prosopagnosia following moderate closed head injury with left hemisphere focal lesion. *Cortex*, **36**, 125–137.

Mazzoni, G. & Nelson, T.O. (eds) (1998). Metacognition and cognitive neuropsychology: monitoring and control processes (pp. 212). Mahwah, NJ: Erlbaum.

McAllister, T.W., Saykin, A.J., Flashman, L.A. et al. (1999). Brain activation during working memory 1 month after mild traumatic brain injury: a functional MRI study. *Neurology*, **121**,1300–1308.

McAndrews, M.P., Glisky, E.L. & Schacter, D.L. (1987). When priming persists: long-lasting implicit memory for a single episode in amnesic patients. *Neuropsychologia*, **25**, 497–506.

McCarthy, R.A. & Warrington, E.K. (1992). Actors but not scripts: the dissociation of people and events in retrograde amnesia, *Neuropsychologia*, **30**, 633–644.

McCauley, S.R. & Levin, H.S. (2000). Prospective memory deficits in children and adolescents sustaining severe closed-head injury. Presentation at the 7th Annual Meeting of the Cognitive Neuroscience Society, San Francisco, CA.

McEwen, B.S. & Wooley, C.S. (1994). Estradial and progesterone regulate neuronal structure and synaptic connectivity in adult as well a developing brain. *Experimental Gerontology*, **29**, 431–436.

McIntosh, T.K. (1993). Novel pharmacologic therapies in the treatment of experimental traumatic brain injury: a review. *Journal of Neurotrauma*, **10**, 215–361.

McIntosh, T.K., Smith, D.H., Voddi, M. et al. (1996). Riluzole, a novel neuroprotective agent, attenuates both neurologic motor and cognitive dysfunction following experimental brain injury in the rat. *Journal of Neurotrauma*, **13**, 767–780.

Metcalfe, J. & Shimamura, A.P. (eds) (1996). *Metacognition: Knowing about Knowing*. Cambridge, MA: MIT Press.

Miller, E.K. (2000). The prefrontal cortex and cognitive control. *Nature Reviews*, **1**, 59–65.

Millis, S.R. (1995). Factor structure of the California Verbal Learning Test in moderate and severe closed brain injury. *Perceptual and Motor Skills*, **80**, 219–224.

Millis, S.R. & Dijkers, M. (1993). Use of the Recognition Memory Test in traumatic brain injury: preliminary findings. *Brain Injury*, **7**, 53–58.

Milner, B., Corkin, S. & Teuber, H.L. (1968). Further analysis of the hippocampal amnesic syndrome: 14-year follow-up study of H.M. *Neuropsychologia*, **6**, 215–234.

Oddy, M. Coughlan, T., Tyerman, A. & Jenkins, D. (1985). Social adjustment after closed head injury: A further follow-up seven years after injury. *Journal of Neurology, Neurosurgery and Psychiatry*, **48**, 564–568.

Ommaya, A.D. & Gennarelli, T.A. (1974). Cerebral concussion and traumatic unconsciousness: correlation of experimental and clinical observations on blunt head injuries. *Brain*, **97**, 633–654.

Parry, F.M., Young, A.W., Saul, J.S.M. & Moss, A. (1991). Dissociable face processing impairments after brain injury. *Journal of Clinical and Experimental Neuropsychology*, **13**, 545–558.

Petrides, M. & Milner, B. (1982). Deficits on subject-ordered tasks after frontal and temporal-lobe lesions in man. *Neuropsychologia*, **20**, 249–262.

Prigatano, G.P., Fordyce, D.J., Zeiner, H.K. et al. (1984). Neuropsychological rehabilitation after closed head injury in young adults. *Journal of Neurology, Neurosurgery, and Psychiatry*, **47**, 505–513.

Rajaram, S. & Roediger, H.L. (1993). Direct comparison of four implicit memory tests. *Journal of Experimental Psychology: Learning, Memory, & Cognition*, **19**, 765–776.

Reed, J.M., Squire, L.R., Patalano, A.L. et al. (1999). Learning about categories that are defined by object-like stimuli despite declarative memory. *Behavioral Neuroscience*, **113**, 411–419.

Reid, D.B. & Kelly, M.P. (1993). Weschler Memory Scale—Revised in closed head injury. *Journal of Clinical Psychology*, **49**, 245–254.

Rey, A.L. (1941). Examen psychologique dans les cas d'encephalopathie traumatique. *Archives de Psychologie*, **28**, 286–340.

Rey, A. (1964). *L' examen clinique en psychologie*. Paris: Presses Universitaires de France.

Ribot, T. (1882). *Diseases of Memory: An Essay in the Positive Psychology*. New York: Appleton.

Richardson, J.T.E. (1979). Mental imagery, human memory, and the effects of closed head injury. *British Journal of Social and Clinical Psychology*, **18**, 319–327.

Richardson, J.T.E. (1984). The effects of closed head injury upon intrusions and confusions in free recall. *Cortex*, **20**, 413–420.

Roediger, H.L. (1990). Implicit memory: retention without remembering. *American Psychologist*, **45**, 1043–1056.

Roediger, H.L. & Blaxton, T.A. (1987). Effects of varying modality, surface features, and retention interval on priming in word-fragment completion. *Memory and Cognition*, **15**, 379–388.

Roediger, H.L., Weldon, M.S., Stadler, M.L. & Riegler, G.L. (1992). Direct comparison of two implicit memory tests: word fragment and word stem completion. *Journal of Experimental Psychology: Learning, Memory, & Cognition*, **18**, 1251–1269.

Roman, M.J., Delis, D.C., Willerman, L. et al. (1998). Impact of pediatric traumatic brain injury on components of verbal memory. *Journal of Clinical and Experimental Neuropsychology*, **20**(2), 245–258.

Ruff R.M., Young D., Levin H.S. et al. (1991). Verbal learning deficits following severe head injury: heterogeneity in recovery over one year. *Journal of Neurosurgery* **75** *(suppl.)*, S50–S58.

Russell, W.R. (1932). Cerebral involvement of head injury. *Brain*, **55**, 549–603.

Russell, W.R. (1971). *The Traumatic Amnesias*. New York: Oxford University Press.

Russell, W.R. & Nathan, P.W. (1946). The traumatic amnesias. *Brain*, **69**, 183–187.

Russell, W.R. & Smith, A. (1961). Post-traumatic amnesia in closed head injury. *Archives of Neurology*, **5**, 4–17.

Saffran, E.M. & Martin, N. (1990). Neuropsychological evidence for lexical involvement in short-term memory. In G. Vallar & T. Shallice (eds), *Neuropsychological Impairments of Short-term Memory* (pp. 145–166). New York: Cambridge University Press.

Sarno, M. (1984). Verbal impairment after closed head injury: report of a replication study. *Journal of Nervous and Mental Disease*, **172**, 475–479.

Schacter, D.L. (1987). Implicit memory history and current status: learning, memory, and cognition. *Journal of Experimental Psychology*, **13**, 501–518.

Schacter, D.L. & Church, B.A. (1992). Auditory priming: Implicit and explicit memory for words and voices. *Journal of Experimental Psychology: Learning, Memory, & Cognition*, **18**, 915–930.

Schacter, D.L. & Crovitz, H.F. (1977). Memory function after closed head injury: a review of the quantitative research. *Cortex*, **8**, 150–176.

Scoville, W.B. & Milner, B., (1957). Loss of recent memory after bilateral hippocampal lesions. *Journal Neurology, Neurosurgery and Psychiary*, **20**, 11–21.

Shallice, T. & Vallar, G. (1990). The impairment of auditory-verbal short-term storage. In G. Vallar & T. Shallice (eds), *Neuropsychological Impairments of Short-term Memory* (pp. 11–53). Cambridge: Cambridge University Press.

Shelton, J.R., Martin, R.C. & Yaffee, L.S. (1992). Investigating a verbal short-term memory deficit and its consequences for language processing. In Margolin, D. I. (ed.), *Cognitive Neuropsychology in Clinical Practice* (pp. 131–167). New York: Oxford University Press.

Shimamura, A.P., Gershberg, F.B., Jurica, P.J. et al. (1992). Intact implicit memory in patients with frontal lobe lesions. *Neuropsychologia*, **30**, 931–937.

Shimamura, A.P., Janowsky, J.S. & Squire, L.R. (1991). What is the role of frontal lobe damage in amnesic disorders? In H.S. Levin, H.M. Eisenberg & A.L. Benton (eds), *Frontal Lobe Function and Dysfunction* (pp.173–195). New York: Oxford University Press.

Shimamura, A.P. & Squire, L.R. (1986). Memory and metamemory: a study of the feeling-of-knowing phenomenon in amnesic patients. *Journal of Experimental Psychology: Learning, Memory, and Cognition*, **12**, 452–560.

Shores, E.A., Marosszeky, J.E., Sandanam, J. et al. (1986). Preliminary validation of a clinical scale for measuring the duration of post-traumatic amnesia. *Medical Journal of Australia*, **144**, 569–572.

Shum, D., Harris, D. & O'Gorman, J.G. (2000). Effects of severe traumatic brain injury on visual memory. *Journal of Clinical and Experimental Neuropsychology*, **22**(1), 25–39.

Shum, D., Jamieson, E., Bahr, M. & Wallace, G. (1999a). Implicit and explicit memory in children with traumatic brain injury. *Journal of Clinical & Experimental Neuropsychology*, **21**, 149–158.

Shum, D., Sweeper, S. & Murray, R. (1996). Performance on verbal implicit and explicit memory tasks following traumatic brain injury. *Journal of Head Trauma Rehabilitation*, **11**, 43–53.

Shum, D., Valentine, M. & Cutmore, T. (1999b). Performance of individuals with severe long-term traumatic brain injury on time-, event-, and activity-based prospective memory tasks. *Journal of Clinical and Experimental Neuropsychology*, **21**(1),49–58.

Sohlberg, M.M. & Mateer, C.A. (1989). *Introduction to Cognitive Rehabilitation. Theory and Practice*. New York: Guilford.

Spikeman, J.M., Berg, I.J. & Deelman, B.G. (1995). Spared recognition capacity in elderly and closed-head-injury subjects with clinical memory deficits. *Journal of Clinical & Experimental Neuropsychology*, **17**(1), 29–34.

Squire, L.R. (1974). Remote memory as affected by ageing. *Neuropsychologia*, **12**, 429–435.

Squire, L.R. (1992). Memory and hippocampus: a synthesis from findings with rats, monkeys and humans. *Psychological Review*, **2**, 195–231.

Squire, L.R. & Slater, P.G. (1975). Forgetting in very long-term memory as assessed by an improved questionnaire technique. *Journal of Experimental Psychology: Human Learning and Memory*, **1**, 50–54.

Squire, L.R. & Zola-Morgan, S. (1988). Memory: brain systems and behavior. *Trends in Neuroscience*, **11**, 170–175.

Stallings, G.A., Hanten, G., Song, J.X. et al. Subject ordered pointing task performance following severe traumatic brain injury in adults. (submitted). Paper presented at the Annual meeting of the International Neuropsychological Association meeting, Denver, CO.

Stein, D.G., Roof, R.L. & Fulop, Z.L. (1999). Brain damage, sex hormones and recovery. In D.T. Stuss, G. Winocur & I.H. Robertson (eds), *Cognitive Neurorehabilitation* (pp. 73–93). Cambridge: Cambridge University Press.

Stuss, D.T., Binns, M.A., Carruth, F.G. et al. (1999). The acute period of recovery from traumatic brain injury: posttraumatic amnesia or posttraumatic confusional state? *Journal of Neurosurgery*, **90**, 635–643.

Sunderland, A., Harris, J.E. & Baddeley, A.D. (1983). Do laboratory tests predict everyday memory? A neuropsychological study. *Journal of Verbal Learning and Verbal Behavior*, **22**, 341–357.

Tate, R.L., Pfaff, A. & Jurjevic, L. (2000). Resolution of disorientation and amnesia during post-traumatic amnesia. *Journal of Neurology, Neurosurgery and Psychiatry*, **68**,178–185.

Teasdale, G. & Jennett, B. (1974). Assessment of coma and impaired consciousness: a practical scale. *Lancet*, **2**, 81–84.

Thoene, A.I. & Glisky, E.L. (1995). Learning of name-face associations in memory impaired patients: a comparison of different training procedures. *Journal of the International Neuropsychological Society*, **1**(1), 29–38.

Timmerman, M.E. & Brouwer, W.H. (1999). Slow information processing after very severe closed head injury: Impaired access to declarative knowledge and intact application and acquisition of procedural knowledge. *Neuropsychologia*, **37**, 467–478.

Tsukiura, T., Otsuka, Y., Miura, R. et al. (2000). Remote memory for items, contents, and contexts: a case study for post-traumatic amnesia. *Brain and Cognition*, **44**, 98–112.

Tulving, E. (1983). *Elements of Episodic Memory*. New York: Oxford University Press.

Vakil, E., Golan. H., Grunbaum, E. et al. (1998). Direct and indirect measures of contextual information in brain-injured patients. *Neuropsychiatry, Neuropsychology, & Behavioral Neurology*, **9**,176–181.

Warrington, E.K. & Weiskrantz, L. (1968). New method of testing long-term retention with special reference to amnesic patients. *Nature*, **217**, 972–974.

Watkins, M.J. & Hanten, G. (unpublished manuscript). Selective remembering in visual short-term memory.

Watt, S., Shores, E.A. & Kinoshita, S. (1999). Effects of reducing attentional resources on implicit and explicit memory after severe traumatic brain injury. *Neuropsychology*, **13**, 338–349.

Wiegner, S. & Donders, J. (1999). Performance on the California Verbal Learning Test after traumatic brain injury. *Journal of Clinical and Experimental Neuropsychology*, **21**, 159–170.

Wilde, M.C. & Boake, C. (1994). Factorial validity of the California Verbal Learning Test in head injury. *Archives of Clinical Neuropsychology*, **9**, 202.

Wilson, B.A. (1997). Semantic memory impairments following non-progressive brain injury: a study of four cases. *Brain Injury*, **11**, 259–269

Wilson, B.A. & Evans, J.J. (1996). Error-free learning in the rehabilitation of people with memory impairments. *Journal of Head Trauma Rehabilitation*, **11**(2), 54–64.

Wilson, B.A. & Moffat, N. (eds) (1984). *Clinical Management of Memory Problems*. Rockville, MD: Aspen.

Wilson, J.T., Wiedmann, K.D., Hadley, D.M. et al. (1988). Early and late magnetic resonance imaging and neuropsychological outcome after head injury. *Journal of Neurology, Neurosurgery, Psychiatry*, **51**, 391–396.

Yeates, K.O., Blumenstein, E., Patterson, C.M. & Delis, D.C. (1995). Verbal learning and memory following pediatric closed-head injury. *Journal of the International Neuropsychological Society*, **1**, 78–87.

Zhu, J., Hamm, R.J., Reeves, T.M. et al. (2000). Postinjury administration of L-deprenyl improves cognitive function and enhances neuroplasticity after traumatic brain injury. *Experimental Neurology*, **166**,136–152.

CHAPTER 4

Psychogenic Amnesia

Michael D. Kopelman

*University Department of Psychiatry and Psychology,
St Thomas' Hospital (Institute of Psychiatry and King's College London), UK*

Psychologically-based amnesia encompasses instances of persistent memory impairment, such as occurs in depression or (in extreme form) in a depressive pseudodementia. Alternatively, it can entail transient or discrete episodes of memory loss. Such transient amnesias can be situation-specific, as occurs in amnesia for offences, fragments of recall in posttraumatic stress disorder, and in amnesia for childhood sexual abuse. In other cases, the transient amnesia can involve a more global memory deficit, often accompanied by a loss of the sense of personal identity, such as occurs in a psychogenic "fugue" state. Whilst these latter instances are the stuff of film and fiction (usually in grossly distorted form), it is important to recognize that situation-specific amnesia is much more commonplace, coming to the attention of clinical and forensic psychologists, psychiatrists and neurologists.

Various forms of terminology are commonly used in discussing this issue. The present writer favours the term "psychogenic amnesia", because it does not make any assumptions about mechanism (as does "dissociative amnesia") or about the degree to which memory loss results from unconscious processes ("hysterical amnesia"), rather than motivated/deliberate/conscious processes ("factitious" or exaggerated amnesia). The term "functional amnesia" is somewhat unsatisfactory in that there are, of course, deficits in function (or "processing") in organic amnesia, and the salient feature of psychogenic amnesia is that, in some sense, it is always "dysfunctional". On the other hand, it can be argued that the term "psychogenic" makes assumptions about underlying aetiology and begs questions about when, and in what circumstances, a psychological stress is sufficient to become "psychogenic". However, similar criticisms can be made in cases of "organic" amnesia, where the markers of pathophysiology are not necessarily clear-cut; and the necessary and sufficient criteria for the attribution of causality to any given "lesion" have been insufficiently addressed in the neuropsychological literature (Kopelman, 2000a, 2002).

The present chapter will discuss examples of situation-specific and global psychogenic amnesia in turn.

The Essential *Handbook of Memory Disorders for Clinicians.* Edited by A.D. Baddeley, M.D. Kopelman and B.A. Wilson.
© 2004 John Wiley & Sons, Ltd. ISBN 0-470-09141-X.

SITUATION-SPECIFIC PSYCHOGENIC AMNESIA

Situation-specific psychogenic amnesia refers to a brief, discrete episode of memory loss, usually relating to a traumatic event in the individual's personal history: this is known as "dissociative amnesia" in DSM-IV (American Psychiatric Association, 2000).

Amnesia for Offences

This is important because, although controversial (Schacter, 1986a, 1986b, 1986c; Kihlstrom & Schacter, 2000), clinical and forensic psychologists, psychiatrists and neurologists are often asked to assess defendants claiming amnesia for their alleged crimes. Whilst there is a burgeoning experimental literature on eyewitness testimony, there is a relative dearth of experimental studies investigating this intriguing form of forgetting.

Amnesia has been reported most commonly in cases of homicide. In six studies conducted between 1948 and 1985, it was found that 23–47% of those convicted of homicide claimed amnesia for the killing (Leitch, 1948; Guttmacher, 1955; O'Connell, 1960; Bradford & Smith, 1979; Taylor & Kopelman, 1984; Parwatikar et al., 1985). In a recent study of all offenders given life sentences in 1994, Pyszora et al. (2003) found that 31% of convicted homicide cases had claimed amnesia at trial. Amnesia also arises following other types of crime, but three studies carried out in very different settings showed a clear relationship with the violence of the offence: these studies were carried out in a maximum security hospital (Hopwood & Snell, 1933), a forensic psychiatry outpatient service in Canada (Lynch & Bradford, 1980), and in a remand prison in the UK (Taylor & Kopelman, 1984). Studies of the victims and eyewitnesses of offences have also revealed that impaired recall is related to the violence of the crime (e.g. Kuehn, 1974; Clifford & Scott, 1978; Yuille & Cutshall, 1986).

In the absence of a substantive, prospective study of this topic, there are conflicting views about the persistence of such amnesia (Leitch, 1948; O'Connell, 1960; Bradford & Smith, 1979). In a retrospective study, Pyszora et al. (2003) found that, at 3-year follow-up, 33% of an amnesic sample were reported to have complete return of memory, 26% had partial return, and 41% no return of memory.

Amnesia for offences appears to occur in four main types of circumstance:

1. *Crimes of passion.* Amnesia appears to be particularly important in homicide cases where the offence was unpremeditated and took place in a state of extreme emotional arousal, the victim usually being closely related to the offender—a wife, lover, close friend or family member. There is often an accompanying diagnosis of depression and occasionally of schizophrenia (Hopwood & Snell, 1933; O'Connell, 1960; Bradford & Smith, 1979; Taylor & Kopelman, 1984).

   > A 40-year-old Egyptian was married to an English woman with two young children. When he discovered that his wife was having an affair with a musician, he became depressed, and he was treated with an antidepressant as an outpatient at his local hospital. During the afternoon of the offence, he had a furious row with his wife, during which he threatened to kill the musician. Later, he could recall going to kiss his daughter good night, but he could not remember anything after that until the police arrived. However, in the meantime, he had telephoned the police, and he was subsequently charged with the murder of his wife by stabbing.

2. *Alcohol abuse and intoxication.* There is commonly a history of chronic alcohol abuse and/or intoxication at the time of the offence in amnesic subjects (O'Connell, 1960; Bradford & Smith, 1979; Taylor & Kopelman, 1984; Parwatikar et al., 1985). In three of these studies, other drugs were also implicated, although the types of substance were not specified. Alcohol could produce amnesia either from a so-called "blackout" or as a state-dependent phenomenon (Goodwin et al., 1969).

> A 20-year-old man had consumed eight or more pints of beer plus three whiskies in the course of an evening. The last thing he could recall was being in a night-club with friends, who had been threatened by a rival gang, and who were then pacified by attendants. Continuous memory returned early the following morning, whilst he was being interviewed in the police station, although there were "islets" of preserved memory in between: peering down from a roof above a shop, being kicked by a policeman whilst up on the roof, being made to descend a ladder with handcuffs on. He had no idea how he had climbed up the roof or why. The accused was charged with assaulting a police officer whilst under the influence of alcohol. Eight months after the offence, there had been some infilling of memory between the "islets", and shrinkage of the amnesic gap from about 6 h to approximately 2 h.

3. *Psychosis/delusional memory.* Some studies report that a small group of patients are found to have committed offences during floridly psychotic episodes (Taylor & Kopelman, 1984). These offences often consist of criminal damage or minor acts of aggression, but the account given of them by their perpetrator, although stated with apparent conviction, is at complete variance with what others had observed. Occasionally, such anomalous or even delusional memories may result in charges being brought inappropriately.

> A young man, who had a history of recurrent hospital admissions for schizophrenia, reported that he had gone into a fish-and-chip shop, that he had looked into the eyes of a Chinese serving woman, and that he had asked for cod roe. He said the lights had then become bright, and that he had fainted, and he could not remember anything else. In fact, there had been no loss of consciousness or altercation—he had suddenly picked up a bar and started smashing the ovens.

4. *Brain disorder/automatism.* As in the case of severe intoxication, this is not "psychogenic" but it is very important to differentiate from the psychogenic forms of memory loss in this context because, in the UK and in many other jurisdictions, amnesias resulting from an organic factor may have important legal implications. Although lawyers are very much aware of this, it should be noted that automatisms are a very rare cause of amnesia for an offence, and they did not feature in at least two surveys of this topic (Bradford & Smith, 1979; Taylor & Kopelman, 1984).

Epileptic automatisms or postictal confusional states occasionally result in crime. When this occurs, EEGs subsequently reveal that the seizure activity has involved the hippocampal and parahippocampal structures bilaterally as well as the mesial diencephalon (Fenton, 1972). As these structures are crucial for memory formation, amnesia for the period of automatic behaviour is always present and is usually complete (Knox, 1968). There is no automatism without amnesia. Consequently, assessment requires a convincing history of both epilepsy and amnesia. Since the case of *R. vs. Sullivan* (reported by Fenwick, 1990), the English courts have regarded epileptic automatisms as a form of "insane automatism", resulting from "intrinsic" brain disease, liable to recur and therefore requiring compulsory psychiatric treatment, often in a secure hospital.

Hypoglycaemia can result from insulin-treated diabetes, alcohol intoxication, insulinoma, insulin abuse, or the "dumping" syndrome. Insulin abuse has been implicated in a number of serious offences, including violent crimes against children (Scarlett et al., 1977; Lancet, 1978). Where hypoglycaemia has resulted from the administration of an "extrinsic" agent such as insulin, the case for a "sane" automatism can be argued, potentially resulting in acquittal (in England and Wales and many other jurisdictions). The present author managed to argue successfully for an acquittal in the case of a young diabetic man who delayed taking a meal after self-administering his insulin because he had become interested in a television programme; subsequently, he killed a friend without any apparent motivation, and he was clearly hypoglycaemic when the police arrived.

Sleepwalking or somnambulism has also been used as grounds for automatism. It occurs most commonly in childhood and adolescence, and occasionally in adult life when precipitated by fatigue, mental stress, sleep deprivation, drugs or alcohol, or a change in the sleeping environment (Kales et al., 1980; Howard & d'Orbán, 1987; Fenwick, 1990). It most commonly occurs within 2 h of falling asleep, and episodes last only a few minutes. There are a substantial number of case-reports in the medical and legal literature of violent attacks during sleepwalking, often involving strangulation, attempted strangulation or the use of available implements as weapons with a sleeping partner as the victim (Howard & d'Orbán, 1987; Fenwick, 1990). Most commonly in these case-reports, there has not been any hostility between the offender and the victim and the behaviour is entirely out of character. Characteristically, episodes of violence accompanying sleepwalking terminate in the subject appearing confused on awakening, recalling relatively little of any accompanying dream, but being aware of a sense of acute dread or terror in such a dream (so-called "night terrors"). This arises because sleepwalking and night terrors characteristically occur in stage 4 of slow-wave sleep, shortly before the transition to rapid-eye-movement (REM) sleep. It used to be thought that violent offences could not occur in association with REM sleep because the subject was paralysed and could not sleepwalk; however, since the identification of REM sleep behaviour disorder (Schenck et al., 1986), episodes of lashing out or more organized violence against a sleeping partner have indeed been reported.

Authentic Amnesia or Deliberate Malingering?

Many observers consider that the amnesia claimed by offenders is a deliberate strategy to try to avoid the legal consequences of their offence (e.g. Schacter, 1986a). In view of this, Hopwood & Snell (1933) conducted a retrospective review of follow-up information in the case-notes of 100 Broadmoor high-security patients who, at the time of their trials, had claimed amnesia for their offences; they concluded that 78% of the amnesias had been "genuine", 14% had been "feigned", and 8% were "doubtful". However, there are a number of other reasons for supposing that many cases of amnesia are authentic, even though this is always hard (if not impossible) to prove.

First, many offenders give a very similar account of their memory loss, viz. a brief "amnesic gap" lasting an hour or less for the period of the offence. Some use phrases somewhat similar to those employed by fugue patients (e.g. Kopelman & Morton, 2001) to describe their memory loss. For example, O'Connell (1960) described amnesic offenders who reported having "buried everything about (the) case" and feeling that recollection would be "so . . . horrifying . . . that I just can't remember anything" or that "there is something in my mind . . . it seems to be forming a picture and then . . . my head hurts . . . [and] it gets all jumbled up again".

Second, many amnesic cases have been described in the literature who either have reported their own crime or failed to take measures to avoid their capture (Hopwood & Snell, 1933; Leitch, 1948; Gudjonsson & Mackeith, 1983; Taylor & Kopelman, 1984; Gudjonsson & Taylor, 1985). This makes an account of amnesia as simulation in order to avoid punishment seem less plausible. This was true of the Egyptian's case-history given above, and Gudjonsson & MacKeith (1983) reported a similar incident:

> A 67-year-old man had apparently battered his wife to death without any obvious motive, before telephoning the police and giving himself up. On their arrival, he reported that he had no memory of the actual attack, but that he recalled standing over the body realizing that he had been responsible for his wife's death. His memory had not cleared by the time of the Court hearing.

Third, it should be noted that the factors which have been associated with amnesia in offenders overlap with those that have been implicated in cases of impaired recall by the victims or eyewitnesses of crime—in particular, violent crime, extreme emotional arousal and alcohol intoxication (e.g. see Kuehn, 1974; Clifford & Scott, 1978; Yuille & Cutshall, 1986; Deffenbacher, 1988; Yuille, 1987). Nobody questions the motivation of eyewitnesses or victims whose recall is impaired.

Fourth, it should be reiterated that, in English law (and in many other, but not all, jurisdictions), amnesia *per se* does not constitute either a barrier to trial or any defence. For amnesia to contribute to the question of responsibility, other issues have to be raised, such as epilepsy or other forms of organic brain disease. Most lawyers are aware of this but, nevertheless, their clients continue to plead amnesia even in instances where recall of what actually happened would be helpful to their cause.

Posttraumatic Stress Disorder (PTSD)

Posttraumatic stress disorder (PTSD) can occur in association with head injury, road traffic accidents, being the victim of a violent crime, or a major disaster (e.g. the sinking of the *Herald of Free Enterprise* at Zeebrugge, or the King's Cross fire in the London Underground). As is well known, it is characterized by intrusive thoughts and memories ("flashbacks") about the traumatic experience, as well as anxiety and avoidance phenomena, a startle reaction, and a variety of other cognitive and somatic complaints (Raphael & Middleton, 1988). However, there may be instances of partial memory loss ("fragmentary" memory), distortions, or even frank confabulations.

Most commonly, there is disorganization in the retrieval of memory for the trauma, evident as gaps in recall and difficulty in producing a coherent narrative: this disorganization may partially explain the tendency for PTSD patients in psychotherapy to recall progressively additional detail of their traumatic experience as therapy progresses (Harvey & Bryant, 2001; Brewin, 2001). With regard to confabulation, the present author saw a victim of the *Herald of Free Enterprise* at Zeebrugge, who described trying to rescue a close friend whilst still on board the ship, when other witnesses reported that this close friend had not been seen from the moment that the ship turned over. Although factors such as head injury or hypothermia may confound the interpretation of such cases, it is of interest that PTSD symptoms have been reported to occur even when the subject appears to have been completely amnesic for the episode (McNeil & Greenwood, 1996; Harvey et al., 2003). Moreover, PTSD victims may show deficits in anterograde memory on formal tasks many years after the original trauma (Bremner et al., 1993), and there are claims that they show a loss of hippocampal volume on MRI brain scan (Bremner et al., 1995), which has been attributed to effects on glucocorticoid levels (Markowitsch, 1996). However, these MRI findings have to be interpreted with caution in view of the rather crude measurements employed, as even the control values were a long way out-of-line with those of most other investigations (Colchester et al., 2001).

A recent review (Brown et al., 1999) documented evidence of amnesia in the victims of lightening flashes, flood disasters, pipeline explosions, earthquakes, concentration camp and holocaust survivors, refugees, and traumatized soldiers from the two world wars and Vietnam. Other reviews have cited instances of kidnap and torture (Van der Kolk & Fisler, 1995). The psychological impact of a road traffic accident may also give rise to amnesia (Harvey, 2000; Kopelman, 2000b), although it may be difficult to separate this from the effects of concussion.

Harvey (2000) reported a personal instance of memory loss for the events of a life-threatening accident in the absence of any apparent concussion or violent accelera-tion/deceleration forces. He concluded that this was a "posttraumatic amnesia in which the trauma was wholly psychological". It is to be noted that he could recall that the front seat passenger was wearing a flowery hat in the car that had swerved across the road in front of him, that the car was a small red Honda saloon, and that a black and white soft toy was dangling in the rear window, but he forgot what happened after he noticed this. It is characteristic that, in trauma, some memories are enhanced, detailed, and may be re-called intrusively thereafter, whereas other items are forgotten. Similarly, in head injury, Russell & Nathan (1946) referred to memories with the quality of "visions" arising from a brief "lucid interval" before the onset of posttraumatic amnesia, e. g. the screech of brakes or the flashing of ambulance lights. In head injury, amnesia predominates and such vivid memories are infrequent, whereas in PTSD intrusive memories predominate and memory lapses are less common. Nevertheless, the two seem to lie at the extremes of a continuum: what is poorly understood in both instances is why certain things are forgotten, whereas others are vividly remembered.

In this connection, Brewin et al. (1996; Brewin, 2001) have produced a dual representation theory of PTSD. According to this, memories of a personally experienced traumatic event can be of two distinct types, stored in different representational formats. One type of format ("verbally accessible memory" or VAM) supports ordinary autobiographical memories that can be retrieved either automatically or using deliberate strategic processes. VAM memories can be edited and interact with the rest of autobiographical memory, so that the trauma is represented within a complete personal context comprising past, present, and future. Such memories contain information that the individual attended to before, during, and after the traumatic event, and which received sufficient conscious processing to be transferred to a long-term memory store in a form that can be deliberately retrieved at a later date, but which are also subject to normal processes of forgetting. The second type of format ("situationally accessible memory" or SAM) supports the specific trauma-related "flashbacks" and dreams that are characteristic of PTSD. The SAM system contains information that has been obtained from more extensive lower-level perceptual processing of the traumatic scene with little conscious processing, including the person's autonomic and motor responses to the scene. This results in flashbacks being more detailed and affect-laden than ordinary memories. Because the SAM system does not use verbal codes, these memories are difficult to communicate to others, and they do not necessarily interact with other autobiographical memories. They are also difficult to control, because people cannot always regulate their exposure to sights, sounds, smells, etc., which act as cues to these flashbacks.

Child Sexual Abuse

The fraught issue of memory for child sexual abuse can be viewed as an aspect of this topic. For many years, child psychologists and child psychiatrists have reported that abused children or adolescents appear amnesic for what has happened, but, in the last decade, this has become a hugely controversial topic. In reviewing the literature, Pope & Hudson (1995) found only four investigations bearing upon this issue, and they criticized these studies on the basis that *either* the original abuse had not been corroborated *or* the findings were heavily dependent upon self-report, in which case a report of past forgetting needed to be corroborated. On the other hand, even the most forthright protagonists of "false memory" have found that 19% of victims of abuse have reported forgetting at some time in the past (Loftus et al., 1994), and Brown et al. (1999) claimed that there was evidence of forgetting in all 68 studies they reviewed on this topic. Whilst there are indeed problems in evaluating self-reports of amnesia for child abuse, some smaller-scale studies have examined the corroborative evidence for the trauma and the subsequent forgetting in some detail (Schooler et al., 1997). Other researchers have suggested that the memories for abuse are never actually completely forgotten, but that they are retained in a vague unelaborated form, poorly located in temporal and spatial context (Schacter, 1996; Shimamura, 1997). Such memories would be vulnerable to the normal processes of decay and interference as well as to conscious avoidance and suppression. Appropriate cueing or triggers might result in the re-retrieval of these memories (Andrews et al., 2000), but the "weak trace" would make them particularly vulnerable to distortion and augmentation.

Trauma as Cause or Coincidence?

More recently, Kihlstrom & Schacter (2000) have queried the nature of the association between trauma and amnesia. In part, their argument reflects the fact that there is a dearth of controlled studies and that, more typically, traumatic memories are held with enhanced intensity. However, they also make the important point that "in the final analysis, the fact that functional amnesia often occurs in association with trauma does not mean that trauma causes amnesia, either directly (like the mental equivalent of a concussive blow to the head) or through some psychological process (like repression or dissociation)".

It is certainly true that trauma does not necessarily cause amnesia: there are many cases where people survive trauma without any memory loss. Against this, it can be pointed out that a severe precipitating stress appears to be a prerequisite for the onset of "fugue" (see below), that amnesia for offences shows characteristic features as described above, and that

PTSD and the resulting disorganization and disruption of memory (as described by Brewin, 2001) appear to be very common phenomena—certainly much more common than multiple personality disorder, which Kihlstrom & Schacter (2000) appear to accept. It needs to be acknowledged, however, that a person's cognitive response to trauma—determining whether or not amnesia develops—is likely to be influenced by factors such as his/her current mood state, past experience of memory loss, and underlying personality traits (see below).

GLOBAL PSYCHOGENIC AMNESIA

Psychogenic Fugue

A "fugue state" refers, in essence, to a syndrome consisting of a sudden loss of all autobiographical memories and the sense of self or personal identity, usually associated with a period of wandering, for which there is a subsequent amnesic gap upon recovery. Kihlstrom & Schacter (2000) point out that there is often a brief delay or lag between the end of the period of wandering and recovery of memory for personal identity. Fugue states usually last a few hours or days only, and they appear to have occurred more commonly earlier in the century, particularly during war time (Hunter, 1964). Where a fugue lasts much longer than this, the possibility of deliberate simulation must be strongly considered. Psychogenic fugues are classified in DSM-IV (American Psychiatric Association, 2000) as "dissociative fugues", and they have also been labelled as "functional retrograde amnesia" (RA) (Schacter et al., 1982).

> Schacter et al. (1982) described a young man who developed "functional RA" after attending the funeral of his grandfather, to whom he had been very close. When asked to retrieve autobiographic memories to cue-words, the median age of his retrieved memories was very brief, relative to both healthy controls and his own subsequent (post-recovery) performance. However, there were some preserved "islands" of autobiographical memory evident when he was "constrained" to produce memories from his earlier life: it emerged that these "islands" of preserved memory came from what he subsequently described as the happiest period of his life. He recovered his memories after seeing a television programme in which a funeral was shown.

> Kopelman et al. (1994a) described a 40-year-old woman who "came round" on the London Underground, unaware of who or where she was. She carried a bag, containing some clothes and an envelope addressed to a name (which subsequently turned out not to be hers). It eventually emerged that, following a marital crisis, this woman had disappeared from her home and had taken a flight across the Atlantic. There was a persistent amnesic gap for a 1 week period, which was thought to reflect an authentic fugue state, although this lady was shown to be at least partially simulating some 3 months after being first seen. During that period, she showed a "reversed" temporal gradient on standardized tests of autobiographical and public event remote memory.

> Kopelman et al. (1994b) described a 55-year-old man who, after being confronted with embezzlements he was alleged to have made from his work place, disappeared from his home the following morning, emerging in the railway station of the city where he grew up (500 miles away) that evening. He also disappeared for a briefer period 3 months later, the day after the police had searched his home. In this case, these episodes of undoubted fugue (in which personal identity was lost) emerged against a background of mild-to-moderate organic memory impairment of vascular aetiology.

Kapur & Abbott (1996) described a 19-year-old male university student who was found in a city park a few days before his university examinations were due to start. In addition to the likely stress resulting from his pending examinations, the patient's grandmother had died 8 months earlier, and the patient had been quite close to her. Witness accounts were obtained from people who had observed the episode from the onset, and the authors monitored the acute stages of recovery of memory function over the next 4 weeks. The memory loss was characterized by impaired performance on both autobiographical and public events memory tests in the context of normal anterograde memory scores. Shrinkage of RA took place over a 4 week period with the autobiographical and public events components of retrograde memory recovering at the same rate.

Markowitsch et al. (1997) described a 37-year-old man who experienced a "fugue" episode lasting 5 days when out bicycling, and who then had a persistent loss of autobiographical memory lasting 8 months or more. During this period, the patient was required to listen to sentences containing information about his past, either preceding or following the onset of amnesia, whilst undergoing a 15-oxygen positron emission tomography (PET) scan. The authors found reduced right hemisphere activation for remote memories, relative to healthy controls performing a similar task.

Reviews of the earlier literature on psychogenic fugue states (Kopelman, 1987, 1995) have suggested that three main factors predispose to such episodes. *First*, fugue states are always preceded by a severe precipitating stress, such as marital or emotional discord (Kanzer, 1939), bereavement (Schacter et al., 1982), financial problems (Kanzer, 1939), a charge of offending (Wilson et al., 1950) or stress during wartime (Sargant & Slater, 1941; Parfitt & Gall, 1944). *Second*, depressed mood is an extremely common antecedent for a psychogenic fugue state. Berrington et al. (1956) wrote:

> In nearly all fugues, there appears to be one common factor, namely a depressive mood. Whether the individual in the fugue is psychotic, neurotic, or even psychopathic, a depression seems to start off the fugue.

For example, Schacter et al.'s (1982) patient was in a depressed mood because he had just attended the funeral of his grandfather, of whom he had been particularly fond. In fact, many patients in a fugue have been contemplating suicide just before the episode, or do so following recovery from it (Abeles & Schilder, 1935; Stengel, 1941); for example, Abeles & Schilder (1935) described a woman who deserted her husband for another man: after a week she determined to return to her family but, as she descended into the railway underground station, she was contemplating suicide. The authors tersely reported that "instead, amnesia developed". The *third* factor which commonly precedes a fugue state is a history of a transient, organic amnesia: Stengel (1941) reported that 10% of his sample had a history of epilepsy, and Berrington et al. (1956) reported that 16 of their 37 cases had previously experienced a severe head injury, and a further three cases had suffered a head injury of unknown severity. In brief, it appears that patients who have experienced a previous, transient organic amnesia and who have become depressed and/or suicidal are particularly likely to go into a fugue in the face of a severe, precipitating stress.

A confounding factor, however, is that several authors have noted that some of their patients appeared to be somewhat unreliable personalities with a possible legal motive for wanting to claim amnesia (Stengel, 1941; Wilson et al., 1950; Berrington et al., 1956). Kopelman (1987) gave the example of a man who reported about 10 or 12 fugue episodes, several of which were well-documented in medical records, and who also had a past history of depression and suicide attempts as well as transient amnesia following epileptic seizures and ECT. This gentleman claimed amnesia for a period of a few hours during which he was involved in a motor accident whilst driving when disqualified, without any insurance, whilst under the influence of alcohol, making assessment (for a medico-legal report) particularly difficult.

The clinical and neuropsychological phenomena of fugue episodes often bear interesting resemblances to organic amnesia, as there may be islets or fragments of preserved memory within the amnesic gap. A woman, who was due to meet her husband to discuss divorce, recalled that she was "supposed to meet someone" (Kanzer, 1939; cf. also Schacter et al., 1982, above). The subject may adopt a detached attitude to these memory fragments, describing them as "strange and unfamiliar" (Coriat, 1907). In many cases, semantic knowledge remains intact (e.g. foreign languages, and the names of streets, towns, and famous people; Kanzer, 1939; Schacter et al., 1982). Consistent with this, IQ scores are characteristically unaffected (Schacter et al., 1982; Kopelman et al., 1994a, 1994b). In other cases, there are suggestions that semantic memory has been affected over-and-above the self-referential component (Kihlstrom & Schacter, 2000), which constitutes the sense of personal identity. Similarly, performance at verbal learning tests has been reported as unaffected (Abeles & Schílder, 1935; Kopelman et al., 1994a), mildly impaired (Schacter et al., 1982), or more severely affected (Gudjonsson & Taylor, 1985). Memory for skills has been relatively little investigated, but appears often to be preserved (e.g. Coriat, 1907). In the Padola hearing in 1959 (Bradford & Smith, 1979), retention of a rudimentary knowledge of aerodynamics and of other skills (e.g. solving jigsaw puzzles) was taken as evidence against an organic amnesia—a frankly erroneous interpretation in the light of contemporary findings demonstrating preserved procedural memory in organic amnesia. Kihlstrom & Schacter (1995, 2000) have provided examples of instances where subjects have appeared to show some "implicit" knowledge of events in the absence of explicit recollection. These included the case described by Christianson & Nilsson (1989), who studied a woman who developed amnesia after an assault and rape. She became extremely upset when taken back to the scene of the assault, even though she did not explicitly remember what had happened or where. In the first edition of this volume, Kopelman (1995) provided a model of hierarchies of awareness in psychogenic amnesia, analogous to that described in normal memory and organic amnesia (see Figure 4.1).

Memory retrieval may be facilitated by chance cues in the environment (e.g. Abeles & Schílder, 1935; Schacter et al., 1982). Kopelman (1995) gave the example of a man who, on seeing the author's name on the spine of a book in a medical ward, remembered that a close friend of that name had recently been admitted to hospital with terminal cancer. On transfer to a psychiatric ward, this same patient remembered that he had been briefly admitted to another psychiatric unit some years earlier. After recovery of these two memories, his other memories rapidly returned. On the other hand, deliberate cueing, such as taking a patient back to the site(s) where he/she had been found or lived or suffered trauma, is often unsuccessful in cueing memory retrieval (Coriat, 1907; Kanzer, 1939; Christianson & Nilsson, 1989; Kopelman et al., 1994a). Hypnosis and/or interview under sodium amylobarbitone (amytal) have commonly been used, but are often disappointing (Lennox, 1943; Adatto, 1949; Kopelman et al., 1994a, 1994b); and there is a dearth of substantive clinical trials supporting their efficacy (Patrick & Howells, 1990). On the other hand, such strategies may be useful to allow a patient to "recover" without loss of face, where there is background information about the patient and some degree of simulation is suspected (Kopelman et al., 1994a).

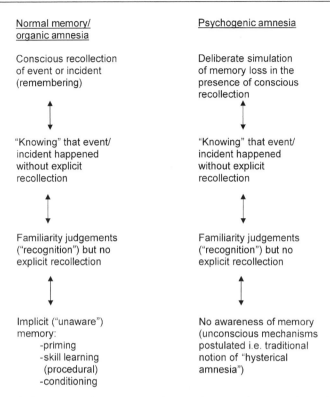

Normal memory/
organic amnesia

Conscious recollection
of event or incident
(remembering)

"Knowing" that event/
incident happened
without explicit
recollection

Familiarity judgements
("recognition") but no
explicit recollection

Implicit ("unaware")
memory:
    -priming
    -skill learning
     (procedural)
    -conditioning

Psychogenic amnesia

Deliberate simulation
of memory loss in the
presence of conscious
recollection

"Knowing" that event/
incident happened
without explicit
recollection

Familiarity judgements
("recognition") but no
explicit recollection

No awareness of memory
(unconscious mechanisms
postulated i.e. traditional
notion of "hysterical
amnesia")

Figure 4.1   Level of awareness in memory and amnesia: normal memory/organic amnesia and psychogenic amnesia

In differentiating psychogenic fugue from a transient organic amnesia, such as transient global amnesia (TGA), clinical factors may be important indicators, such as the rate and the circumstances of the onset of the memory loss, whether there is loss of the sense of personal identity (rare in organic amnesia except for advanced dementia), and whether new learning is affected (often spared in psychogenic amnesia, although not necessarily). In TGA and organic confusional states, repetitive questioning (e.g. "Where am I?" or "What am I doing here?") is a characteristic feature, whereas personal identity is seldom lost (Hodges & Ward, 1989). By contrast, in psychogenic fugue, personal identity is lost but repetitive questioning is rare (Kopelman et al., 1994c). If TGA attacks are frequent and brief (an hour or less), they are likely to have an epileptic basis (Hodges & Warlow, 1990), which Kapur (1990) has termed "transient epileptic amnesia" (TEA). On the other hand, TGA episodes are preceded by a precipitating stress in 14–33% of cases (Hodges & Ward, 1989; Miller et al., 1987), and it is misleading to assume that such stressors mean that an amnesia must necessarily be psychogenic. An important feature, although seldom assessed clinically, is the slope (temporal gradient) of the remote memory curve during the attack. Kritchevsky et al. (1997) obtained a pronounced recency effect on a cued autobiographical memory task in nine patients with "functional RA" (cf. Kopelman et al., 1994a), whereas TGA patients showed a conventional Ribot temporal gradient (i.e. sparing of early memories) during an attack.

Psychogenic Focal Retrograde Amnesia

This is a contentious topic, which has given rise to recent debate (Kopelman, 2000a, 2000c; Kapur, 2000). However, the present author would argue that many of these cases are likely to have had a psychogenic origin, even where there has been some evidence of organic brain pathology. Kapur (1999) has also acknowledged that psychogenic retrograde amnesia can occur in either the absence or the presence of concomitant brain pathology, and Kapur (2000) was brave and honest enough to acknowledge that psychological factors now appeared contributory in a patient previously described as having focal RA as a result of definite brain pathology (Kapur et al., 1992). Since this latter case was one of the better-described cases in the literature, the discovery of these putatively psychogenic factors must raise question marks about other cases in whom all physical investigations have been normal, but in whom underlying organic pathology was inferred (Stracciari et al., 1994; Lucchelli et al., 1995; De Renzi et al., 1995).

In focal RA, the subject characteristically loses memories for the entirety of his/her previous life. However, current new learning is preserved, and these patients often show only minor impairments on formal measures of anterograde amnesia. There is not necessarily any loss of the sense of personal identity, nor is there a period of wandering, although occasionally focal RA may follow a more typical "fugue" episode (Kopelman et al., 1994a; Markowitsch et al., 1997). However, the present author has noted that it seems to be very common, at least in the early stages, for these patients to complain that they cannot recognize their spouses and/or other close family members and, later, they say that they have "relearned" whom these people are. Two features make these patients particularly difficult to diagnose and manage. First, the underlying stressor or stressors are often not clearly apparent, as the patient and/or family are often reluctant to discuss them. The family may indeed reinforce the patient's adopting and maintaining a "sick role". Only later, after the patient's trust has been engaged, and new information has emerged, will underlying issues become evident, as in Kapur's (2000) case (see also Kopelman, 2000a). Second, as already mentioned, there may be concomitant brain pathology. This is usually minor, and the disorder often seems to follow mild concussion (Kopelman, 2000a), but occasionally it can be more serious (Stuss & Guzman, 1988; Binder, 1994).

> Barbarotto et al. (1996) described a 38-year-old woman who slipped and fell in her office, losing consciousness for an unknown period of time and who, upon recovery, showed an apparently complete loss of explicit autobiographical memory. The authors favoured the possibility that this was "a psychogenic block in a person with a hysterical personality structure", but emphasized that the patient was able to show implicit knowledge of information to which she apparently lacked explicit access—as demonstrated on tests requiring familiarity judgements and in her rate of relearning facts about her past.

> Della Sala et al. (1996) described a 33-year-old man who suffered a loss of autobiographical memory following a fall down some stairs at his parent-in-laws' home, resulting in concussion. Despite this patient's severe loss of explicit, autobiographical recall, and an initial loss of personal identity as well as a failure to recognize his wife, relatives and friends, there was substantial evidence of preserved implicit/procedural memories, including the ability to access secret codes on his computer. The authors considered the possibility of a psychogenic amnesia, although they favoured the more neutral term "functional amnesia". It is of interest that, although no formal psychiatric disorder was diagnosed, the patient had shown progressively less interest in his young wife over the preceding months, joined an unusual role-playing group from which he excluded his wife, started to collect sadomasochistic pornography, became involved in a homosexual relationship, and subsequently pursued a divorce.

Papagno (1998) described a 26-year-old man who fell from a scaffold no higher than 2 metres. He briefly lost consciousness, but he could not remember his name, what he was doing there, or any autobiographical detail. He failed to recognize his relatives, including his mother. He appeared unconcerned by his memory loss. There were no focal neurological signs; CT scan and MRI were normal; an EEG showed mild left temporal changes only. Although "no abnormalities" were detected during a psychiatric interview, there was a history that his girlfriend had broken off their relationship the previous December, leaving him very depressed, irritable, and quarrelsome with everybody. He made every possible attempt to meet his ex-girlfriend again, whilst she tried to avoid him. On one occasion, he had left home suddenly without warning; 3 days later he telephoned his ex-girlfriend from Rome, saying he was sleeping on the road and out of money. On his return, his mother described him as "out of his mind", threatening to kill his girlfriend as well as threatening suicide. One night he awoke and broke some of his home furniture. Apparently, he had stopped speaking about his girlfriend a month before the present accident and he "seemed" to have accepted the situation. Papagno postulated a primary retrieval deficit, i.e. "an inhibition (psychogenic and/or organic) of retrieval without a storage deficit". It should be noted that, in this case, psychological factors were present and acknowledged by the author, despite a report that there were "no pathological traits" by a psychiatrist.

MacKenzie Ross (2000) described a 56-year-old woman who, following a minor head injury at work, developed a profound RA for both public events and autobiographical memories spanning her entire life. The accident occurred shortly after the patient had returned to England to live with a fiancé, only to discover that he was already living with someone else. MacKenzie Ross emphasized that hospital and general practitioner records described repeated complaints of anxiety and depression, going back many years, and a "tendency to make mountains out of molehills". Mackenzie Ross argued for a "functional" disorder of memory retrieval, whilst acknowledging the putative importance of psychological factors in this case.

Kopelman (2000a) described a 55-year-old man who collapsed at work during early 1998 with a transient left-sided weakness and a complete loss of autobiographical memory. At initial admission, this patient was disorientated in time and place as well as person, and there was a mild loss of power in the left arm and leg with an equivocally upgoing left plantar response. A CT scan was normal, but an MRI brain scan showed evidence of a few pinpoint regions of altered signal bilaterally, consistent with a history of previously diagnosed hypercholesteraemia and diabetes. However, the physicians attending this man felt confident that his memory loss was entirely disproportionate to his neurological signs, which rapidly resolved. The patient did not recognize his wife, and he could not remember the names and ages of his children. He claimed to have "relearned" language and mental calculation, and that "each day I remember more of the day before". On formal tests, he showed severe and extensive autobiographical and remote memory loss with intact anterograde memory. When first seen, he and his family were extremely angry at any suggestion that there might be a psychological component to his memory loss. However, during the succeeding weeks, his wife provided information about an emotionally deprived childhood, abuse, and subsequent psychological problems. The initial onset had occurred after the patient had been confronted about "moonlighting" in two employments, from which he had been dismissed. After being seen on a regular basis for several weeks, he was more willing to accept a psychological contribution to his RA and, following an amytal interview, virtually all of this patient's memories were recovered.

There is evidence that the implicit component of memory may be relatively intact in such patients:

Campodonico & Rediess (1996) administered a measure of indirect remote memory to a patient with "profound psychogenic retrograde amnesia". The patient showed more rapid learning of famous identities relative to novel ones, comparable with controlled subjects, despite having been unable to name the famous faces at baseline. She also recalled the names and occupations of famous people better than she did those for novel items. The authors interpreted these findings as evidence for preserved "implicit" remote semantic knowledge.

One further study pointed to possible underlying brain mechanisms:

> Costello et al. (1998) described a man in his 40s who, following a left superior dorsolateral prefrontal haemorrhage, developed a dense RA for 19 years preceding the stroke. However, the authors considered that "a purely organic account of the condition does not seem very plausible". They carried out a PET activation study, in which the subject attempted to recall events using family photographs as stimuli in three conditions— events for which he was amnesic but at which he had been present, events from the amnesic period at which he was not present, and events outside the amnesic period. In the "amnesic-present" condition, activation was increased in the precuneus, but diminished in the right posterior ventrolateral frontal cortex and a region close to the site of haemorrhage. The finding of reduced right ventrolateral frontal activation was broadly consistent with Markowitsch et al.'s (1997) finding of diminished right hemisphere activation (see above).

This last finding indicates that psychogenic phenomena may produce their effect upon mechanisms operating in normal memory retrieval, which can of course also be affected by brain damage. Kopelman (2000a) proposed a model of how psychosocial factors and brain systems may influence autobiographical memory retrieval and personal identity (Figure 4.2) (cf. Markowitsch, 1996). The relevant psychosocial factors are indicated in the ovals, and are derived largely from the literature on fugue. The brain systems are indicated in the rectangular boxes. The model postulated that psychosocial stresses affect frontal control/executive systems, such that there is inhibition in the retrieval of autobiographical and episodic memories. As indicated in the model, this inhibition will be exacerbated, or made more likely, when a subject is extremely aroused or very depressed, or when there is a past "learning experience" of transient amnesia (see above, p. 77). When such stresses are severe, the inhibition may even affect a "personal semantic belief system", resulting in a transient loss of knowledge of self and identity (dashed arrow). Despite this suppression of autobiographical memory retrieval by these frontal inhibitory mechanisms, anterograde learning (and "new" episodic memory retrieval) can occur from "normal" environmental stimuli via the intact medial temporal/diencephalic system.

Multiple Personality Disorder

Multiple personality disorder (MPD), known as "dissociative identity disorder" in DSM-IV, has been described as the "crown jewel of the dissociative disorders and also of the functional amnesias" by Kihlstrom & Schacter (2000). By contrast, Merskey (1992, 1995) regarded the widely varying geographical prevalence of this disorder as almost certainly reflecting differences in the reinforcing behaviour of doctors, psychologists, and the outside world. Kihlstrom & Schacter (2000) noted that, of almost 2000 papers on this topic, approximately two-thirds appeared between 1989 and 2000. However, these authors themselves acknowledged that "the features of amnesia observed in experimental studies of MPD patients may be influenced to varying degrees by iatrogenic and sociocultural factors".

According to Kihlstrom & Schacter (2000), a cardinal symptom of this disorder is the between-personality amnesia. The amnesia often appears to be asymmetrical, in that at least

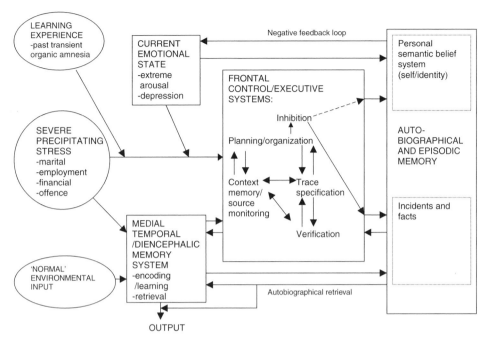

Figure 4.2 Social factors and brain systems influencing autobiographical memory retrieval and personal identity. The relevant social and psychological factors are indicated in the ovals. The brain systems are indicated in the rectangular boxes. Severe stress affects frontal control/executive system, thereby inhibiting the retrieval of autobiographical/episodic memories. This is more likely if the subject is extremely aroused, very depressed, or if there is past experience of a transient organic amnesia. If the stress is severe, there may even be a transient loss of knowledge of self and identity (dashed arrow). Reproduced from Kopelman (2000a)

one personality shows dense amnesia for the experiences of the others, while one or more personalities typically have unimpaired access to the experience of some or all the other personalities. Kihlstrom & Schacter (1995, 2000) have described a number of experimental studies in such patients.

Nissen et al. (1988) examined a 45-year-old woman with 22 diagnosed personalities. The authors focused upon eight mutually amnesic personalities who could each be elicited in response to an appropriate request by the experimenter. Target materials were studied by one personality (elicited by the patient's psychiatrist) and, after retention intervals of approximately 5–10 min, another personality was elicited for memory testing. Little or no evidence of between-personality explicit memory was observed across a variety of tests. However, on a word-fragment completion test, one personality's performance was indeed facilitated or primed by previous exposure of the words to another personality, and similar cross-personality implicit memory effects were observed on other tasks which required perceptual identification of briefly exposed words.

Schacter et al. (1989) studied I.C., a 24-year-old married woman, who manifested four other personalities. The authors used a variant of the Crovitz procedure, previously employed in a fugue patient (Schacter et al., 1982). In marked contrast to the performance of age-matched control subjects, I.C. produced almost no memories from the first 14 years of her life, and her earliest recollection was dated to age 12. When instructed to confine her responses to childhood, all of her memories were dated from years 10–12, again in marked contrast to controls. The authors suggested that I.C.'s current personality had, in fact, first emerged around the time of adolescence.

Eich et al. (1996) examined nine patients with MPD. Explicit tests of free and cued recall gave strong evidence of interpersonality amnesia. However, implicit memory was spared on a test of picture-fragment completion, but not on a test of word-fragment completion, indicating that implicit memory is not always or uniformly spared in such patients.

Such patients are rare, and they may be particularly vulnerable to suggestions from clinicians and researchers. The present author has noted that some of his fugue patients have used their fugue episode as a means of adopting a new way of life (Kopelman et al., 1994a; Kopelman & Morton, 2001) and several fugue patients have asked the author whether he "believes in" multiple personality disorder—as if they were seeking ways of experimenting with other alternatives.

THE NATURE OF PSYCHOGENIC AMNESIA

Leaving aside deliberate simulation, various mechanisms have been proposed to account for psychogenic amnesia. These include repression, dissociative states, failure of initial encoding, an encoding–retrieval interaction, and state or context-dependent retrieval deficits. These various theories can be grouped into those that place emphasis on the failure of memory at the time of initial encoding, which may be particularly true of amnesic offenders where severe alcohol or drug intoxication is implicated, and those that place emphasis on a failure of memory retrieval. The latter is possibly more true of those unpremeditated homicide cases, which take place in a state of extreme emotional arousal, although compromised encoding and avoidance of rehearsal (cf. O'Connell, 1960) may also be important factors contributing to subsequent difficulties in retrieval. Figure 4.2 has provided a model in which frontal control mechanisms, operating within a particular psychosocial environment, inhibit the retrieval of autobiographical memories and even of personal identity, whilst new learning remains intact. Anderson & Green (2001) have recently reported evidence that executive mechanisms can indeed be recruited to prevent unwanted memories from entering awareness, and that repeated use of this strategy inhibits the subsequent recall of the suppressed memories.

In the present author's experience, a complete absence of any recollection is very rare, where organic brain disease, intoxication, or obvious simulation have been excluded. On detailed assessment, subjects often show some degree of "knowledge" or "recognition" of certain memories without explicit recollection, in a manner analogous to that seen in studies of amnesic patients or healthy controls who have failed to remember something (Gardiner & Parkin, 1990; see also Figure 4.1). For example, as discussed above, O'Connell (1960) pointed to the qualitative similarities between what he called the "passive disregard" of those who deliberately put an unpleasant or traumatic memory to the back of their mind, and those subjects who, although claiming amnesia, described the memory as being on the verge of "forming a picture". The Egyptian homicide case, cited above, and Gudjonsson & Mackeith's (1983) case both "knew" that they must have committed their respective offences (although, in part, this was from the evidence before their eyes). Patient A.T. (Kopelman et al., 1994a) "recognized" a hotel she had stayed in when she was taken back there, but she could recollect nothing about her time there, even after recovery of most of her earlier memories. Kihlstrom & Schacter (1995, 2000) have given examples of other evidence of preserved implicit memory in the absence of explicit recollection.

CONCLUSIONS

In summary, psychogenic amnesia encompasses situation-specific and global forms of memory loss. The former includes amnesia for offences and memory loss (or "fragmentation") arising in PTSD and for childhood sexual abuse. The latter entails fugue episodes, cases of psychogenic focal retrograde amnesia, and cases of multiple personality disorder (even though the last may often be iatrogenically determined). Knowledge of the circumstances in which amnesia for an offence arises is important for its assessment; and investigations of PTSD are beginning to shed light on why certain images show enhanced recall, whilst other features are forgotten. Studies of fugue episodes and psychogenic focal retrograde amnesia indicate features in common with organic amnesia—such as preserved memory "fragments" and some evidence of preserved implicit and semantic components—although the temporal gradient is characteristically "reversed" (a strong recency effect in psychogenic amnesia; a Ribot gradient in TGA and other forms of organic amnesia). It seems likely that psychosocial influences exert their effects upon brain mechanisms that have been implicated in studies of normal memory and organic amnesia (Kopelman, 2002): the present chapter has provided a model to take account of this phenomenon.

ACKNOWLEDGEMENT

Professor Kopelman's research has been supported by grants from the Wellcome Trust.

REFERENCES

Abeles, M. & Schílder, P. (1935). Psychogenic loss of personal identity. *Archives of Neurology and Psychiatry*, **34**, 587–604.

Adatto, C.P. (1949). Observations on criminal patients during narcoanalysis. *Archives of Neurology and Psychiatry*, **62**, 82–92.

American Psychiatric Association (2000). *Diagnostic and Statistical Manual of Mental Disorders (DSM-IV)*. Washington, DC: APA.

Anderson, M.C. & Green, C. (2001). Suppressing unwanted memories by executive control. *Nature*, **410**, 366–369.

Andrews, B., Brewin, C.R., Ochera, J. et al. (2000). The timing, triggers and qualities of recovered memories in therapy. *British Journal of Clinical Psychology*, **39**, 11–26.

Barbarotto, R., Laiacona, M. & Cocchini, G. (1996). A case of simulated, psychogenic or focal pure retrograde amnesia: did an entire life become unconscious? *Neuropsychologia*, **34**, 575–585.

Berrington, W.P., Liddell, D.W. & Foulds, G.A. (1956). A revaluation of the fugue. *Journal of Mental Science*, **102**, 281–286.

Binder, L.M. (1994). Psychogenic mechanisms of prolonged autobiographical retrograde amnesia. *Clinical Neuropsychologist*, **8**, 439–450.

Bradford, J. & Smith, S.M. (1979). Amnesia and homicide: the Padola case and a study of thirty cases. *Bulletin of the American Academy of Psychiatry and the Law*, **7**, 219–231.

Bremner, J.D., Scott, T.M., Delaney, R.C. et al. (1993). Deficits in short-term memory in posttraumatic stress disorder. *American Journal of Psychiatry*, **150**, 1015–1019.

Bremner, J.D., Randall, P., Scott, T.M. et al. (1995). Memory-based measurement of hippocampal volume in patients with combat-related posttraumatic stress disorder. *American Journal of Psychiatry*, **152**, 973–981.

Brewin, C.R. (2001). A cognitive neuroscience account of posttraumatic stress disorder and its treatment. *Behavioural Research and Therapy*, **39**, 373–393.

Brewin, C.R., Dalgleish, T. & Joseph, S. (1996). A dual representation of posttraumatic stress disorder. *Psychological Review*, **103**, 670–686.

Brooks, D.N. (1984). Cognitive deficits after head injury. In D.N. Brooks (ed.), *Closed Head Injury: Psychological, Social and Family Consequences* (pp. 44–73). Oxford: Oxford University Press.

Brown, D., Scheflin, A.W. & Whitfield, C.L. (1999) Recovered memories: the current weight of the evidence in science and in the courts. *Journal of Psychiatry and Law*. **27**, 5–156.

Campodonico, J.R. & Rediess, S. (1996). Dissociation of implicit and explicit knowledge in a case of psychogenic retrograde amnesia. *Journal of the International Neuropsychological Society*, **2**, 146–158.

Christianson, S-A. & Nilsson, L.G. (1989). Hysterical amnesia: a case of aversively motivated isolation of memory. In T. Archer & L.G. Nilsson (eds), *Aversion, Avoidance, and Anxiety* (pp. 289–310). Hillsdale, NJ: Erlbaum.

Clifford, B.R. & Scott, J. (1978). Individual and situational factors in eyewitness testimony. *Journal of Applied Psychology*, **63**, 852–859.

Colchester, A., Kingsley, D., Lasserson, D. et al. (2001). Structural MRI volumetric analysis in patients with organic amnesia, 1: methods and comparative findings across diagnostic groups. *Journal of Neurology, Neursurgery, and Psychiatry*, **71**, 13–22.

Coriat, I.H. (1907). The Lowell case of amnesia. *Journal of Abnormal Psychology*, **2**, 93–111.

Costello, A., Fletcher, P.C., Dolan, R.J. et al. (1998). The origins of forgetting in a case of isolated retrograde amnesia following a haemorrhage: evidence from functional imaging. *Neuroscase*, **4**, 437–446.

Deffenbacher, K. (1988). Eyewitness research: the next ten years. In M. Gruneberg, P. Morris & R. Sykes (eds), *Practical Aspects of Memory*, Vol. 1 (pp. 20–26). Chichester: Wiley.

Della Sala, S., Freschi, R., Lucchelli, F. (1996). Retrograde amnesia: no past, new life. In P.W. Halligan & J.C. Marshall (eds), *Method in Madness: Case Studies in Cognitive Neuropsychiatry* (pp. 209–233). Hove: Psychology Press.

De Renzi, E., Lucchelli, F., Muggia, S. & Spinnler, H. (1995). Persistent retrograde amnesia following a minor trauma. *Cortex*, **31**, 531–542.

Eich, E., McCaulay, D., Lowenstein, R.J. & Dihle, P.H. (1996). Memory, amnesia, and dissociative identity disorder. *Psychological Science*, **8**, 417–422.

Fenton, G.W. (1972). Epilepsy and automatism. *British Journal of Hospital Medicine*, **7**, 57–64.

Fenwick, P. (1990). Automatism, medicine and the law. *Psychological Medicine Monographs*, suppl. 17. Cambridge: Cambridge University Press.

Gardiner, J.M. & Parkin, A.J. (1990). Attention and recollective experience. *Memory and Cognition*, **18**, 579–583.

Goodwin, D.W., Crane, J.B. & Guze, S.E. (1969). Phenomenological aspects of the alcoholic "blackout". *British Journal of Psychiatry*, **115**, 1033–1038.

Gudjonsson, G.H. & MacKeith, J. (1983). A specific recognition deficit in case of homicide. *Medicine, Science and the Law*, **23**, 37–40.

Gudjonsson, G.H. & Taylor, P.J. (1985). Cognitive deficit in a case of retrograde amnesia. *British Journal of Psychiatry*, **147**, 715–718.

Guttmacher, M.S. (1955). *Psychiatry and the Law*. New York: Grune & Stratton.

Harvey, P. (2000). Fear can interrupt the continuum of memory. *Journal of Neurology, Neurosurgery and Psychiatry*, **69**, 431–432.

Harvey, A.G. & Bryant, R.A. (2001). Reconstructing trauma memories: a prospective study of "amnesic" trauma survivors. *Journal of Traumatic Stress*, **14**, 277–282.

Harvey, A.G., Brewin C.R., Jones, C. & Kopelman, M.D. (2003). Co-existence of post-traumatic stress disorder and traumatic brain injury: towards a resolution of the paradox. *Journal of the International Neuropsychological Society*, **9**, 663–676.

Hodges, J.R. & Ward C.D. (1989). Observations during transient global amnesia: a behavioural and neuropsychological study of the five cases. *Brain*, **112**, 595–620.

Hodges, J. & Warlow, C.P. (1990). The aetiology of transient global amnesia. *Brain*, **113**, 639–657.

Hopwood, J.S. & Snell, H.K. (1933). Amnesia in relation to crime. *Journal of Mental Science*, **79**, 27–41.

Howard, C. & d'Orbán, P.T. (1987). Violence in sleep: medico-legal issues and two case reports. *Psychological Medicine*, **17**, 915–925.

Hunter, I.M.L. (1964). *Memory.* Harmondsworth: Penguin.

Kales, A., Soldatos, C.R., Caldwell, A.B. et al. (1980). Somnambulism. *Archives of General Psychiatry*, **37**, 1406–1410.

Kanzer, M. (1939). Amnesia: a statistical study. *American Journal of Psychiatry*, **96**, 711–716.

Kapur, N. (1990). Transient epileptic amnesia: a clinically distinct form of neurological memory disorder. In H.J. Markowitsch (ed.), *Transient Global Amnesia and Related Disorders.* Lewiston, NY: Hogrefe and Huber.

Kapur, N. (1999). Syndromes of retrograde amnesia: conceptual and empirical synthesis. *Psychological Bulletin*, **125**, 800–825.

Kapur, N. (2000). Focal retrograde amnesia and the attribution of causality: an exceptionally benign commentary. *Cognitive Neuropsychology*, **17**, 623–637.

Kapur, N. & Abbot, P. (1996). A study of recovery of memory function in a case of witnessed functional retrograde amnesia. *Cognitive Neuropsychiatry*, **1**, 247–258.

Kapur, N., Ellison, D., Smith, M. et al. (1992). Focal retrograde amnesia following bilateral temporal lobe pathology: a neuropsychological and magnetic resonance study. *Brain*, **116**, 73–86.

Kihlstrom, J.F. & Schacter, D. (1995). Functional disorders of autobiographical memory. In A.D. Baddeley, B.A. Wilson & F.N. Watts (eds), *Handbook of Memory Disorders*, 1st edn (pp. 337–364). Chichester: Wiley.

Kihlstrom, J.F. & Schacter, D.L. (2000). Functional amnesia. In L. Cermak (ed.), *Handbook of Neuropsychology*, 2nd edn, Vol. 2. (pp. 409–427). Amsterdam: Elsevier Science.

Knox, S.J. (1968). Epileptic automatism and violence. *Medicine, Science and the Law*, **8**, 96–104.

Kopelman, M.D. (1987). Amnesia: organic and psychogenic. *British Journal of Psychiatry*, **150**, 428–442.

Kopelman, M.D. (1995). Assessment of psychogenic amnesia. In A.D. Baddeley, B.A. Wilson & F.N. Watts (eds), *Handbook of Memory Disorders*, 1st edn (pp. 427–448). Chichester: Wiley.

Kopelman, M.D. (2000a). Focal retrograde amnesia and the attribution of causality: an exceptionally critical review. *Cognitive Neuropsychology*, **17**, 585–621.

Kopelman, M.D. (2000b). Editorial commentary: fear can interrupt the continuum of memory. *Journal of Neurology, Neurosurgery and Psychiatry*, **69**, 431–432

Kopelman, M.D. (2000c). Comments on focal retrograde amnesia and the attribution of causality: an exceptionally benign commentary by Narinder Kapur. *Cognitive Neuropsychology*, **17**, 639–640.

Kopelman, M.D. (2002). Disorders of Memory. *Brain*, **125**, 2152–2190.

Kopelman, M.D., Christensen, H., Parfitt, A. & Stanhope, N. (1994a). The Great Escape: a neuropsychological study of psychogenic amnesia. *Neuropsychologia*, **32**, 675–691.

Kopelman, M.D., Green, R.E.A., Guinan, E.M. (1994b). The case of the amnesic intelligence officer. *Psychological Medicine*, **24**, 1037–1045.

Kopelman, M.D. & Morton, J. (2001). Psychogenic amnesia—functional memory loss. In G. Davies & T. Dalgleish (eds), *Recovered Memories: The Middle Ground.* Chichester: Wiley (pp. 219–243).

Kopelman, M.D., Panayiotopoulos, C.P. & Lewis, P. (1994c). Transient epileptic amnesia differentiated from psychogenic "fugue": neuropsychological, EEG and PET findings. *Journal of Neurology, Neurosurgery, and Psychiatry*, **57**, 1002–1004.

Kritchevsky, M., Zouzounis, J. & Squire, L. (1997). Transient global amnesia and functional retrograde amnesia: Contrasting examples of episodic memory loss. *Philosophical Transactions of the Royal Society of London, Series B, Biological Sciences*, **352**, 1747–1754.

Kuehn, L.L. (1974). Looking down a gun barrel: person perception and violent crime. *Perceptual and Motor Skills*, **39**, 1159–1164.

Lancet (1978). Editorial: Factitious hypoglycaemia. *Lancet*, **I**, 1293.

Leitch, A. (1948). Notes on amnesia in crime for the general practitioner. *Medical Press*, **219**, 459–463.

Lennox, W.G. (1943). Amnesia, real and feigned. *American Journal of Psychiatry*, **99**, 732–743.

Loftus, E.F., Polonsky, S. & Fullilove, M.T. (1994). Memories of childhood sexual abuse: remembering and repressing. *Psychology of Women*, **18**, 67–84.

Lucchelli, F., Muggia, S. & Spinnler, H. (1995). The "Petites Madeleines" phenomenon in two amnesic patients. Sudden recovery of forgotten memories. *Brain*, **118**, 167–183.

Lynch, B.E. & Bradford, J.M.W. (1980). Amnesia—its detection by psychophysiological measures. *Bulletin of the American Academy of Psychiatry and the Law*, **8**, 288–297.

Markowitsch, H.J. (1996). Organic and psychogenic retrograde amnesia: two sides of the same coin? *Neurocase*, **2**, 357–371.

Markowitsch, H.J., Fink, G., Thone, A. et al. (1997). A PET study of persistent psychogenic amnesia covering the whole life span. *Cognitive Neuropsychiatry*, **2**, 135–158.

MacKenzie Ross, S. (2000). A process of discovery: profound retrograde amnesia following mild head injury: organic or functional? *Cortex*, **36**, 521–538.

Merskey, H. (1992). The manufacture of personalities: the production of multiple personality disorder. *British Journal of Psychiatry*, **160**, 327–340.

Merskey, H. (1995). Multiple personality disorder and false memory syndrome. *British Journal of Psychiatry*, **166**, 281–283.

McNeil, J.E. & Greenwood, R. (1996). Can PTSD occur with amnesia for the precipitating event? *Cognitive Neuropsychiatry*, **1**, 239–246.

Miller, J.W., Petersen, R.C., Metter, E.J. et al. (1987). Transient global amnesia: clinical characteristics and prognosis. *Neurology*, **37**, 733–737.

Nissen, M.J., Ross, J.L., Willingham, D.B. et al. (1988). Memory and awareness in a patient with multiple personality disorder. *Brain and Cognition*, **8**, 21–38.

O'Connell, B.A. (1960). Amnesia and homicide. *British Journal of Delinquency*, **10**, 262–276.

Papagno, C. (1998). Transient retrograde amnesia associated with impaired naming of living categories. *Cortex*, **34**, 111–121.

Parfitt, D.N. & Gall, C.M.C. (1944). Psychogenic amnesia: the refusal to remember. *Journal of Mental Science*, **90**, 511–527.

Parwatikar, S.D., Holcomb, W.R. & Meninger, K.A. (1985). The detection of malingered amnesia in accused murderers. *Bulletin of the American Academy of Psychiatry and the Law*, **13**, 97–103.

Patrick, M. & Howells, R. (1990). Barbiturate-assisted interviews in modern clinical practice. *Psychological Medicine*, **20**, 763–765.

Pope, H.G. & Hudson, J.I. (1995). Can memories of childhood sexual abuse be repressed? *Psychological Medicine*, **25**, 121–126.

Pyszora, N., Barker, A. & Kopelman, M.D. (2003). Amnesia for criminal offences: a study of life sentence prisoners. *Journal of Forensic Psychiatry and Psychology*, in press.

Raphael, B. & Middleton, W. (1988). After the horror. *British Medical Journal*, **296**, 1142–1144.

Russell, W.R. & Nathan, P.W. (1946). Traumatic amnesia. *Brain*, **69**, 280–300.

Sargant, W. & Slater, E. (1941). Amnesic syndromes in war. *Proceedings of the Royal Society of Medicine*, **34**, 757–764.

Scarlett, J.A., Mako, M.E., Rubenstein, A.H. et al. (1977). Factitious hypoglycaemia. *New England Journal of Medicine*, **297**, 1029–1032.

Schacter, D.L. (1986a). Amnesia and crime: how much do we really know? *American Psychologist*, **41**, 286–295.

Schacter, D.L. (1986b). On the relation between genuine and simulated amnesia. *Behavioural Sciences and the Law*, **4**, 47–64.

Schacter, D.L. (1986c). Feelings-of-knowing ratings distinguish between genuine and simulated forgetting. *Journal of Experimental Psychology: Learning, Memory and Cognition*, **12**, 30–41.

Schacter, D.L., Wang, P.L., Tulving, E. & Freeman, M. (1982). Functional retrograde amnesia: a quantitative case study. *Neuropsychologia*, **20**, 523–532.

Schacter, D.L. (1996). *Searching for Memory: the Brain, the Mind, and the Past*. New York: Basic Books.

Schacter, D.L., Kihlstrom, J.F., Kihlstrom, L. & Berren, M. (1989). Autobiographical memory in a case of multiple personality disorder. *Journal of Abnormal Psychology*, **98**, 508–514.

Schenck, C.H., Bundlie, S., Ettinger, M. & Mahowald, M. (1986). Chronic behaviour disorders of human REM sleep: a new category of parasomnia: *Sleep*, **9**: 293–308.

Schooler, J.W., Bendiksen, M. & Ambadar, Z. (1997). Taking the middle line: can we accommodate both fabricated and recovered memories of sexual abuse? In M.A. Conway (ed.), *Recovered Memories and False Memories*. New York: Oxford University Press.

Shimamura, A.P. (1997). Neuropsychological factors associated with memory recollection: what can science tell us about reinstated memories? In J.D. Read & D.S. Lindsay (eds), *Recollections of Trauma: Scientific Research and Clinical Practice* (pp. 253–272). New York: Plenum.

Stengel, E. (1941). On the aetiology of the fugue states. *Journal of Mental Science*, **87**, 572–599.

Stracciari, A., Ghidoni, E., Guarino, M. et al. (1994). Post-traumatic retrograde amnesia with selective impairment of autobiographic memory. *Cortex*, **30**, 459–468.

Stuss, D. & Guzman, D. (1988). Severe remote memory loss with minimal anterograde amnesia: a clinical note. *Brain and Cognition*, **8**, 21–30.

Taylor, P.J. & Kopelman, M. (1984). Amnesia for criminal offences. *Psychological Medicine*, **14**, 581–588.

Van der Kolk, B.A. & Fisler, R. (1995). Dissociation and the fragmentary nature of traumatic memories: overview and exploratory study. *Journal of Trauma and Stress*, **8**, 505–525.

Wilson, G., Rupp, C. & Wilson, W.W. (1950). Amnesia. *American Journal of Psychiatry*, **106**, 481–485.

Yuille, J.C. (1987). The effects of alcohol and marijuana on eyewitness recall. Paper presented at the Conference on Practical Aspects of Memory, Swansea, UK (unpublished).

Yuille, J.C. & Cutshall, J.L. (1986). A case study of eye-witness memory of a crime. *Journal of Applied Psychology*, **71**, 291–301.

CHAPTER 5

Developmental Amnesias and Acquired Amnesias of Childhood

Christine M. Temple

Developmental Neuropsychology Unit, University of Essex, Colchester, UK

BACKGROUND ISSUES

Selective impairments of literacy or language in children of otherwise good intelligence have been well documented in both acquired and developmental forms. There has also been recognition that there are other selective impairments of cognitive development which may coexist with intact intelligence and may be manifest in developmental or acquired form, for example disorders of face recognition (de Haan & Campbell, 1991; Temple, 1992a; Young & Ellis, 1989) or disorders of executive skill (Marlowe, 1992; Williams & Mateer, 1992; Temple, 1997a). The first detailed case analyses were presented 10–15 years ago of both acquired amnesia in childhood (Ostergaard, 1987) and developmental amnesia (De Renzi & Lucchelli, 1990), with both individuals displaying normal intelligence. There was relatively limited discussion of these conditions in the 1990s, but there is now an expanding literature that indicates not only that these disorders may be more common than had been recognized but also that they have interesting implications for discussions of memory systems in adults as well as children. They provide models of memory development with unusual constraints, which affect theorizing about distinctions between component processes in adult memory systems; for example, there are issues in the adult literature about the relationship between episodic and semantic memory. Dissociations may be seen in childhood that are not evident in adulthood but are directly relevant to such issues. Disorders of memory in childhood also provide information about the normal development of memory and are relevant to theoretical debates about prescribed or emergent modularity in development (Bishop, 1997; Temple, 1997a, 1997b). They are also significant from a more applied perspective, since children with amnesia yet normal intelligence constitute a group whose education is being accommodated within normal classrooms, despite limited recognition of the form of their difficulties.

The idea that memory impairments might be present in those of limited intellectual skills gained earlier credence than the idea that they might occur in those of normal intelligence.

The Essential *Handbook of Memory Disorders for Clinicians*. Edited by A.D. Baddeley, M.D. Kopelman and B.A. Wilson.
© 2004 John Wiley & Sons, Ltd. ISBN 0-470-09141-X.

Ribot (1882, cited by Maurer, 1992) argued that "idiots", "imbeciles" and some "cretins" have "a general debility of memory". More explicitly, it has been suggested that in children with general learning disabilities, the later stages of memory may be intact but the ability to code information effectively for storage may be impaired. However, as Maurer (1992) emphasizes, memory can also seem to be well developed in some "idiots savants" who are able to use efficient mnemonic strategies. The apparent dissociation of memory skills from many aspects of intellectual development becomes evident, however, in the cases of developmental and acquired amnesia that are discussed below.

There are a variety of potential aetiologies for memory impairments in childhood. Traditionally, disorders in children are divided into those that are acquired and those that are developmental (Temple, 1992b). In acquired disorders, a child has a normally developing skill, then sustains injury or disease and the development of the skill or its subsequent progress is impaired. In developmental disorders, the child has never learnt the skill and has not sustained a known injury, the disorder simply becoming manifest as the child acquires and develops cognitive competence.

In practice, this division for memory impairments, as for other disorders in childhood, may not be straightforward; for example, epilepsy, which is often associated with memory impairments, may be a developmental or an acquired disorder. Recently, Vargha-Khadem et al. (1997) and Gadian et al. (2000) have also discussed children with memory impairments who have had hypoxic-ischaemic episodes at or shortly after birth. These children are referred to as having acquired amnesias and the disorders are acquired, in the sense that there has been injury or disease and pathology is identified in the hippocampus. However, the children have not had a period of normal skill development that has been interrupted, and their development from the outset is with an impaired substrate for memory. Within child neuropsychology, it has not simply been the occurrence of an acquired lesion that has led to a classification as an acquired disorder. In Landau–Kleffner syndrome, so-called "acquired aphasia of childhood", there is a period of normal development followed by declining and then severely impaired language function but no episode of injury or disease.

Thus, we see classification as an acquired disorder in childhood either where there is a known lesion or where a period of normal development is followed by decline and impairment. The issue of classification becomes significant if developmental amnesias and acquired amnesias of childhood differ in their characteristics and if the pattern of memory impairment differs, dependent upon the age of onset of the impairment. Effects of age of onset would be predicted by a number of developmental models, within which systems evolve but would be predicted less by developmental frameworks which incorporate more preformist views of the underlying functional architecture.

Acquired memory impairments in children may follow closed head injury or encephalitis, exhibiting similar symptomatology to adults (Herkowitz & Rosman, 1982). However, additional cognitive impairments are common in these cases, which may sometimes make the study of the effect of the memory impairments itself difficult to disentangle form other cognitive loss. Cases of more selective acquired amnesia have been described following anoxia, to which it appears that the large mitochondria of the hippocampi may be particularly vulnerable, and in temporal lobe epilepsy similar circuitry may be affected. Developmental amnesias may occur in association with epilepsy, family history suggesting a genetic vulnerability, or in the absence of any explicit predisposing factor.

In the analysis of memory impairments in children, an issue arises that differs from their study in adulthood. This relates to the potential effects of memory impairments upon the acquisition of skill or knowledge in other cognitive domains, for example adults with classical amnesia typically have normal language skills. In contrast, if a child acquires amnesia before language is fully established or has developmental amnesia, then the memory impairment itself could affect the subsequent development of semantic or other memory stores which may underpin language. Thus, for example, Julia (Temple, 1997a), discussed below in the section on developmental amnesia, also had a developmental anomia, which was a disorder resulting from failure to establish knowledge of vocabulary items, rather than a straightforward retrieval difficulty. Thus, children with developmental disorders of memory provide knowledge not only about the structure of developing memory systems but also about the relationship between memory and other skills, as learning and development take place.

In disorders of naming in childhood, a distinction has been drawn between *semantic representation anomia* (Temple, 1997a), in which naming difficulties are associated with apparent failure to establish a semantic representations for the word, reflected in similarly impaired receptive vocabulary, and *semantic access anomia* (Van Hout, 1993; Temple, 1997a), in which there is evidence of an intact representation for the word but difficulties with lexical retrieval of its name. The former disorder may be associated with more generalized memory impairments. The latter disorder has been described by Van Hout (1993) in parallel developmental and acquired forms.

ACQUIRED AMNESIA IN CHILDREN

An early case of acquired amnesia in a child, following ECT, is reported by Geschwind (1974). The 10-year-old child had normal language prior to the ECT but subsequently developed both memory and language impairment. Geschwind attributed the language impairment to a retrograde amnesia which extended back into the period of language acquisition. An alternative explanation would be that the acquired amnesia and acquired dyphasia were distinct disorders. However, Geschwind argued that an acquired memory impairment in childhood may not only affect the acquisition of subsequent skills, as discussed above, but may also affect skills that have been previously acquired if the amnesia disrupts the storage, consolidation or subsequent retrieval of previously learnt material.

Ostergaard (1987) presented the first detailed analysis of a child with acquired amnesia. The 10-year-old child, C.C., developed amnesia following an episode of anoxia following water intoxication in the treatment of diabetic ketoacidosis, resulting in severe left hippocampal damage and at least partial right hippocampal damage. The child remained of normal intelligence but many memory skills were impaired. Ostergaard (1987) made the first attempt to determine the components of memory that might be affected and spared in such cases. He argued that the distinction between the skills that were impaired and those that were intact related to a procedural–declarative dimension, with declarative memory impaired and procedural memory intact.

Within declarative memory, both semantic and episodic memory was impaired. Knowledge of semantic memory for facts was impaired, as reflected by scores on the Information subtest of the WISC-R (Wechsler, 1974). The impairment in semantic memory also extended to vocabulary skills in tasks of lexical decision, semantic classification and verbal fluency. In lexical decision, accuracy was good, indicating development of lexical representations, but responses were very slow, suggesting access difficulties, and there was a significantly elevated priming effect of a related preceding word. In semantic classification, Ostergaard (1987) divided words by age of acquisition into three groups, 0–4 years, 4–8 years and over 8 years. He found a much sharper than normal temporal gradient to performance in terms of response speed, with words acquired early being responded to more quickly than those acquired later. He argued that this reflected a retrograde amnesia with a temporal gradient.

Impaired episodic memory was seen on immediate and delayed story recall, design recall and delayed free recall of word lists, although immediate free recall of words was within the normal range. Reading and spelling were also impaired and there was the suggestion of some retrograde loss, with teachers reporting normal reading prior to illness, yet reading and spelling ages 6 months after illness were found to be 9–14 months below chronological age at time of illness.

However, like cases of acquired amnesia in adulthood, C.C. had intact procedural memory for skills, such as learning a computer video-attack game. Like acquired amnesic patients, Ostergaard (1987) also showed that C.C. could learn and retain skills on the Gollin incomplete pictures tests, where pictures depicting an item become progressively more complete. Repeat testing 24 h later showed much improved skills for both C.C. and controls and the improvement was sustained on further retesting 8 days later. Follow-up at age 15 indicated a similar pattern, with a distinction between declarative and procedural memory skills. There was some limited progress in reading and spelling but much less than would be expected from a normal child.

Vargha-Khadem et al. (1992) reported, in an abstract, a case of acquired amnesia in a child, J.L., where they also found impaired performance in declarative memory but normal performance on procedural memory. J.L. developed amnesia after surgery for a craniopharyngioma. There was ventral diencephalic pathology encompassing the mammillary bodies. Some scholastic skills were nevertheless attained and reading developed to age level.

A further case of acquired amnesia is described in a 9-year-old child, T.C., who had acute encephalopathy, possibly as a result of herpes simplex encephalitis, resulting in diffuse cerebral injury (Wood et al., 1982, 1989). T.C. had severely impaired semantic memory in relation to facts about the world and severely impaired episodic memory impairment affecting both story recall and autobiographical day-to-day memory. However, Woods et al. (1987) argued that their case did not conform to the procedural–declarative distinction of the Ostergaard case, since T.C. made some scholastic progress through the school years, although a dense amnesia remained in both clinical and psychometric terms. However, Ostergaard & Squire (1990) argued, in response, that some scholastic progress would be expected in the absence of declarative memory on the basis of automated procedures or conceptual development. They also emphasized that the distinction they had proposed was based upon relative rather than absolute impairment, with studies of even acquired amnesia in adults discussing "differential susceptibility of these systems to amnesia" (Squire & Cohen, 1984). C.C.'s declarative skills were severely impaired and were much more impaired than procedural memory skills. Similarly, for T.C., declarative knowledge at age 20 remained severely impaired, with inability to report events of the last hour and memory for verbal and visual material "essentially absent", but there were some miminal skills, for example with some words recalled on repeated exposure with the Rey Auditory Verbal Learning task. Ostergaard & Squire (1990) argued that minimal residual declarative skills in C.C. or T.C. could enable some limited acquisition of skills contributing to scholastic progress, without difficulty for the Ostergaard (1987) proposal. They point out that in the cases of both C.C. and T.C. scholastic progress in literacy and arithmetic was abnormally slow, although the Vargha-Khadem et al. (1992) case of J.L., mentioned above, illustrates that impairment in literacy is not a necessary concomitant of a declarative impairment.

Subsequent to this debate, Brainerd & Reyna (1992) argued that children's logical and mathematical skills and ability to make pragmatic inferences are not dependent upon memory in terms of reactivation of previously encoded traces. This would permit progress in these scholastic areas despite memory impairment. Wood et al. (1989) had reported above-average skills for T.C. in general problem-solving ability on the Porteus mazes, and a further pattern of this sort was confirmed by Broman et al. (1997), who reported the case of a child, M.S., with an acquired amnesia that followed respiratory arrest and consequent anoxic encephalopathy at the age of 8 years. MRI indicated loss of volume in bilateral hippocampal and medial temporal grey areas, with no evidence of amygdala atrophy.

The child was followed up into adulthood and assessed in detail at the age of 28. Intelligence on Progressive Matrices was normal. In contrast, declarative memory was severely impaired. His profile on the Wechsler Intelligence Scales indicated that as an adult his weakest subtest scores were attained on Information, which assesses the factual general knowledge established in semantic memory, and on Vocabulary, which assesses the knowledge of words established in semantic memory. On further formal testing, he was impaired in episodic recall of words, stories and patterns. He was also impaired in learning paired associates and delayed recall of a route. His memory impairment extended to both anterograde and retrograde loss as he was unable to remember any events more than 6–9 months prior to the anoxia.

Recognition memory for words, faces and doors on the WRMB (Warrington, 1984) and the Doors and People Test (Baddeley et al., 1994) was impaired but immediate recognition memory for patterns on Benton's Visual Retention Test was normal. Short-term memory, as assessed by digit span, was also normal. Consistent with the view of Brainerd & Reyna (1992), some mathematical and logical skills had become established, i.e. he developed algorithms to derive the multiplication tables he was unable to memorise by rote. With lengthy perseverance, he could solve puzzles like Rubic's cube and some computer games. On the Wechsler Intelligence Scales, Picture Completion, Object Assembly and Block Design were entirely normal, indicating intact skills of logical analysis, nonverbal reasoning and construction. He could also assemble items in real life, for example a canopy tent, and he could recite the tune and lyrics to the signature songs for his favourite television programmes. Thus, some automated and procedural memory skills had also been acquired. Within language, comprehension of syntax of varying complexity and comprehension of the sentences comprising the verbal ideational material taken from the BDAE (Goodglass & Kaplan, 1983), which incorporate adult logical complexity, were both at an average level for an adult. In contrast, receptive vocabulary was impaired and was at an average 9-year-old level; naming was also impaired to the expected level relative to his receptive vocabulary. Thus, he has a semantic representation anomia as discussed above. Reading and spelling remained at an 8-year-old level, hence whilst syntactic and logical reasoning skills in language had developed to an adult level, knowledge of word meanings and ability to read or spell words had remained severely impaired.

Broman et al. (1997) noted the difference in the patterns of deficit in the reported cases of acquired amnesia in childhood with respect to language and literacy development, with the degree of reading difficulty for M.S. being more extreme than that of C.C. (Ostergaard, 1987) or T.C. (Woods et al., 1982, 1989). Reviewing the identified lesions, he proposed that for those cases involving the hippocampus and its circuitry, language development and skills were also affected to a degree, which might vary dependent upon the degree of the amnesia. In cases like that of J.L (Vargha-Khadem et al., 1992), where the damage was to the diencephalic structures including the mammillary bodies, language and reading appear to develop normally, since reading was at the expected level for chronological age.

However, in contrast to this view, Vargha-Khadem et al. (1997) reported a further three cases of amnesic impairment in children following early hippocampal pathology. In each case they argued that language and literacy were in the low-average to average range and that episodic memory was much more significantly affected than semantic memory. Despite the bilateral hippocampal pathology, they argue for the development of semantic skills. These are the first cases of acquired amnesia in childhood in which it is argued that semantic skills are normal for both knowledge of words and factual knowledge of the world, and that some declarative skills are intact despite episodic impairment.

The first of Vargha-Khadem et al.'s (1997) three cases was a 14-year-old girl, Beth. After birth Beth remained without a heartbeat for 7–8 min before resuscitation. Memory difficulties were noticed on entrance into mainstream school. The second case, Jon, was a 19-year-old boy. He had been delivered prematurely at 26 weeks, had breathing difficulties and was in an incubator, on a ventilator, for 2 months. At the age of 4, he had two protracted seizures. Memory difficulties were noted by his parents at age 5.5 years. The third case was a 22-year-old, Kate, who for 3 days at the age of 9 had received a toxic dose of theophylline, a drug being given for her asthma. This led to respiratory arrest and loss of consciousness. Upon physical recovery, she displayed amnesia.

In support of competent semantic skills, Vargha-Khadem et al. (1997) discuss both the Information and Vocabulary subtests on the WISC-III (Wechsler, 1992) and predicted reading and spelling skills on the basis of IQ. They argue that there is a pronounced disparity between attainments on these measures and a severe amnesia for everyday life. In relation to the Information subtest, Beth and Jon attain normal scaled scores, although Kate has a scaled score of 6, indicative of a degree of impairment and equivalent to the level of performance taken to indicate impairment in the Ostergaard (1987) study. Scores on Vocabulary for all three children were within the normal range. Reading scores for all three children were commensurate with predictions from IQ, although for Beth, where intellectual skills were a standard deviation below average, these attainments were equivalently below average. Spelling was similarly at the predicted level for Beth and Kate, although this was more markedly impaired for Jon. Thus, whilst semantic memory is not intact for all skills in all three cases, there is clear evidence that it is has developed to a substantive degree.

For all three cases, immediate episodic memory for a word list was normal, as was digit span and Corsi span. Thus, short-term memory appeared normal. However, delayed recall of both verbal and nonverbal material was severely impaired. There was also parental complaint of severe difficulties with day-to-day memory to a degree that significantly affects their day-to-day abilities. This was confirmed for all three children by their very weak scores on the Rivermead Behavioural Memory Test (Vargha-Khadem et al., 1997). Thus, episodic memory is severely impaired and is much less well developed than semantic memory skills.

This inequality of sparing might result from independent storage, with the more significant impact upon episodic rather than semantic stores in these cases of bilateral hippocampal pathology, being similar to that seen in acquired amnesia. Another possibility that Vargha-Khadem et al. (1997) discuss is that, whilst episodic memory is impaired, it might be sufficiently preserved to enable the acquisition of knowledge to which there is repeated exposure in different contexts, and therefore enable context-free linguistic and factual knowledge. This would enable preservation of the theory of acquired amnesia for both adults and children, and would argue that both episodic memory and semantic memory are a single process mediated by the hippocampal system. However, Vargha-Khadem et al.'s (1997) proposal is that the underlying semantic memory functions of the perirhinal and entorhinal cortices may be sufficient to support context-free semantic memories, but not context-rich episodic memories, for which hippocampal circuitry is required. For both semantic and episodic memory to be affected severely, the hippocampi and underlying cortices would then require to be damaged.

Both Beth and Jon (Vargha-Khadem et al., 1997) had hypoxic–ischaemic episodes at or shortly after birth without showing any subsequent hard neurological signs. A further three similar cases are also presented by Gadian et al. (2000). In each of these five cases, the authors argue for the relative preservation of semantic memory over episodic memory. In each case, the Information and Vocabulary subtest scores on the WISC-III (Wechsler, 1992) are normal, and in each case basic reading is in line with IQ, episodic memory in terms of delayed story recall, delayed recall of listed words and delayed recall of the Rey figure is very poor, and day-to-day memory is impaired, based on both parental report and psychometric assessment. MRI scans indicate visible bilateral hippocampal atrophy in all cases and quantitative measures also indicate reduced grey matter in the putamen, with abnormality in the thalamus and midbrain.

Of further interest in the Gadian et al. (2000) paper is the parental comment, "Although his understanding of language is good, his use of language is often simplistic and he gropes for words". This suggests possible anomic difficulties in the use of language and, whilst name retrieval has not been explored in the cases of acquired amnesia discussed above, it has been found to be impaired in some of the cases of developmental amnesia outlined below (Temple, 1997a; Casalini et al., 1999).

A more detailed investigation of Jon, one of the hypoxic–ischaemic cases of Gadian et al. (2000), is given by Baddeley et al. (2001). Baddeley et al. (2001) established that, despite the very weak episodic recall skills, recognition memory for both visual and verbal material might nevertheless be normal. Recognition skills at a normal level were demonstrated on a range of tasks, including those which involved different speeds of presentation and those involving recognition after a 2 day delay. The only example of good recall came from material presented on a newsreel studied four times over a 2 day period, the conditions most like those involved in the acquisition of semantic memory. As Baddeley et al. (2001) note, Jon is an intelligent and highly motivated subject, so an above-average level of performance might have been expected. Thus, they do not argue that recognition is definitely normal but they do demonstrate convincingly that recognition is very significantly better than recall, even when scores are scaled to take account of the generally greater ease of recognition over recall. The enhancement of recognition over recall for Jon is of a degree that would not be typical of peer performance or the performance of adults with memory disorders.

Thus it would appear, from cases such as Jon's, that memory is being encoded and stored and that whilst the recollective process of episodic memory is impaired, this is not necessary for the acquisition of semantic knowledge or for recognition memory. This negates the view that semantic memory is simply the derivative of many episodes (e.g. Baddeley, 1997; Squire, 1992), a view derived from adult studies, where impaired episodic memory generally coexists with failure to update semantic memory, although Tulving (1972; Tulving & Markovitch, 1998) has argued otherwise for many years. It also indicates a more focal pattern of impairment in these cases of developmental amnesia than is typically seen in acquired amnesia. In acquired amnesia, recognition is usually, although not always, impaired (Aggleton & Brown, 1999; Holdstock et al., 2000) and, whilst semantic memory for facts acquired prior to injury is intact, there is difficulty in upgrading semantic information. In amnesic cases like Jon, recognition memory is good and semantic memory stores are upgraded, despite severe episodic memory impairment.

The idea of a developmental disorder being more focal than a similar acquired disorder in adulthood is interesting, given the view often argued that abnormalities in development have a pervasive and generalized impact because the system is adapting and formulating without prespecified functional architecture. Jon's case of amnesia from an early age demonstrated the potentially focal impact of a developmental memory impairment, with a pattern of performance entirely consistent with a modular view of the developing memory system.

Tulving (1985) defined episodic memory in a more focal way than it is often used now. He stressed the subjective experience of recollection in episodic memory. Thus, he distinguished between "remembering" and simply "knowing". Recognition memory is also argued to reflect these two processes of "remembering" and "knowing" (Tulving, 1985). Baddeley et al. (2001) argue that when Jon recognizes information, he "knows" he has seen it before but he does not "remember" the experience of having seen it before. In their terms, he lacks the ability to recollect the contextual detail which would be necessary for a "remember" response. Thus, the memory impairment is truly episodic in the original Tulving (1972, 1985) meaning of the term.

A further case of acquired amnesia, in which there are retrieval difficulties of a more unusual form, is described by Vargha-Khadem et al. (1994) in a 14-year-old boy, Neil. The amnesia followed successful treatment the preceding year with radiotherapy and chemotherapy for a tumour in the pineal region of the posterior third ventricle. Neil retained normal verbal intelligence, attaining scores of 111/109 on the verbal scale of the Wechsler Intelligence Scales. Although Performance IQ was significantly impaired, block design scores were normal. Retrograde memory was normal but episodic memory was impaired. Memory assessed on the Wechsler Memory Scales was very poor, with a MQ of 59 attained. Neil could copy a complex design well but delayed recall was severely impaired. With spoken verbal response, the verbal memory impairment appeared to be pervasive. There was also both agnosia and alexia. Although he could recognize familiar objects when they were in their customary place in his home, he was unable to recognize any of them when they were placed on a table directly in front of him. Yet, he could produce precise and intricate drawings of imagined objects and scenes and had intact and detailed visual memories for these items. Writing was also intact and he could produce accurate written responses for some information that he could not access in oral form, thereby indicating some ability to learn and retain new information. He was not always aware of his correct written responses. Thus, the recall is not linked to explicit awareness.

These abilities argued for separate stores and/or retrieval modalities for verbal material, one oral and one orthographic. His ability to use orthographic output included information taught in a verbal format at school but also included recall of day-to-day events. In the case of Jon (Baddeley et al., 2001), overt recall was problematic but recognition was much better. In the case of Neil (Vargha-Khadem et al., 1994), overt oral recall is problematic but written recall is much better. In both cases, it appears that memory is being encoded and stored but the recollective process of episodic memory is impaired and, without that episodic process, one may "know" rather than "remember", as in the case of Jon (Baddeley et al., 2001), or one may not have conscious awareness of "knowing", as in the case of Neil (Vargha-Khadem et al., 1994), despite explicit response accuracy with orthographic output.

REYE'S SYNDROME

A seemingly quite different form of acquired memory impairment despite intact intellectual skills is documented as a consequence of Reye's syndrome (RS; Quart et al., 1987). RS is most common in children aged 5–15 years (Nelson et al., 1979). It occurs in children who have previously been healthy. The child may appear to have a viral infection from which he/she seems to be recovering. RS has also been linked to ingestion of 5-aminosalicylates (5-ASA), or to both viral infection and 5-ASA ingestion. The child then develops a serious acute encephalopathy linked to liver disease and severe disturbance of intracellular metabolism (Meekin et al., 1999). Behaviourally, there is vomiting, lethargy, personality change and disorientation. The disease differs in severity from mild personality changes in an otherwise oriented child (Stage 1) to coma (Stage 5) (Lovejoy et al., 1974). Changes to the brain include astrocyte swelling, myelin bleb formation and damage to neuron mitochondria (Partin et al., 1978). There is diffuse encephalopathy with cerebral oedema and raised intracranial pressure, causing tissue displacement and reduced cerebral perfusion pressure. This occasionally leads to death (Sarnaik, 1982) but more commonly there is recovery, with intact intelligence but specific neuropsychological impairment (Quart, 1984).

The position of the temporal lobes is thought to make them particularly vulnerable to the effects of oedema and raised intracranial pressure in RS and elsewhere (Quart et al., 1987). However, a single MRI case study indicated compressed ventricles and lesions of the thalamus, mesencephalon and pons, with the thalamic lesion persisting for 2 months as the others resolved. When the age of onset is below a year, the incidence of neurological impairment is higher (Meekin et al., 1999). Thus, in similar fashion to Landau–Kleffner syndrome with language (Bishop, 1985), earlier onset is associated with poorer prognosis (Davidson et al., 1978), the reverse of the normal expectation from developmental plasticity.

Quart et al. (1987) report a study of 26 children with RS, with a mean age of 12.9 and a range of 7–18 years. They were aged at least 3 when they became ill. Controls were matched by age, race, sex, socioeconomic status and receptive vocabulary score on the PPVT, which provided an estimate of intelligence levels. The children with RS were significantly poorer than controls on the children's version of the Wechsler Memory Scales. The mean IQ–MQ difference for the RS group was also significantly greater than for controls. No details are given about semantic memory skills, except that since PPVT scores are normal, it appears that semantic memory for words has developed normally. The memory impairment for the children with RS included verbal and visual episodic memory, as reflected in immediate and delayed recall of stories and designs. Working memory as assessed by digit span forward was also impaired. In contrast, paired associate learning was not significantly different from normal.

Quart et al. (1987) carried out a "levels of processing" experiment. In the face section, 30 unfamiliar faces were presented and the children either had to make a "superficial" judgement by indicating whether the person was "male" or "female", or they had to engage in "deep" processing and indicate whether the person was "nice" or "not nice". For a parallel words version, the superficial judgement was whether the word was printed in "small letters" or "capitals", and the deep processing occurred in indicating whether the thing was "alive" or "not alive". On the face section, there was no difference between the groups. However, on the word section, whilst there was no difference in responses for the items which had been superficially cued, the RS group missed significant words that had been deeply processed. Only the control group benefited from deep processing. Semantic activation did not assist the verbal memory of the children with RS.

A further difference between the children with RS and controls was in the use of other memory techniques. None of the children with RS outwardly demonstrated the use of mnemonic strategies, whereas nine of the 26 controls used techniques such as chunking, rehearsing digits and words, drawing designs in the air when the design card was exposed and verbalizing associations to go with difficult pairs of words. Quart et al. (1987) suggest that there is less active involvement in the effort to retain information. They also suggest that the children with RS are less good as organizing visual designs, with almost half failing to perceive the overall design, in contrast to 15% of the control group. These failures in encoding and organization of memory are reminiscent of the discussion of frontal amnesia by Luria (1966, 1973), discussed further by Warrington & Weiskrantz (1982).

In acquired amnesia in adults and in some of the cases of acquired amnesia in children, with onset later than infancy, there is evidence that memory is intact for events before a point in time and impaired for subsequent points. Maurer (1992) suggests that in such cases registration is normal but retention abnormal. In the cases of Jon and Neil, discussed above, both registration and retention appear to be normal but there is difficulty with episodic retrieval and normal free recall. However, with diffuse pathology, such as Reye's syndrome, there may be impairment in registration as well as retention and recall (Lishman, 1987; Maurer, 1992).

TEMPORAL LOBECTOMIES AND TEMPORAL LOBE SURGERY

Temporal lobectomies in children are carried out for the relief of intractable epilepsy, in cases where there is a temporal lobe focus. Dennis et al. (1988) report a study of the effects of temporal lobectomies in adolescent and young adults. Those with left-sided lobectomies showed impairments in verbal recognition memory. However, Dennis et al. (1988) also found complex interactions between side of surgery, age at onset and seizure type which are difficult to interpret. Meyer et al. (1986) also report complex effects of surgery in a study of 50 children aged under 18 years. IQ was not significantly affected by the surgery. Overall, there were no significant effects in memory scores. However, boys were significantly more likely to show memory impairment after surgery and girls were significantly more likely to show memory improvement. Sex differences in memory skill have received little attention in other studies.

Temporal lobe surgery is also carried out for lateralized tumours of the temporal lobes. Cavazzutti et al. (1980) discuss a study in which 60% of the subjects were aged 3–19. Those who had left temporal lobe surgery had increased verbal dysfunction and reduced verbal memory quotient but had improved nonverbal memory. Those who had right temporal lobe surgery had improved verbal skills and verbal learning. The improvements in skill were interpreted as reflecting the removal of the inhibitory effects of the pathological areas upon intact systems in the contralateral hemisphere via the commissural connections.

Carpantieri & Mulhern (1993) also reported memory impairments in 50% of children surviving temporal lobe tumours. They found that the earlier the age of diagnosis, and therefore presumably the earlier the tumour developed, the more severe the long-term memory deficits. However, the greatest memory impairments were seen in those who had radiation therapy, and in such cases memory impairments were probable, even if intelligence was well-preserved. Reading and spelling were significantly correlated with verbal memory performance.

Memory impairment following radiation treatment at the age of 5.6 for a tumour of unspecified location is also reported by Morrow et al. (1989). They briefly described a child, K.I., whose memory for the time around the treatment was intact, as was the knowledge that she had at that time, suggesting intact semantic memory. However, she became "almost completely unable to encode or retrieve long-term memories . . . she became unable to add new information", suggesting severely impaired episodic memory. Although intellectual development was age-appropriate, a year and a half after treatment it failed to rise as fast as chronological age, so that by the age of 8.3 her mental age on the WISC-R was below expectation at 7.2. By the age of 12.8, there had been essentially no intellectual development and, if anything, a slight decline. Mental age on the WISC-R had dropped to 6.8. Cognitive measures had plateaued. Thus, although intelligence seemed age-appropriate immediately after treatment, impairment became more evident over time. It is not clear whether such a pattern relates to long-term effects of the memory impairment itself or to the more generalized impairment to the substrate for cognition, caused by the radiation treatment.

DEVELOPMENTAL AMNESIA

Maurer (1992) described a child, N.S., with developmental amnesia, which he termed "congenital amnesia". CT scan at the age of 9 years revealed low-density areas in both temporal fossae, indicating absence of the left temporal lobe and the pole and mesial parts of the right temporal lobe. These abnormalities were thought to result from prenatal events, possibly as the result of a stroke *in utero*. The memory impairment of N.S. is described as resembling H.M. (Scoville & Milner, 1957). Since in H.M. there is a disorder of declarative memory but procedural memory is intact, Maurer (1992) attempted remediation based on embedding responses within actions that were trained as habits. The information that N.S. was to learn was embedded in stimulus–response sets of pairings, which were then trained by repetition day after day. N.S. had difficulty in learning the names of the people she met everyday. Every time she met the person she was cued to say "Hello" and then the name of the person. The remediation was effective and N.S. was able to learn some names. Moreover, she was then able to use these names effectively in other contexts. Using similar procedures, which are not given in detail, Maurer (1992) reports that she was taught to read.

Vargha-Khadem et al. (1994) report brief details in an abstract of a case, J.F., of developmental amnesia in childhood. The child had seizures from the age of 4. A memory difficulty was recognized at the age of 8 years. There was no mention of any loss of previously acquired skills. MRI showed bilateral mesial temporal sclerosis and intact mammillary bodies. The development of some verbal skills and reading was impaired.

The first extensive analysis of a case of developmental amnesia is given by De Renzi & Lucchelli (1990), who describe a 22-year-old man, M.S. M.S. was born early at 7 months of gestation with a birth weight of 2500 g. CT scan was normal but EEG indicated bilateral bursts of theta and delta waves, with a left frontotemporal prevalence. He was of normal intelligence, with a Verbal IQ of 110 and a Performance IQ of 111. Oral language, visual perception, praxis and attention were normal. M.S. complained that he had had memory difficulties since earliest childhood. He complained of extreme difficulty in remembering the names of familiar people, places, foreign language words and mathematical formulae and tables. He had never managed to learn the lyrics of a song or a poem by heart. He also reported that he had difficulty in remembering faces and his day-to-day memory created everyday problems for him.

On formal assessment, semantic memory for past events and famous names was impaired, as was recognition memory for famous faces. However, vocabulary levels were normal. M.S. was also found to have severe impairment of episodic memory, with difficulty in learning new verbal or nonverbal material. Story recall and paired associate learning were at an amnesic level. In relation to automated series, he was unable to recite the alphabet or the months of the year. There was also difficulty in recognition memory for newly learnt, previously unfamiliar faces. There was a severe reading and spelling difficulty throughout development, which persisted into adulthood, when reading remained slow and laborious. Memory for recurring items was impaired for verbal material but surprisingly unimpaired for nonverbal material.

A further case of developmental amnesia, Julia, was reported by Temple (1997a). Julia was born at 40 weeks' gestation. She smiled at 6 weeks, walked at 13 months and could dress herself at 2 years, indicating good milestones. There was a family history of convulsions and specific learning difficulties with language and reading. All of the family was right-handed but Julia was left-handed. Both memory difficulties and delayed language development were noted in the preschool years. At the age of 3.9, naming skills were at the first centile for age. At the age of 6, temporal lobe epilepsy developed. CT scan was normal. Difficulties with both word recognition and word finding were noted in the speech therapist's report at this time. When she was 7, Julia's class teacher noted that she "sometimes has difficulty remembering words or what a word actually means". Assessed at the age of 12, on the WISC-R, there was a wide scatter in subtests with half in the 7–10 score range, i.e. within 1 SD of the mean for age. The weakest subtests were Information, reflecting established semantic memory for facts about the world (scaled score 1), and Vocabulary, reflecting established semantic knowledge of word meanings (scaled score 3). She was also unable to answer correctly any factual questions about contemporary events that would have been familiar to most children. The impairment of semantic memory encompassed both factual general knowledge about the world and knowledge of words. Language was characterized by an anomia, such that at the age of 12.8 her naming age was 5.3. Further analysis of this anomia indicated a pattern of consistency in the items found to be difficult, with identical errors being generated across trials in many cases. Further, receptive vocabulary was no better than naming skills. There was no significant difference in Julia's ability to comprehend the names of clothes, animals and foodstuffs than her ability to name these items. The naming impairment was not thus a modality-specific access difficulty. Further, it seemed to reflect impaired establishment of knowledge of words, i.e. a *semantic representation anomia* (Temple, 1997a). There was also impairment in episodic memory and the acquisition of new verbal and nonverbal material. She was impaired in story recall, both when a story was read to her and when she read the story herself. She was also impaired in the recall of patterns and designs. Procedural knowledge, as reflected by knowledge and recall of automated sequences, counting, alphabet and days of the week, was normal, quick and accurate. Recognition memory for words on Warrington's Recognition Memory Battery [WRMB] was very good, with a score of 49/50, which is near ceiling. In contrast, recognition memory for faces was entirely random, with a score of 25/50 in this forced-choice paradigm.

Thus, in Julia's case, there is a severe semantic memory impairment for both facts and word meanings. There is episodic memory impairment for both verbal material and designs. Procedural memory appears intact, as does recognition memory for words, but recognition memory for faces is very impaired. There is an immediate contrast between M.S. (De Renzi & Lucchelli, 1990) and Julia (Temple, 1997a). Whilst both cases have severe impairment of semantic and episodic memory, M.S. has developed normal language, although he continues to have difficulty in learning proper names and foreign language words. Thus, for M.S. the semantic memory impairment does not extend to semantic memory for the majority of vocabulary. For Julia there is a marked anomia, which takes the form of a semantic representation anomia, in which the semantic memory for words is impoverished. A further contrast between the two cases lies in procedural memory, as assessed by memory of automated series. There is impairment and failure to learn these series for M.S. but development of automated series is intact for Julia.

Casalini et al. (1999) report a further case of developmental amnesia, in a 9-year-old girl, O.N. There were no neurological symptoms but there was a positive family history, with O.N.'s father reported to have similar difficulties. Her semantic memory was impaired, with poor established knowledge for facts. Like Julia, discussed above, O.N. also had difficulties in naming, which affected spontaneous speech, and there was poor semantic knowledge of vocabulary. There was also episodic memory impairment, with difficulty in learning new verbal material. Autobiographical memory for past events was also poor. However, there were some material-specific effects; since nonverbal learning and memory were unimpaired. Thus, whilst O.N. is like Julia in having a semantic memory impairment which extends to knowledge of vocabulary, she is unlike Julia in having intact nonverbal memory skills.

The possibility that developmental amnesia may be relatively common and found in the normal classroom population has been explored recently in a study from our Unit (Temple & Richardson, in press). Normal children were screened for both semantic knowledge reflected in knowledge of facts about the world, using the *Information* subtest of the WISC-III (Wechsler, 1992), and for episodic memory, using a word recall task; 3–4% of the children screened were found to have memory difficulties (see Table 5.1). Children were also identified who had normal average intelligence, defined strictly as an IQ within 1 SD of the mean (i.e. 85–115), but who nevertheless had selective impairments of either semantic or episodic memory (see Table 5.1). These children had average IQs but scored below the 5th centile

Table 5.1 Incidence of memory difficulties in a sample of normal children

	8–9 Years	11–12 Years
Children screened (*n*)	239	70
Memory difficulties (%)	3.4	4.3
Average children (*n*) (IQ 85–115)	134	52
Average children with specific memory difficulties (%)	5.9	5.8

on the memory screening tests. Temple & Richardson (in press) describe the pattern of memory development in one of these screened cases for whom no explicit aetiology is known. C.L. was aged 8.11. He was compared to 10 control children who also had IQs in the 85–115 range but who had memory screening scores within 1 SD of the mean. C.L. was therefore matched to the controls for age and IQ, yet he was significantly impaired in comparison to them in terms of semantic memory for facts. Despite this impairment, given forced-choice response of possible alternatives, C.L. was no longer significantly different from normal, indicating a retrieval difficulty in semantic memory. There was also impairment in semantic knowledge of words, with significant impairment in both lexical decision and receptive vocabulary. In oral fluency, there was a sharp dissociation between retrieval on the basis of initial letters, where's C.L. performance was at the mean level for controls, and retrieval on the basis of semantic category, where performance was significantly impaired.(C.L., 26; controls, 45.6; SD, 6.13; range, 38–56). Unlike all the other cases of developmental amnesia discussed above, episodic recall and recognition was normal. Paired associate learning was also normal. Autobiographical memory was normal and Behavioural Memory on the Rivermead was normal. Procedural memory showed normal learning on the first few trials, although later in the series the skill tailed off and performance levels fell, whilst controls improved.

The picture was thus of a selective semantic memory impairment with other memory systems intact. The pattern of semantic impairment but intact episodic skill is a new dissociation in developmental amnesia and forms a double dissociation to the cases of Gadian et al. (2000), where episodic skill is impaired but semantic knowledge is intact. C.L. was also dyslexic, with significant impairment in word recognition skills in comparison to controls. The pattern of reading was that of surface dyslexia, with normal reading of nonwords, impaired reading of irregular words and homophone confusion. This pattern of reading is typically interpreted as reflecting impairment of the lexico–semantic reading route, and in this case the impairment within this route would be localized to retrieval from the semantic system itself.

MEMORY IN EPILEPSY

The areas of the brain within which it is most likely that an epileptic seizure will be sustained are the temporal lobes, which has been attributed to their proximity to the hippocampus. Invasive EEG monitoring has indicated that idiopathic temporal lobe seizures are predominantly of hippocampal origin (Spencer et al., 1990; Wyler et al., 1988). Thus, the most epileptogenic areas of the brain are those known to be intimately involved in memory and it is possible that the underlying characteristics which make them appropriate for memory encoding and storage are also characteristics that make them susceptible to seizures. In both cases, distributed networks are involved and critical steady states are attained (Temple, 1997a). However, when the steady states associated with the occurrence of seizures are active, they prohibit the generation of the steady states required for memory encoding or consolidation.

Memory impairments are common in those who suffer from epilepsy (Loiseau et al., 1988), particularly those who have temporal lobe epilepsy (TLE), who comprise one-third of those who have epilepsy. There are at least four reasons why those with epilepsy may have memory impairments. First, there may be underlying pathology in the temporal lobes or the hippocampi which lie beneath them, which leads to an impaired substrate for memory encoding and storage and which also leads to less stable circuitry more prone to generate seizures. Thus, underlying pathology may create both memory impairment and seizures; for example hippocampal sclerosis is evident in medial TLE (Engel, 1996) and may contribute to both seizures and memory impairment.

Secondly, ongoing seizures or subclinical interictal activity may interfere with the processes of memory consolidation (Glowinski, 1973; O'Connor et al., 1997). In the case of J.T. (O'Connor et al., 1997), retention for hours and days was accurate for new material but there was then rapid forgetting. Increased seizures increased the forgetting, and medication that reduced seizures reduced the forgetting. O'Connor et al. (1997) argue that this provides evidence that consolidation occurs over a long period of time. A similar case is described by Kapur et al. (1997). Their patient with TLE displayed normal episodic retention on immediate and half-hour delay measures, but 40 days later had dense amnesia for the information, whereas controls could remember much of it. Behaviourally, their patient complained of amnesia for events 3–24 months previously. MRI scans and EEG maps showed left temporal pathology and a possible left anterior hippocampus focus. Kapur et al. (1997) argued that the data support a long-term consolidation process, rather than a single-stage unitary consolidation process.

A third reason for memory impairment in epilepsy is that anticonvulsive medication, such as phenobarbital, phenytoin and primidone, may exacerbate impairments in memory (Trimble & Reynolds, 1976). Finally, repeated seizures in which there are extended periods of status epilepticus may cause structural damage to the areas affected by the seizures, thereby damaging one of the substrates employed in memory (Reynolds et al., 1983).

A specific memory impairment has been found in children with TLE, in contrast to normal memory skills in centrencephalic epilepsy. Early studies demonstrated that children with left TLE are worse than those with right TLE on memory for factual material (e.g. Fedio & Mirsky, 1969). In particular, medial left TLE, which begins around the age of 4–8 years (Adam et al., 1996), is linked to verbal memory impairment. In contrast, those with right TLE have poorer delayed recall for unfamiliar faces than those with left TLE (Beardsworth & Zaidel, 1994) and poorer spatial memory (Abrahams et al., 1999). Using combined data from TLE and temporal lobectomies. Helmstaedter et al. (1997) argue that material-specific acquisition is mediated by neocortical structures, which demonstrate laterality effects, whilst long-term consolidation/retrieval is mediated by temporomesial structures, which are material-nonspecific.

EXECUTIVE IMPAIRMENT IN MEMORY

Cornoldi et al. (1999) report impairment in strategic memory in children with ADHD. They found that, in comparison to controls, children with ADHD had weak recall and many intrusion errors. However, when they were given a strategy to use, their performance improved to become as good as controls. They had to be shown how to use the strategy, as otherwise their recall remained poor. Cornoldi et al. (1999) interpreted these results as reflecting an executive impairment in memory. They also gave the children with ADHD and controls other executive tasks to perform and found that performance on the other executive tasks predicted memory skills. These strategic difficulties with memory may be similar to some of the difficulties discussed above in relation to Reye's syndrome.

MATERIAL-SPECIFIC IMPAIRMENT OF MEMORY

Temple (1992b) described Dr S., an intelligent and highly educated lady, who had sustained no neurological injury or disease and was in good health. However, throughout her life she had experienced severe difficulties with memory for faces and visual patterns. Another member of her family is also reported to have similar difficulties. Dr S. had high academic attainments, reflecting good semantic memory. She also had a well-developed vocabulary. Further, her episodic memory for the stories in the Wechsler Memory Battery was very good. However, she had a severe impairment in memory for faces, houses, buildings and visual patterns. The impairment in memory for faces produced a specific form of developmental prosopagnosia. The pattern of her difficulties on face processing was interpreted in relation to the model of Bruce & Young (1986). In relation to this model, it was suggested that Dr S. had specific difficulty in retaining or making use of the face recognition units needed to activate person identity information. Since verbal memory is good, she thus has a material-specific impairment in memory affecting visuospatial material. This focal impairment has been a lifelong deficit coexisting with a successful professional career.

Bishop et al. (2000) described material-specific memory impairments in Turner's syndrome (TS). TS is a genetic disorder in females, in which the second X chromosome is absent or abnormal. Intelligence spans the normal range but there is a set of specific learning difficulties. Cerebral glucose metabolism studies of brain activation and MRI studies suggest bilateral, parietal and occipital lobe involvement in TS (Clark et al., 1989; Elliott et al., 1996; Murphy et al., 1993; Reiss et al., 1993). However, Murphy et al.'s (1993) study also indicated bilateral involvement of the hippocampi. In a MRI study of monozygotic twins discordant for TS, Reiss et al. (1993) concurred with the parieto–occipital locus on the right with a parietal–perisylvian locus on the left. However, in addition, they found marked discrepancies between the twins in right prefrontal areas.

Impairment in visual memory has been documented in a number of studies (Alexander et al., 1966; Clark et al., 1989; Lahood & Bacon, 1985; Lewandowski et al., 1985; Riess et al., 1993; Rovet & Netley, 1981; Silbert et al., 1977; Waber, 1979). Pennington et al. (1985) reported either a verbal or a nonverbal memory deficit in 8/10 cases of TS. Surprisingly, since some theoretical interpretations of TS have implicated the right hemisphere, Pennington et al. (1985) found that 7/10 cases had episodic verbal memory impairments, whilst impairment in nonverbal episodic memory was found in only 4/10.

However, Bishop et al. (2000) argue that the pattern of memory performance varied, depending upon whether the single X came from the mother (X^m) or the father (X^p). She reported that for immediate verbal recall, both TS groups obtained significantly higher scores than control boys, and the X^p group also outscored control girls. This result is consistent with a number of studies indicating elevated verbal skills in TS (Shaffer, 1962; Lahood & Bacon, 1985; Temple, 1996, 2002; Temple & Carney, 1996). However, in relation to the elevated immediate recall level, the X^m group showed enhanced verbal forgetting. Thus, although both immediate and delayed recall scores were in the normal range, Bishop et al. (2000) argued that the relationship between the two was abnormal, with the $45X^m$ group showing elevated immediate recall but then disproportionate forgetting with delay. In a visual memory task, both groups performed poorly on the initial copy of a design, and both were significantly impaired on delayed recall of the design. However, Bishop et al. (2000) argued that the X^p group, who appeared marginally better than the X^m on the initial copy, had nevertheless forgotten a disproportionate amount with delay interpreted as enhanced spatial forgetting.

As Maurer (1992) pointed out, many learning disabilities can be recast as disorders of material-specific memory. Exploring this idea within the framework of developmental cognitive neuropsychology provides a number of examples. Temple (1986, 1995) described the case of a developmental anomic, John, who had particular difficulty in naming animals in comparison to indoor objects. The impairment with animals was pervasive across tasks and at least part of his difficulty appeared to arise from a failure to establish effective semantic representations for animals, and may therefore be thought of as a selective impairment of the semantic system and thereby memory.

The reading disorder, surface dyslexia (e.g. Coltheart et al., 1983; Castles & Coltheart, 1993, 1996), is characterized by relatively good phonological reading skills and ability to read nonwords but poor development of the lexico–semantic reading route employed in the reading of irregular words and the reading of highly familiar established words. This difficulty could be characterized as a difficulty in developing the memory that enables word recognition. The surface dyslexic fails to recognize words that would be recognized with ease by his peers.

Similarly, in surface dysgraphia, there can be well-developed phonological spelling systems associated with using the sound of the word to analytically determine its spelling. In contrast, there is difficulty with the memory for spelling patterns, which is essential for the spelling of irregular words in English and for spelling the many words for which the representation of the vowel is ambiguous with multiple possibilities.

Number fact dyscalculia (Temple, 1991, 1994, 1997b) is a selective impairment which affects the development of factual knowledge about arithmetic and tables, with intact development of number processing and knowledge of arithmetic procedures. This could be considered a material-specific impairment of memory for arithmetical facts. Other aspects of semantic memory can be quite normal (Temple, 1997a).

However, formulating these selective disorders as material-specific impairments of memory is, to some extent, simply redescribing their problems without addressing anything more fundamental. It may be more constructive to continue to discuss such disorders in relation to the cognitive domain within which they occur.

CONCLUDING COMMENTS

At the outset it was suggested that the study of developmental amnesia may provide evidence relevant to: (a) models of normal development; (b) theorizing about adults; and (c) education of children with memory difficulties. It is evident from the work discussed above that there are many forms that the developmental amnesias and acquired amnesias of childhood may take.

In relation to both models of normal development and theorizing about adults, one may ask: are there any double dissociations evident? In the studies of Vargha-Khadem et al. (1997) and Gadian et al. (2000), semantic memory is intact but episodic memory is impaired. In the developmental anomic, C.L. (Temple & Richardson, in press), episodic memory is intact but semantic memory is impaired. In both cases, memory has been abnormal throughout development. In neither case has memory been partially established with subsequent impairment. The contrasting patterns argue for the relative independence of episodic and semantic memory during development and further argue that neither is critically dependent upon the other.

Within semantic memory, semantic knowledge for facts may be impaired and may coexist with impaired or intact semantic knowledge about words. A double dissociation would require semantic representation anomia in the absence of semantic memory impairment for facts, a dissociation not yet reported and hence not explored.

There is a double dissociation between M.S. (De Renzi & Lucchelli, 1990) and Julia (Temple, 1997a) between semantic knowledge for words and procedural knowledge, indicating an unsurprising distinction between these systems in development. With the exception of M.S., in almost all the cases of amnesia reported procedural memory is intact.

There are further single dissociations that justify Tulving's proposal for episodic memory, where there is a sense not only of "knowing" but also of "remembering" specific elements of the personal experience.

There are also distinctions in the memory processes that may be impaired. There appears to be impairment of memory encoding in Reye's syndrome (Quart et al., 1987), memory storage as a result of failure of consolidation in TLE, and impairment of retrieval processes for Jon (Baddeley et al., 2001), where recognition memory is intact, and for Neil (Vargha-Khadem et al., 1994), where orthographic retrieval is superior to oral.

In relation to classroom implications, the results are less clear, for it seems that the developmental amnesias and acquired amnesias of childhood do not take one prescribed form for which a specialized remedial programme could be recommended. Rather, the disorders have a variety of forms, and the pattern of intact skills to be utilized in establishing new strategies and impaired skills to be targeted in remedial learning vary sharply from case to case, and require individual case analysis for their identification.

REFERENCES

Abrahams, S., Morris, R.G., Polkey, C.E. et al. (1999). Hippocampal involvement in spatial and working memory: a structural MRI analysis of patients with unilateral mesial temporal lobe sclerosis. *Brain & Cognition*, **41**, 39–65.

Adam, C., Clemenceau, S., Semah, F. et al. (1996). Variability of presentation in medial temporal lobe epilepsy: a study of 30 operated cases. *Acta Neurolica Scandinavica*, **94**, 1–11.

Aggleton, J.P. & Brown, M.W. (1999). Episodic memory, amnesia and the hippocampal–anterior thalamic axis. *Behavioural & Brain Sciences*, **22**, 425–490.

Alexander, D., Ehrhardt, A. & Money, J. (1966). Defective figure drawing, geometric and human in Turner's syndrome. *Journal of Nervous & Mental Diseases*, **142**, 161–167.

Baddeley, A., Emslie, H. & Nimmo-Smith, I. (1994). *The Doors & People Test*. Bury St. Edmunds: Thames Valley Test Company.

Baddeley, A. (1997). *Human Memory: Theory & Practice* (revised edn). Hove: Psychology Press.

Baddeley, A., Vargha-Khadem, F. & Mishkin, M. (2001). Preserved recognition in a case of developmental amnesia: implications for the acquisition of semantic memory. *Journal of Cognitive Neuroscience*, **13**, 357–369.

Beardsworth, E.D. & Zaidel, D.W. (1994). Memory for faces in epileptic children before and after brain surgery. *Journal of Clinical & Experimental Neuropsychology*, **16**, 589–596.

Bishop, D.V.M. (1985). Age of onset and outcome in acquired aphasia with convulsive disorder (Landau–Kleffner syndrome). *Developmental Medicine & Child Neurology*, **27**, 705–712.

Bishop, D.V.M. (1997). Cognitive neuropsychology and developmental disorders: Uncomfortable bedfellows. *Quarterly Journal of Experimental Psychology*, **50A**, 899–923.

Bishop, D.V.M., Canning, E., Elgar, K. et al. (2000). Distinctive patterns of memory function in subgroups of females with Turner syndrome: evidence for imprinted loci on the X-chromosome affecting neurodevelopment. *Neuropsychologia*, **38**, 712–721.

Brainerd, C.J. & Reyna, V.F. (1992). Explaining "memory free" reasoning. *Psychological Science*, **3**, 332–339.

Broman, M., Rose, A.L., Hotson, G. & Casey, C.M. (1997). Severe anterograde amnesia with onset in childhood as a result of anoxic encephalopathy. *Brain*, **120**, 417–433.

Bruce, V. & Young, A. (1986). Understanding face recognition. *British Journal of Psychology*, **77**, 305–327.

Carpantieri, S.C. & Mulhern, R.K. (1993). Patterns of memory dysfunction among children surviving temporal lobe tumors. *Archives of Clinical Neuropsychology*, **8**, 345–357.

Casalini, C., Brizzolara, D., Cavallaro, M.C. & Cipriani, P. (1999). Developmental dysmnesia: a case report. *Cortex*, **35**, 713–727.

Castles, A. & Coltheart, M. (1993). Varieties of developmental dyslexia. *Cognition*, **47**, 149–180.

Castles, A. & Coltheart, M. (1996). Cognitive correlates of developmental surface dyslexia: a single case study. *Cognitive Neuropsychology*, **13**, 25–50.

Cavazzutti, V., Winston, K., Baker, R. & Welch, K. (1980). Psychological changes following surgery for tumours in the temporal lobes. *Journal of Neurosurgery*, **53**, 618–626.

Clark, C., Klonoff, H. & Hayden, M. (1990). Regional cerebral glucose metabolism in Turner's syndrome. *The Canadian Journal Neurological Sciences*, **17**, 140–144.

Coltheart, M., Masterson, J., Byng, S. et al. (1983). Surface dyslexia. *Quarterly Journal of Experimental Psychology*, **35**, 469–496.

Cornoldi, C., Barbieri, A., Gaiani, C. & Zocchi, S. (1999). Strategic memory deficits in attention deficit disorder with hyperactivity participants: the role of executive processes. *Developmental Neuropsychology*, **15**, 53–71.

Davidson, P.W., Wiloughby, L.A., O'Tuama, L.A. et al. (1978). Neurological and intellectual sequelae of Reye's syndrome. *American Journal of Mental Deficiencies*, **82**, 535–541.

De Haan, E. & Campbell, R. (1991). A fifteen year follow-up of a case of developmental prosopagnosia. *Cortex*, **27**, 489–509.

Dennis, M., Farrell, K., Hoffman, H.J. et al. (1988). Recognition memory of item, associative and serial-order information after temporal lobectomy for seizure disorder. *Neuropsychologia*, **26**, 55–65.

De Renzi, E. & Lucchelli, F. (1990). Developmental dysmnesia in a poor reader. *Cortex*, **113**, 1337–1345.

Dupont, S., Van de Moortele, P., Samson, S. et al. (2000). Episodic memory in left temporal lobe epilepsy: a functional MRI study. *Brain*, **123**, 1722–1732.

Elliott, T.K., Watkins, J.M., Messa, C. et al. (1996). Positron emission tomography and neuropsychological correlations in children with Turner's syndrome. *Developmental Neuropsychology*, **12**, 365–386.

Engel, J. (1996). Surgery for seizures. *New England Journal of Medicine*, **334**, 647–652.

Fedio, P. & Mirsky, A. (1969). Selective intellectual deficits in children with temporal lobe or centrencephalic epilepsy. *Neuropsychologia*, **3**, 287–300.

Gadian, D.G., Aicardi, J., Watkins, K.E. et al. (2000). Developmental amnesia associated with early hypoxic-ischaemic injury. *Brain*, **123**, 499–507.

Geschwind, N. (1974). Disorders of higher cortical function in children. In N. Geschwind (ed.), *Selected Papers on Language and the Brain. Boston Studies in the Philosophy of Science*, Vol. XVI. Boston: Reidel.

Glowinski, H. (1973). Cognitive deficits in temporal lobe epilepsy: an investigation of memory functioning. *Journal of Nervous & Mental Diseases*, **157**, 129–137.

Goodglass, H. & Kaplan, E. (1983). *The Assessment of Aphasia and Related Disorders*, 2nd edn. Philadelphia, PA: Lea & Febiger.

Helmstaedter, C., Grunwald, T., Lehnertz, K. (1997). Differential involvement of left temporolateral and temporomesial structures in verbal declarative learning and memory: evidence from temporal lobe epilepsy. *Brain & Cognition*, **35**, 110–131.

Herkowitz, J. & Rosman, N.P. (1982). *Pediatrics, Neurology and Psychiatry—Common Ground: Behavioural, Cognitive, Affective and Physical Disorders in Childhood and Adolescence.* New York: Macmillan.

Holdstock, J.S., Mayes, A.R., Cezayirli, E. et al. (2000). A comparison of egocentric and allocentric spatial memory in a patient with selective hippocampal damage. *Neuropsychologia,* **38**, 410–425.

Kapur, N., Millar, J., Colbourn, C. et al. (1997). Very long-term amnesia in association with temporal lobe epilepsy: evidence for multiple-stage consolidation processes. *Brain & Cognition,* **35**, 58–70.

Lahood, B.J. & Bacon, G.E. (1985). Cognitive abilities of adolescent Turner's syndrome patients. *Journal of Adolescent Health Care,* **6**, 358–364.

Lewandowski, L., Costenbader, V. & Richman, R. (1985). Neuropsychological aspects of Turner's syndrome. *International Journal of Clinical Neuropsychology,* **7**, 144–147.

Lishman, W.A. (1987). *Organic Psychiatry: The Psychological Consequences of Cerebral Disorder,* 2nd edn. Oxford: Blackwell Scientific.

Loiseau, P., Strube, E. & Signoret, J.-L. (1988). Memory and epilepsy. In M.R. Trimble & E.H. Reynolds (eds), *Epilepsy, Behaviour and Cognitive Function.* Stratford-upon-Avon: Wiley.

Lovejoy, F.H., Smith, A.L., Bresnan, M.J. et al. (1974). Clinical staging in Reye's syndrome. *American Journal of Diseases in Children,* **128**, 36–41.

Luria, A.R. (1966). *The Higher Cortical Function of Man.* New York: Basic Books.

Luria, A.R. (1973). *The Working Brain.* New York: Penguin.

Marlowe, W.B. (1992). The impact of a right prefrontal lesion on the developing brain. *Brain & Cognition,* **20**, 205–213.

Maurer, R.G. (1992). Disorders of memory and learning. In S.J. Segalowitz & I. Rapin (eds), *Handbook of Neuropsychology, Vol. 7: Child Neuropsychology.* Amsterdam: Elsevier.

Meekin, S.L., Glasgow, J.F.T., McCusker, C.G. & Rooney, N. (1999). A long-term follow-up of cognitive, emotional and behavioural sequelae to Reye syndrome. *Developmental Medicine & Child Neurology,* **41**, 549–553.

Meyer, F., Marsh, R., Laws, E. & Sharborough, F. (1986). Temporal lobectomy in children with epilepsy. *Journal of Neurosurgery,* **64**, 371–376.

Morrow, J., O'Connor, D., Whitman, B. & Accardo, P. (1989). CNS Irradiation and memory deficit. *Developmental Medicine & Child Neurology,* **31**, 690–692.

Murphy, D., DeCarli, C., Daly, E. et al. (1993). X-chromosome effects on female brain: a magnetic resonance imaging study of Turner's syndrome. *Lancet,* **342**, 1197–1200.

Nelson, D.B., Sullivan-Bolyai, J.Z., Marks, J.S. et al. (1989). Reye's syndrome: an epidemiologic assessment based on national surveillance, 1977–1978 and a population-based study in Ohio 1973–1977. In J.F.S. Croker (ed.), *Reye's Syndrome II* (pp. 33–49). New York: Grune & Stratton.

O'Connor, M., Sieggreen, M.A., Ahern, G. et al. (1997). Accelerated forgetting in association with temporal lobe epilepsy. *Brain & Cognition,* **35**, 71–84.

Ostergaard, A.L. (1987). Episodic, semantic and procedural memory in a case of amnesia at an early age. *Neuropsychologia,* **25**, 341–357.

Ostergaard, A.L. & Squire, L. (1990). Childhood amnesia and distinctions between forms of memory: a comment on Wood, Brown & Felton. *Brain & Cognition,* **14**, 127–133.

Partin, J.S., McAdams, J.J., Partin, J.C. et al. (1978). Brain ultrastructure in Reye's disease II. *Journal of Neuropathology & Experimental Neurology,* **37**, 796–819.

Pennington, B.F., Heaton, R.K., Karzmark, P. et al. (1985). The neuropsychological phenotype in Turner syndrome. *Cortex,* **21**, 391–404.

Quart, E.J. (1984). Memory and attention in children recovering from Reye's syndrome. *Dissertation Abstracts International,* **45**, 711-B (University Microfilms No 22185).

Quart, E.J., Buchtel, H.A. & Sarnaik, A.P. (1987). Long lasting memory deficits in children recovering from Reye's syndrome. *Journal of Clinical & Experimental Neuropsychology,* **10**, 409–420.

Reiss, A.L., Freund, L., Plotnick, L. et al. (1993). The effects of X monosomy on brain development: monozygotic twins discordant for Turner's syndrome. *Annals of Neurology,* **34**, 95–107.

Reynolds, E.H., Elwes, R.D.C. & Shorvon, S.D. (1983). Why does epilepsy become intractable? Prevention of chronic epilepsy. *Lancet,* **2**, 952–954.

Ribot, T.R. (1882). Diseases *of Memory.* New York: Appleton & Co.

Rovet, J. & Netley, C. (1981). Turner syndrome in a pair of dizygotic twins: a single case study. *Behavior Genetics,* **11**, 65–72.

Sarnaik, A. (1982). Diagnosis and management of Reye's syndrome. *Comprehensive Therapy*, **8**, 47–53.

Scoville, W.B. & Milner, B. (1957). Loss of recent memory after bilateral hippocampal lesions. *Journal of Neurology, Neurosurgery & Psychiatry*, **20**, 11–21.

Shaffer, J. (1962). A specific cognitive deficit observed in gonadal aplasia (Turner's syndrome). *Journal of Clinical Psychology*, **18**, 403–406.

Silbert, A., Wolff, P.H. & Lilienthal, J. (1977). Spatial and temporal processing in patients with Turner's syndrome. *Behaviour Genetics*, **7**, 11–21.

Spencer, S.S., Spencer, D.D., Williamson, P.D. & Mattson, R. (1990). Combined depth and subdural electrode investigation in uncontrolled epilepsy. *Neurology*, **40**, 74–79.

Squire, L. (1992). Declarative and non-declarative memory: multiple brain systems supporting learning and memory. *Journal of Cognitive Neuroscience*, **4**, 232–243.

Squire, L.R. & Cohen, N.J. (1984). Human memory and amnesia. In G. Lynch, J.L. McGaugh & N.M. Weinberger (eds), *Neurobiology of Learning and Memory*. New York: Guilford.

Temple, C.M. (1986). Anomia for animals in a child. *Brain*, **109**, 1225–1242.

Temple, C.M. (1991). Procedural dyscalculia and number fact dyscalculia: double dissociation in developmental dyscalculia. *Cognitive Neuropsychology*, **8**, 155–176.

Temple, C.M. (1992a). Developmental and acquired disorders in children. In S.J. Segalowitz & I. Rapin (eds), *Handbook of Neuropsychology, Vol 7: Child Neuropsychology*. Amsterdam: Elsevier.

Temple, C.M. (1992b). Developmental memory impairment: faces and patterns. In R. Campbell (ed.) *Mental Lives: Case Studies in Cognition* (pp. 199–215). Oxford: Blackwell.

Temple, C.M. (1994). The cognitive neuropsychology of the developmental dyscalculias. *Cahiers de Psychologie Cognitive/ Current Psychology of Cognition*, **133**, 351–370.

Temple, C.M. (1995). The kangaroo's a fox. In R. Campbell (ed.), *Broken Memories* (pp. 383–396). Oxford: Blackwell.

Temple, C.M. (1996). Language ability and disability in Turner's syndrome. Paper presented at the XXVI International Congress of Psychology, Montreal. *International Journal of Psychology*, **31**, 3644 [Abstract].

Temple, C.M. (1997a). *Developmental Cognitive Neuropsychology*. Hove: Erlbaum.

Temple, C.M. (1997b). Cognitive neuropsychology and its application to children. *Journal of Child Psychology & Psychiatry*, **38**, 27–52.

Temple, C.M. (2002). Oral fluency and narrative production in children with Turner's syndrome. *Neuropsychologia*, **40**, 1419–1427.

Temple, C.M. & Carney, R. (1996). Reading skills in children with Turner's Syndrome: an analysis of hyperlexia: *Cortex*, **32**, 335–345.

Temple, C.M. & Richardson, P. (in press). Developmental amnesia: a new pattern of dissociation with intact episodic memory. *Neuropsychologia*.

Trimble, M.R. & Reynolds, E.H. (1976). Anticonvulsant drugs and mental symptoms. *Psychological Medicine*, **6**, 169–178.

Tulving, E. (1972). Episodic and semantic memory. In E. Tulving & W. Donaldson (eds), *Organization of Memory* (pp. 381–403). New York: Academic Press.

Tulving, E. (1985). Memory and consciousness. *Canadian Psychologist*, **26**, 1–12.

Tulving, E. & Markovitch, H.J. (1998). Episodic and declarative memory: the role of the hippocampus. *Hippocampus*, **8**, 198–204.

Vargha-Khadem, F., Isaacs, E.B. & Watkins, K.E. (1992). Medial temporal lobe vs. diencephalic amnesia in childhood. *Journal of Clinical & Experimental Neuropsychology*, **14**, 371–372.

Vargha-Khadem, F., Gadian, D.G., Watkins, K.E. et al. (1997). Differential effects of early hippocampal pathology on episodic and semantic memory. *Science*, **277**, 376–380.

Vargha-Khadem, F., Isaacs, E.B. & Mishkin, M. (1994). Agnosia, alexia and a remarkable form of amnesia in an adolescent boy. *Brain*, **117**, 683–703.

Van Hout, A. (1993). Acquired aphasia in childhood and developmental dysphasias: are the errors similar? Analysis of errors made in confrontation naming tasks. *Aphasiology*, **7**, 525–531.

Waber, D. (1979). Neuropsychological aspects of Turner's Syndrome. *Developmental Medicine & Child Neurology*, **31**, 58–70.

Warrington, E.K. (1984). *Recognition Memory Battery*. Windsor: NFER, Nelson.

Warrington, E.K. & Weiskrantz, L. (1982). Amnesia: a disconnection syndrome. *Neuropsychologia*, **20**, 233–249.

Wechsler, D. (1974). *Wechsler Intelligence Scale for Children—Revised*. New York: Psychological Corporation.

Wechsler, D. (1992). *Wechsler Intelligence Scale for Children*, 3rd edn (UK edn). London: Psychological Corporation.

Williams, D. & Mateer, C.A. (1992). Developmental impact of frontal lobe injury in middle childhood. *Brain & Cognition*, **20**, 196–204.

Wood, F.B., Brown, I.S. & Felton, R.H. (1989). Long-term follow-up of a childhood amnesic syndrome. *Brain & Cognition*, **10**, 76–89.

Wood, F.B., Ebert, V. & Kinsbourne, M. (1982). The episodic–semantic memory distinction in memory and amnesia: clinical and experimental observations. In L.S. Cermak (ed.), *Human Memory and Amnesia*. Hillsdale, NJ: Erlbaum.

Wyler, A.R., Walker, G., Richey, E.T. & Hermann, B.P. (1988). Chronic subdural strip electrode recording for difficult epileptic problems. *Journal of Epilepsy*, **1**, 71–78.

Young, A.W. & Ellis, H.D. (1989). Childhood propospagnosia. *Brain & Cognition*, **9**, 16–47.

CHAPTER 6

The Memory Deficit in Alzheimer's Disease

James T. Becker
and
Amy A. Overman
Western Psychiatric Institute and Clinic, University of Pittsburgh, PA, USA

Patients diagnosed with Alzheimer's disease (AD) suffer from a devastating and progressive loss of memory (APA, 1987; McKhann et al., 1984). At the earliest stages of the illness, the patient may forget day-to-day events, misplace money or car keys, fail to pay bills on time, or even to remember the day of the week, all of which significantly affects their daily lives. The failure to establish and retrieve these personally relevant, context-dependent memories—so-called *episodic* memories (Tulving, 1972)—is one of the hallmarks of AD. Although this loss of episodic memories is common among progressive dementias of the elderly, it is by no means the only memory dysfunction suffered by these patients. Perhaps equally important in terms of functional adaptation is the loss of what Tulving referred to as *semantic* memory—the lexicon of facts, words, concepts and ideas that form the basis of our world knowledge and language. Defects in the retrieval of semantic memories can affect not only communication (both expressive and receptive) but also the patient's sense of self.

Episodic memory is the result of the encoding, storage and retrieval of temporally and spatially defined events, and the temporal and spatial relationships among them (Tulving, 1984). The study of these kinds of engrams has been, and probably will remain, the focus of most research on memory (Tulving, 1972) and memory disorders. By contrast, semantic memory is that information necessary for language, a "mental thesaurus" including not only lexical information (i.e. word meaning and concepts) but also facts and general world knowledge. Although Tulving (1987) assumed that episodic and semantic memory are functionally independent systems, others suggest that while these concepts are useful heuristic devices, the evidence that they are independent functional systems is less compelling (Baddeley, 1986; Baddeley et al., 1986; Squire, 1992; Squire & Zola-Morgan, 1991). It is now clear from a variety of neuropsychological studies that these systems interact a great deal, especially at the encoding and retrieval stages. Nevertheless, for the sake of this discussion, we assume that these are functionally distinct systems, and that their dysfunction in AD results from the breakdown of anatomically independent systems.

The Essential *Handbook of Memory Disorders for Clinicians.* Edited by A.D. Baddeley, M.D. Kopelman and B.A. Wilson.
© 2004 John Wiley & Sons, Ltd. ISBN 0-470-09141-X.

There is, however, a third memory system that plays a key role in our understanding of the memory loss in AD—working memory. Unlike other models of memory that were popular in the late 1960s and early 1970s (e.g. Atkinson & Shiffrin, 1968), Baddeley & Hitch (1974) concluded that a system of *active* processors (i.e. a *working* memory, WM) was needed for the encoding and retrieval of information over short delays. Memory is, in their view, a set of multiple, interacting processes and WM has a role in cognition generally, rather than only in "memory" itself (Baddeley, 2000).

At the core of the WM model are two verbal subsystems, and a system dedicated to the processing of nonverbal, imagery-based information. The verbal subsystems, the articulatory loop and phonological input store, are thought of as relatively automatic processors which can thus function without much direct control; the visuospatial scratchpad was thought of as the nonverbal analog of the two verbal systems. Neuropsychological data suggest that these systems are, indeed, interdependent and interactive (Baddeley & Wilson, 1988; Farah et al., 1985; Shallice & Warrington, 1970; Vallar & Baddeley, 1984). However, in addition to these apparently automatic information processors, the model also proposes the existence of a central executive system (CES), similar to the supervisory attentional system of Norman & Shallice (1980), that provides attentional control to WM.

Although the WM system has been successful in accounting for a wide variety of data in cognitive psychology, neuropsychology and cognitive neuroscience, there were a range of phenomena not so easily explained (for review, see Baddeley, 2000). The problems could largely be subsumed under the general notion of the need for a storage system that was intimately associated with WM but was not the phonological loop. Although earlier versions of the model had ascribed some limited capacity storage to the CES, this had been rejected (Baddeley et al., 1999; Baddeley, 1986). Recently, however, Baddeley (2000) has proposed the concept of the *episodic buffer* (EB) to serve as a processor that acts as a kind of intermediary between WM and the component subsystems, and long-term memory (cf. Ericsson & Kintsch, 1995). The EB is thought to integrate information from WM and long-term memory, but is of limited capacity. It has a role in binding information from separate cognitive systems (and, it is assumed, different sensory and perceptual representations) into a coherent whole. The CES plays an important role in this binding process, but needs the EB to maintain such complex representations. Thus, the EB is also accessible to the CES, and the CES can affect the content of the store by attending to a different source of information (either as an external percept or as a representation from one of the subsystems of WM or from long-term memory). This concept of a binding process (and of a neuroanatomical structure needed for the process) is strongly reminiscent of the theories of McClelland and colleagues as they relate to the hippocampus (McClelland, 1998). The EB might therefore be seen not only as a bridge between WM and long-term memory, but also between frontal/parietal systems and the mesial temporal lobe.

Thus, WM has a role not only in the short-term processing and retention of incoming information but also in the longer-term memory processes. It may very well then serve, to some extent, as a link between the more permanent episodic memories and semantic memory. Thus, each of the memory systems interacts with the other, and their breakdown results in the characteristic memory loss of AD. By understanding the pattern of cognitive dysfunction and the neuroanatomical abnormalities that lead to them, we will have a better understanding of the neuropsychology of AD.

THE MEMORY DEFICIT IN ALZHEIMER'S DISEASE

Working Memory in AD

The verbal subsystems of working memory appear to function normally in AD patients. Although performance is clearly poorer than normal, the qualitative aspects of performance suggest that the same factors that influence the performance of healthy subjects also influence that of AD patients. Thus, the phonological store and articulatory loop appear intact in AD patients (Morris, 1986; Morris & Baddeley, 1988). The CES, by contrast, does *not* appear to function normally in AD patients, especially when their performance is compared with that of old and young normal control subjects on concurrent tasks (Baddeley et al., 1986). The subjects were required first to demonstrate a stable level of performance on a manual tracking task and a digit span task. After having established the baseline performance, the subjects were then required to perform the two tasks concurrently. The older control subjects were no less competent than the younger controls at combining the two tools. By contrast, the AD patients were dramatically impaired. Their performance on both the tracking and repetition tasks fell significantly, and the authors interpreted these data to suggest that the AD patients were suffering from a CES defect. (In practice, many although not all patients will trade off their performance on one of the tasks to "protect" the performance of the other (A.D. Baddeley, personal communication)). However, when the executive defect is sufficiently severe, this sort of trade-off does not occur and the patient seems at a loss as to how to proceed (J.T. Becker, unpublished observation).

Based on these data and the previous suggestions by Morris & Kopelman (1986), we tested the hypothesis that AD patients suffer from two independent syndromes, an "amnesic syndrome", identical to that seen in patients with focal amnesic syndromes, and a "dysexecutive syndrome", resulting from a defective CES (Becker et al., 1988, 1992a). We argued, on the basis of the pattern of impairment in AD patients, that we should be able to identify individual patients with "focal" amnesic and dysexecutive syndromes. We analyzed the performance of 194 AD patients on measures of verbal fluency (Benton 1968; Benton et al., 1983), verbal similarities (Wechsler, 1945), card sorting (Weigl, 1927) and letter cancellation (Diller et al., 1979) relative to their performance on secondary episodic memory tasks (paired-associate learning and free recall). We were able to identify eight patients with dysexecutive syndromes and 24 with amnesic syndromes (Becker et al., 1992a), confirming an observation that this functional dissociation is possible (Becker, 1988). Baddeley et al. (1991) independently identified patients with relatively focal impairments in memory or executive function. These studies also demonstrated that these dissociations were not merely the result of the random assortment of symptoms, but rather followed the predictions of the two-component model. However, Baddeley et al. (1991) also found other dissociations, and certainly careful neuropsychological assessment can reveal a variety of such differential patterns of impairment (e.g. Williams et al., 1996; see also discussion of other such groups, below).

Episodic Memory in Alzheimer's Disease

The earliest symptoms of AD include an impairment in episodic memory (Huff et al., 1987; Kaszniak, 1988; Kaszniak et al., 1986; Kopelman, 1985b; Welsh et al., 1992). One influential neuropathological model of the progression of the senile plaques and neurofibrillary tangles in AD has emphasized that early in the disease it is the mesial temporal regions, including the hippocampal formation and related structures, that are most heavily affected (Braak & Braak, 1991). Among patients with mild cognitive impairment (Morris et al., 2001; Petersen et al., 1999) it is hippocampal atrophy that distinguishes these patients from healthy controls (independently of symptoms of memory loss) (Jack et al., 1999, 1997; Johnson et al., 1998), whereas among AD patients the neuropathology has progressed to include perihippocampal temporal neocortex and, to a lesser extent, the parietal lobes (Ouchi et al., 1998; Stout et al., 1999). Indeed, it is likely that a disconnection of these brain regions from associated cortex is responsible for the episodic memory loss (Geula, 1998; Hyman 1984, 1986, 1990).

Functional and structural neuroimaging studies emphasize the association between the integrity of these mesial temporal regions and episodic memory function in AD; for example, Ouchi et al. (1998) noted both structural and metabolic abnormalities in AD patients relative to controls, and Stout et al. (1999) reported correlations between verbal memory test scores and the volume (i.e. inverse of atrophy) of both the mesial temporal and diencephalic gray matter. In a separate study comparing probable AD with "questionable" AD, Johnson et al. (1998) noted lower cerebral perfusion values (using SPECT imaging) in the hippocampal–amygdaloid area of the probable AD cases. Again, there was a significant association between perfusion values and memory test scores. Furthermore, consistent with other data (Ouchi et al., 1998), these investigators noted decreased perfusion of the temporoparietal region *only* in the probable AD cases, emphasizing the importance of the mesial temporal pathology at the earliest stage of the dementia.

Because of the prominent temporal lobe damage early in AD and the resulting impairment in episodic memory, much attention has focused on this symptom cluster. Indeed, the ability to learn and remember new information is a highly sensitive marker of dementia (Delis et al., 1991; Huff et al., 1987; Kaszniak et al., 1986). In one of the first reports to arise from the Center to Establish a Registry of Alzheimer's Disease, Welsh and associates reported that delayed recall memory testing was a highly accurate method for differentiating mildly demented subjects from normal elderly (Welsh et al., 1991). Indeed, memory measures are consistently better at such case identification than measures of other cognitive functions (Flicker et al., 1991; Morris et al., 1991; Troster et al., 1993).

The episodic memory defect in AD is similar to that of patients with other types of memory disorders, but differs qualitatively from patients with dementia syndromes arising from pathology in subcortical regions (e.g. Huntington's disease, Parkinson's disease, progressive supranuclear palsy, Lewy body dementia). In AD, the extent of the memory deficit is evident from the virtually flat learning curves in any list-learning procedures; the relatively little information that is remembered usually comes from working memory, with little if any information more permanently encoded (e.g. Buschke & Fuld, 1974; Moss et al., 1986; Wilson et al., 1983b). For example, early in AD the primacy effect in free recall is minimized as less information is transferred into longer-term storage and sensitivity to interference effects increases (Miller, 1971; Pepin & Eslinger, 1989; Wilson et al., 1983b). As the disease progresses, the primacy effect is virtually eliminated and the recency effect is also reduced. Estimates of the *capacity* of primary or working memory in AD patients remain stable even into the moderate stage of severity (i.e. 2.5–3.5 items).

A striking qualitative difference between the memory loss in AD and that seen in other dementias was first documented by Delis et al. (1991). These investigators found that although the overall *quantitative* performance of AD and Huntington's disease (HD) patient subgroups were similar using many standard measures (e.g. delayed recall), there were certain *qualitative* features that could distinguish them. Specifically, the rate of intrusion errors (i.e. reporting a word that was not on the to-be-remembered list) was higher among the AD patients and recognition memory test performance was poorer. The latter measure is particularly important, since recognition memory testing minimizes the retrieval demands of the task and thus it is often interpreted as a more direct measure of memory storage. The reliability and validity of this qualitative analysis has been demonstrated by, among other methods, showing that patients with dementia disorders due to conditions other than AD or HD can be meaningfully classified. Thus, HIV/AIDS patients with impaired California Verbal Learning Test (CVLT) performance are classified as having the HD-like pattern of retrieval failure (Becker et al., 1995), and Salmon et al. (1996) reported the subcortical pattern of performance in patients with Lewy body dementia. It should be noted that while many authors will describe these qualitatively different patterns of memory abnormalities as "cortical" (typical AD) or "subcortical" (as in HD or Parkinson's disease), it is probably more helpful (and at least as accurate) to consider the one pattern to reflect more of an encoding and storage deficit (with less effect on retrieval) as compared with a deficit primarily in memory retrieval (with less effect on encoding and storage). Obviously, these neuropsychological patterns are not "process pure" and neither is the neuropathological substrate of the respective dementia syndromes (Whitehouse, 1986).

In spite of the fact that intrusion errors are relatively common in AD, the specificity of the error type to this disease is not high (Butters et al., 1986a, 1986b; Fuld et al., 1982; Kopelman, 1985a; Kramer et al., 1988), i.e. patients with memory disorders arising from other conditions can also have increased rates of intrusion errors. For example, AD patients remember few facts and make numerous prior-story and extra-story intrusion errors when recalling a short prose passage (Butters et al., 1986b). However, patients with amnesic Korsakoff's syndrome (KS) also produce intrusion errors, show an increased sensitivity to proactive interference and manifest perseverative errors on a letter fluency test. The parallel performance of AD and KS patients led Butters et al. (1986b) to suggest this was due to an anatomical lesion that was common to both diseases, namely damage to the nucleus basalis of Meynert. Further, in the majority of AD patients, senile plaques and neurofibrillary tangles are found in the mammillary bodies, hypothalamus and dorsomedial nucleus of the thalamus (Grossi et al., 1989), which are structures heavily affected in KS (Mair et al., 1979; Victor et al., 1971). Thus, the overlap in neuropsychological symptoms between AD and KS—in this case, errors of intrusion—are likely due to common disruptions of the circuits responsible for normal memory retrieval processes. These findings thus presaged the neuroimaging studies that showed that subcortical structures—specifically the midline thalamus—are involved in memory processes in an important way in AD (Stout et al., 1999).

One aspect of episodic memory in AD that has received considerable attention has to do with the rate at which information is lost over time: AD patients were given a recognition memory test for photographs and their performance was compared to that of normal controls immediately after presentation of the list (Kopelman, 1985a). The exposure to the pictures had been adjusted (i.e. lengthened) so that the AD patients performed as well as the controls at the short interval (i.e. 5 min), and their recognition memory was re-evaluated up to 24 h later. Under these conditions, the rate of decay of information from long-term memory was normal. In a separate study, we examined the ability of patients to remember a short 18 item story and a modified 24 item Rey–Osterreith complex figure (Becker et al., 1987). The rate of decay of information from immediate to delayed recall did not differ between the patients and controls; i.e. they did not have an abnormally rapid rate of forgetting (Becker et al., 1987). However, the AD patients did lose significantly more information between the figure copy and immediate recall conditions, suggesting a deficit in the encoding of the stimulus. This would be consistent with Kopelman's suggestion that any accelerated forgetting in AD occurs very soon after stimulus presentation (i.e. 2–3 s) and that the rate of loss is normal thereafter (Greene et al., 1996; Kopelman, 1985a, 1989; cf. Christensen et al., 1998).

At least some of the difficulty that AD patients have with long-term episodic memory is due to processing defects earlier in the chain of events, and several lines of evidence support this conclusion. Unlike control subjects, AD patients' secondary memory is significantly correlated with their primary memory capacity (Kramer et al., 1989; Wilson et al., 1983b), i.e. the ability (or inability) of the patients to maintain information in primary memory limits their performance on the secondary memory component of the task. Morris (1986) and Morris & Kopelman (1986) reached a similar conclusion, that AD patients suffer from a defect in the ability to transfer information from primary memory into secondary memory, due at least in part to an abnormally rapid rate of decay from primary memory. Greene et al. (1996) assessed episodic memory in 33 AD patients using a variety of measures, including recall of a prose passage, word list learning, and the Doors and People test. Detailed data analysis revealed that defects in primary memory played a substantial role in the AD patient's difficult time with immediate memory. Furthermore, these investigators did not find that memory was more disrupted using recall, as opposed to recognition procedures, suggesting that the AD patient's difficulties occur due to weaknesses in the initial learning of the items.

Reductions in elaborative stimulus encoding by AD patients severely limits their recall of newly learned information. Granholm & Butters (1988) presented subjects with associative cues during encoding and retrieval of word lists. Unlike HD patients and normal controls, AD patients only benefited from the use of strong associative cues at the time of recall (and not at input), suggesting not only that the patients failed to encode and/or utilize the semantic association of the to-be-remembered words and the cue words, but that when they did appear to use these links, it was based almost exclusively on free associations with cue words. Several reports of performance on verbal recognition memory tasks also support the hypothesis that poor initial encoding and the severity of language impairment may account for some of the deficit in verbal memory in AD patients (Kaszniak et al., 1986; Wilson et al., 1983a, 1983b). These findings indicate that impairments in semantic memory limit the verbal encoding and make a significant contribution to the word recognition impairment. By contrast, face recognition performance seemed not to be affected by verbal semantic limitations (Wilson et al., 1982). All of these findings are consistent with the growing body of evidence from functional neuroimaging studies about the importance of mesial temporal lobe structures, including the hippocampus, parahippocampal gyrus and fusiform cortex, for the initial encoding of stimulus materials (e.g. Schacter et al., 1999; Wagner et al., 1998; see also Martin & Chao, 2001). Given that it is these structures that are affected early in AD, it is not surprising to find that these encoding defects occur early in AD.

Of particular relevance to understanding the clinical manifestations of the episodic memory loss in AD is the notion of subgroups of patients (Jorm, 1985); these consist of individuals with islands of preserved function in the context of a syndrome that meets the criteria for probable AD. The importance of this type of analysis has been discussed in detail by Martin (1990) and it is important to emphasize that these patterns are not simply the result of random co-occurances of cognitive impairments but that they likely relate to the underlying neuroanatomical disruption caused by the disease. There are specific subgroups of AD patients (Becker, 1988; Becker et al., 1992a, 1992b; Becker & Lopez, 1992; Butters et al., 1996); not only can subgroups of AD patients be defined based on differences in degree of impairment *between* cognitive domains (e.g. visuospatial and language; Becker et al., 1988; Martin, 1987; Martin et al., 1986), but these subgroups exist *within* domains (e.g. memory) (Becker et al., 1992b). Thus, a "global" degenerative disease such as AD can have breakdowns in cognition that affect one cognitive domain more than another, and these patterns of breakdown can inform us about the basis of the memory disorder (e.g. Martin et al., 1985).

Of particular interest to this review, because it involves the breakdown of both episodic and semantic memory, was the identification of the "temporal lobe variant" of AD (Butters et al., 1996). These are patients who present for evaluation with complaints of progressive memory loss. Careful neuropsychological examination reveals that memory is impaired: delayed recall of pictures and stories is abnormal. Semantic memory is also affected: visual confrontation naming and word fluency are reduced. However, other cognitive functions are either normal (e.g. visuospatial) or only mildly affected (e.g. executive functions). Thus, temporal lobe functions are prominently affected, but cognitive functions normally localized outside of the temporal lobes are not. What is important about these patients is that their rate of decline over time is very slow. Families typically describe changes over a matter of 3–5 years, rather than the more typical 12–18 months.

These findings of subgroups of AD patients motivated a novel statistical analysis of the neuropsychological test performances of 180 AD patients and 1010 normal elderly subjects (Salthouse & Becker, 1998). The purpose of that study was to determine whether the cognitive dysfunction seen in AD was the additive effect of several independent domain-specific impairments (as would be predicted by the subgroup analyses), or whether there was a single core element that could account for the variability in patterns of impairment. The analysis technique, called single common factor analysis (SCFA), essentially determined what all of the neuropsychological tests had in common and then, after controlling for this common factor, determined the relationship between each test variable and group (i.e. patient or control). Because all of the variables had moderate-to-high loadings on the common factor, this indicated that they shared substantial variance and were not independent. However, a subset of the tests also had a substantial independent relationship, and these tests shared the feature that they all involved episodic memory. These findings not only emphasize the importance of the episodic memory loss in AD as a core component of the syndrome, but also that once the common factor is accounted for, there are no further effects of importance on 75% of the test variables. The results of this analysis do not invalidate the subgroup analyses reported above but do suggest that, for the majority of patients, there is but a single common factor that plays a critical role in the cognitive expression of the disease.

Functional Neuroimaging Studies of Episodic Memory in Alzheimer's Disease

Over the past decade, the use of functional neuroimaging techniques as tools for the neuropsychological evaluation of cognitive dysfunction has flourished. Although the field is still in its infancy, functional neuroimaging has greatly aided our understanding of disordered cognition. In one series of studies (Becker et al., 1994b, 1996; Herbster et al., 1996), we documented the changes in brain regional activation that occurs in AD while the patients were performing a verbal free recall task. Although crude by current technological standards (due to improvement in both PET scanning technology and data analysis procedures) these studies pointed out that, at least early in the disease, AD patients had a normal pattern of brain regional activity during verbal free recall. Indeed, the patients had what appeared to be a paradoxical hyperactivation of the functional network during recall of three- and eight-word lists of words. Initially, we interpreted this finding as a compensatory reallocation of resources to allow the patients the opportunity to perform the task regardless of the level of performance. However, the development of latent structure statistical analysis techniques led us to other conclusions.

In order to understand the relationships *among* the brain regions activated during the performance of memory tasks, and whether there were differences in these relationships between AD patients and normal elderly subjects, we examined the functional connectivity among brain regions (Friston, 1997; Friston & Frith, 1995; Friston et al., 1993; Herbster et al., 1996). Whereas *t*-tests are useful for determining regional activity that occurs above a given threshold (*functional specialization*), a network of functionally associated regions may exist within the dataset that can be revealed by analyses that emphasize *functional integration* (Friston et al., 1993). We used an analysis that focused on the pattern of regional covariation of relative cerebral blood flow, a procedure similar to principal components analysis. We extended this analysis to find the pattern of distributed brain activity that was most prevalent in one subject group and least prevalent in the other (Friston, 1997; Friston & Frith, 1995). The pattern of connectivity that maximally differentiated the AD patients and controls reflected, in general, the memory circuits displayed by the normal controls, i.e. the difference in functional connectivity between the patients and controls on the verbal episodic memory recall tasks is related not to the connections themselves but rather to the extent to which they are expressed. As such, the functional network is normal, but is simply differentially active in the two study groups. Indeed, as we noted previously (Herbster et al., 1996), the patients expressed the matrix *more than* the controls. This finding is important because it suggests that, at least for this episodic memory functional network, the basic structure is intact.

In retrospect, the functional activation that we observed, especially in the eight-word recall condition, was more related to the retrieval aspects of the task than to encoding. In addition, the dorsal parietal and prefrontal circuit that was identified seems to suggest a high degree of attentional load, even though the task was auditory (and that loop is usually associated with visual attention) (Posner & Petersen, 1990). Thus, further research is needed to determine the nature and extent of any compensatory response in AD patients using cognitive probes that more carefully dissect the memory circuits.

Semantic Memory Loss in AD

The performance of AD patients on tests that require semantic memory, such as visual confrontation naming or word generation, is often severely impaired (Hodges et al., 1990), whereas the performance of patients with some other dementias (e.g. HD) is relatively normal (Butters et al., 1988). Thus, consistent with the growing body of neuropsychological, behavioral, neurological and neuroimaging data, the loss of semantic knowledge may be peculiar to those pathological states that affect the functional integrity of the temporal lobes (Hodges & Patterson, 1995; Hodges et al., 1999). This position is supported by the descriptions of *semantic dementia*, a condition occurring in the context of a progressive aphasia and marked by a profound loss of semantic knowledge (e.g. Graham et al., 1997a, 1997b; Hodges et al., 1992; Neary et al., 1993; Snowden et al., 1992). Structural and functional imaging studies demonstrate that these conditions are associated with severe disruption of the function of the language-dominant temporal lobe (Mummery et al., 1999, 2000).

Early in the course of their dementia, AD patients have difficulty performing many tests that rely on semantic memory (Nebes & Brady, 1989); even "minimally" impaired patients have significant impairments in category fluency, confrontation naming, naming to description, and answering questions about semantic features (Hodges & Patterson, 1995) (although some mild AD patients can have normal semantic memory, cf. Becker et al., 1988; Martin et al., 1986). However, it is still not clear whether these difficulties reflect a disruption of the patients' semantic knowledge (i.e. an actual loss of information), a disruption of their ability to access or use that knowledge base, or both. As noted by Perry & Hodges (1996), there is considerable variability in the nature and extent of semantic memory dysfunction, especially early in the course of the dementia (Hodges & Patterson, 1995), and there is evidence to support models that differentially emphasize storage loss, retrieval defects and alterations in the basic structure of semantic memory (Bayles et al., 1991; Chan et al., 1995b; Chertkow & Bub, 1990).

Although early in AD visual confrontation naming can be relatively preserved, as the disorder progresses patients have more and more difficulty with this function (Becker et al., 1994a, 1988). Typically, the use of semantic cues is not helpful to AD patients, whereas a phonemic cue can elicit the correct response (at least early in the disease course). In terms of word generation, category fluency (e.g. animals) is typically more impaired than letter fluency (e.g. CFL) early in the disease, but with increasing severity this distinction is blurred. If a patient is asked about subcategories (e.g. birds or dogs) he/she can also have a significant defect, even when the superordinate (i.e. animals) was not appreciably affected. Even with a general category cue (e.g. the Supermarket Task from the Mattis (1976) dementia rating scale) it is possible to show that there are fewer exemplars from subcategories (e.g. meat, vegetables/fruits; Martin & Fedio, 1983). By contrast, patients with frontal lobe lesions are quantitatively similar to AD patients (i.e. same total number of words generated), but they achieve this by sampling from fewer subcategories and generating more words from each. This finding, as well as the *relative* sparing of letter (vs. category) fluency in AD, emphasizes the importance of the temporal lobe pathology (as opposed to any frontal system dysfunction) in explaining the nature of the semantic memory loss.

It is reasonable to ask whether the poor performance of AD patients on a given semantic memory task is the result of an actual semantic memory deficit, or stems from a problem in more general information-processing operations; for example, is the visual naming defect that is so characteristic of AD patients due to knowledge lost about the semantic features that define different lexical referents (Bayles & Tomoeda, 1983), or is it because AD patients cannot carry out the needed perceptual analysis of the object (Kirshner et al., 1984), or cannot access the name (Barker & Lawson, 1968)? Although the first of these potential mechanisms would involve a deficit in semantic knowledge, the latter two would represent situations in which a failure on a "semantic" test would result from limitations in *non*semantic cognitive operations necessary for the appropriate use of an intact semantic knowledge base.

A number of investigators have suggested that AD patients' knowledge of concept meaning is impaired (Chertkow et al., 1989; Huff et al., 1986; Martin & Fedio, 1983; Troster et al., 1989). They claim that although AD patients usually retain knowledge of the semantic category to which a concept belongs, they lose information about its specific attributes. In confrontation naming, AD patients often misname objects, using their category names or the names of other items from the same category. They also have a great deal of difficulty recognizing the name of a pictured object in a multiple-choice task when the distractors are drawn from the same category as the target object, but not when they are drawn from other categories (Chertkow et al., 1989; Huff et al., 1986). This pattern of performance may reflect a preservation of category information, coupled with a loss of those specific attributes that make it possible to differentiate semantically related objects—hence the confusion with other items from the same category. Perhaps the most impressive evidence for a loss of specific attribute information in AD comes from several studies that have asked subjects direct questions about an item's category membership and its attributes. AD patients can accurately answer a question about an object's category but have a great deal of difficulty in answering questions about its physical features or functions (Martin & Fedio, 1983). Even when given multiple-choice questions (e.g. "Do you use this object to lift things or to cut things?"), AD patients are much more impaired on questions about an object's attributes than on questions about its category membership (Chertkow et al., 1989).

Other evidence suggests that AD patients *retain* their knowledge of the semantic attributes of concepts. Demented patients can be quite accurate (95% correct) when asked to recognize features that were attributes of a target (Grober et al., 1985). Nebes & Brady (1988) used a task in which they measured the time it took normal elderly and AD patients to decide whether a given stimulus word was related to a target word. If AD patients have actually lost knowledge of the features and functions of objects, or find such knowledge differentially difficult to access, then they should be slower and less accurate in making decisions about a target's features and actions than about its category membership and associations. However, the difference in response time between AD patients and the normal elderly was, if anything, smaller for decisions about features and actions than for decisions about categories and associates. The AD patients made very few errors, and there was no evidence that decisions about a concept's action or feature were significantly more difficult. These results, unlike others (Chertkow et al., 1989; Martin & Fedio, 1983), suggest that AD patients are aware of the relationship between concepts and their attributes.

Innovative work by Chan and colleagues, however, has shown that the structure of the semantic networks is perturbed in AD. These studies used a variety of latent structure techniques, including multidimensional scaling, to analyze the organization of information in semantic memory; in other words, using the method of triads (and a multidimensional scaling analysis), they compared and contrasted the semantic organization of the concept of "animal" in AD patients and elderly controls (Chan et al., 1993a, 1993b, 1995a). AD patients and normal controls used the same dimensions to distinguish among the animals (i.e. domestic, predatory, size); however, the patients tended to use the more concrete concept of physical size in their categorization, whereas the controls primarily used the more abstract concept of domestication. In addition, relationships among the stimuli along the multidimensional axes also differed between the patients and controls.

How are we to reconcile these contradictory conclusions about concept knowledge in AD? Nebes (1992) has argued that one possible source for this discrepancy lies in the differing cognitive demands imposed by the experimental tasks. When AD patients are asked a direct question about a concept's attributes, they perform poorly; by contrast, if they are asked merely to decide whether a concept and one of its attributes are related, they do very well. Therefore, what appears in some studies to be an impairment in the structure of semantic memory in AD (i.e. a loss of knowledge of concept attributes or their relative importance) may instead reflect a failure of more general-purpose cognitive operations, such as those involved in intentionally accessing and evaluating information (e.g. response search and response selection). If the need for these cognitive operations is minimized, AD patients may show a pattern of performance similar to that seen in normal control subjects. Thus, before we attribute poor semantic memory in AD to an actual semantic deficit, it is important to be sure that performance is not limited by a nonsemantic processing impairment.

In their longitudinal study of semantic memory in AD, Hodges & Patterson tested knowledge about specific items using a variety of different techniques in different test modalities. While not minimizing the nonsemantic processing demands of individual tasks, consistent findings across several tasks would point toward a degradation of semantic knowledge. Indeed, their data demonstrate a high reliability between tests (and within items); for example, if an AD patient was unable to spontaneously name an object, he/she was also unlikely, to be able to describe it or to pick it out using a multiple choice format (Hodges et al., 1996; Lambon-Ralph et al., 1997).

In sum, there is evidence for a multicomponent breakdown in semantic memory in AD. This may reflect, in part, the multifactorial aspects of semantic memory, and may also reflect the fact that various aspects of semantic memory function are subsumed in different neuroanatomical regions. The heterogeneity of symptoms and symptom clusters may reflect both cognitive and pathological variation.

Neuroimaging Studies of Semantic Memory in AD

There have been relatively few studies of the functional neuroanatomical basis of semantic memory function and dysfunction in AD patients. Indeed, there have been relatively few published functional neuroimaging studies involving AD patients at all (e.g. Becker et al., 1996; Herbster et al., 1996; Hirono et al., 2001; Kessler et al., 1991, 1996; Rombouts et al., 2000) and fewer that use fMRI to study semantic memory in AD (Saykin et al., 1999b; cf. Mummery et al., 1999). However, these data all suggest that there are abnormalities in the functional networks involved in semantic memory retrieval in AD. Saykin et al. (1999a) reported the differences in brain regional activation between AD patients and normal controls when performing two semantic decision tasks relative to a phonological decision task. Although the AD patients were selectively impaired in performing the semantic tasks relative to the phonological task, it was nevertheless possible to obtain meaningful data. Both AD patients and controls activated the left inferior frontal cortex, but the patients had additional activation in the left dorsolateral prefrontal cortex and the superior temporal gyrus. As we had reported earlier for episodic memory tasks (Becker et al., 1996; Herbster et al., 1996), these investigators found that the spatial extent of the activations by the patients were greater than those observed in the controls for their semantic memory task. This finding, coupled with a specific association between right medial prefrontal activation and performance in the patients but not the controls, is further evidence for some form of compensatory response in the AD patients.

One way to examine the pathological locus responsible for a specific cognitive defect in AD is to study structure–function relationships with structural neuroimaging data. In

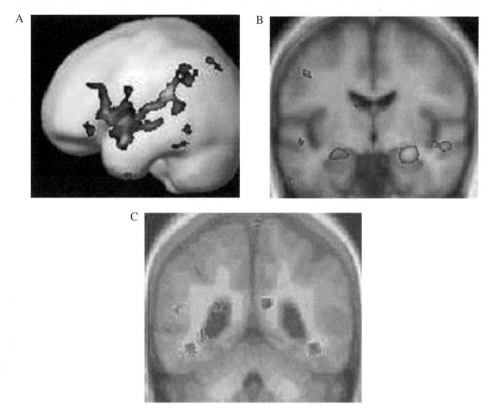

Figure 6.1 Brain structural differences between probable AD patients and normal controls. (A) Cortical atrophy in the left hemisphere, with typical gray matter loss. (B) Coronal plane view showing tissue loss in the inferior temporal lobe and hippocampus. (C) Errors/no errors.

our own studies of the neuroanatomical basis of the semantic memory loss in AD, we have adopted the voxel-based morphometry methods used by Mummery et al. (1999) in their studies of semantic dementia. High-resolution structural MR images are spatially normalized using a nonlinear algorithm and then segmented into gray matter and white matter images (Ashburner & Friston, 1997; Mazziotta et al., 1997). For our studies, the focus is on the grey matter and these images are smoothed (using a 3-D Gaussian filter) and analyzed using a between-group analysis to identify the voxels with significant differences in intensity, reflecting differences in brain volumes (see also Sowell et al., 1999).

Figure 6.1 (top) shows the results of an analysis comparing the brain structural differences between probable AD patients and normal, elderly control subjects (S.B. McGinty, personal communication). The left-hand image shows the cortical atrophy in the language-dominant left hemisphere, with the typical temporoparietal gray matter loss. The right-hand image shows a view in the coronal plane, demonstrating the tissue loss in the inferior temporal lobe and hippocampus.

In the bottom pair of images, we show the results of an analysis of AD patients who were divided into two groups based on their object-naming performance: those who made no naming errors, and those who did make naming errors on the relevant section of the AD Assessment Scale. There were no significant differences between groups in education or on overall cognitive impairment, but the groups did differ significantly on age.

The analysis revealed a significant difference in the gray matter volume of several temporal lobe structures. In particular, Brodmann area 37 in the posterior temporal lobe showed a significant reduction in volume in the AD patients with poor visual naming, compared with patients with good visual naming. In addition, middle inferior regions of the temporal lobe, the fusiform gyrus and parahippocampal gyrus, also had significant differences in density between groups, such that the patients with poor naming had reduced volumes relative to those with good naming.

These structural data are consistent with the existing functional neuroimaging and neuropsychological studies that have demonstrated the critical role of the temporal lobe in the processes needed to execute semantic memory tasks. There is reliable functional activation of the left temporal lobe during object-naming tasks (Martin et al., 1996; Vandenberghe et al., 1996; Zelkowicz et al., 1997), and structural imaging studies have shown that temporal lobe volume is abnormal in AD patients compared with the normal aged (Jernigan et al., 1991; Killiany et al., 1993). Knowing that AD patients have these structural changes not only helps explain the basis of their naming impairment, but also helps understand the functional basis of visual object naming.

The results in this study extend those of Mummery et al. (1999), who found that in semantic dementia the site of significant atrophy was the anterolateral temporal lobe. However, a functional neuroimaging analysis of a semantic task revealed activity in the left posterior inferior temporal gyrus, and they suggested that the decreased functional activation found in these patients was due to lack of input from the atrophied anterior temporal lobe to the posterior inferior temporal gyrus, and not due to atrophy of the posterior inferior temporal gyrus. Our data suggest, therefore, that the anatomical basis for the naming impairment in AD is different from that seen in semantic dementia, which is commonly associated with Pick's disease and other variants of frontotemporal lobe dementia (FTD), i.e. the more posterior temporal regions may be directly involved in the semantic processing of visual objects, and these are directly affected in AD, but only indirectly affected in FTD (by virtue of disruption of upstream connections from the anterior temporal lobe). Thus, while there appears to be a common final pathway to explain the naming defect, the *cause* of that defect differs between diseases.

Analysis of the neuroanatomical abnormalities in patients with language disturbance associated with frontotemporal dementia (Snowden et al., 1992) reveals the different functional loci that can produce impaired processing in dementia. For example, patient G.C. has a semantic dementia syndrome (Graham et al., 1997a; Hodges et al., 1992), and has been followed by our group for more than 5 years. Figure 6.2 shows the brain regional atrophy (projected onto an average brain image) in G.C. relative to controls (top row of images). What is striking is the significant left temporal lobe atrophy. Specifically, superior and middle temporal cortex are affected, as well as the hippocampus and peri-hippocampal regions. When this is compared with the atrophy seen in AD patients relative to controls (Figure 6.1), the focal nature of the defect in semantic dementia can be appreciated.

Patient S.M., by contrast, has little impairment in semantics *per se*, but rather has significant abnormalities in word retrieval and word production. He is able to perform a variety of tasks that require semantic memory (e.g. the Vocabulary subtest of the Wechsler Adult Intelligence Scale—Revised; Pyramids and Palm Trees (Howard & Patterson, 1992),

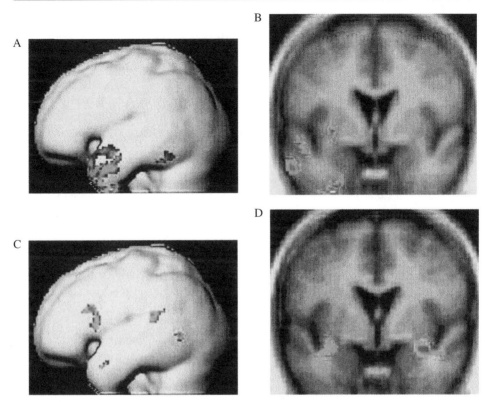

Figure 6.2 (A, B) Neuroanatomical abnormalities in a patient (G.C) with language disturbance associated with frontotemporal dementia, showing brain in regional atrophy. In patient S.M. (C, D), there are significant abnormalities in word retrieval and word production; the figures show a small region of atrophy in left frontal cortex near Broca's area, with no significant atrophy in the temporal lobe.

word-picture matching (Kay et al., 1992), but has significant impairments when required to generate words (e.g. visual naming, fluency tasks). A voxel-based morphometric analysis of his MRI scan (relative to age- and education-appropriate normal elderly) revealed a small region of significant atrophy in the left frontal cortex, around Broca's area (see bottom row, Figure 6.2), with no significant atrophy in the temporal lobe.

The results of these three morphometric analyses allow several conclusions about the functional basis of the semantic memory loss in AD. First, the inferior temporal lobe, and perhaps most importantly the parahippocampal gyrus, is critical for the ability to successfully name objects. However, the ability to effectively retrieve the names of objects appears to be related to atrophy in the frontal cortex, BA44/45. The data further imply, although this has not been directly tested, that even early in AD there is sufficient atrophy in the frontal cortex to explain at least part of AD patients' defects in verbal fluency. Finally, as was shown by G.C., the extent of temporal atrophy can be quite profound, but this nevertheless does not affect cognitive processes that do not require the extensive memory functions subsumed by these brain regions.

SUMMARY

Although the cognitive dysfunction associated with AD is often described as generalized, it is perhaps more accurate and meaningful to describe it as multifocal; the development of CNS dysfunction in AD appears to progress such that some cognitive systems are more or less affected than others. Thus, at various points during the progression of the disease, the neuropsychological profile will reflect the relative impairments and sparing of cognitive functions, based on the underlying patterns of neuropathological change. These patterns of impairments should, and do, follow the "natural fracture lines of behavior" (Thomas et al., 1968), reflecting the way in which normal memory processes are organized. By understanding better the nature of the breakdown of these multiple processes, it will be possible to inform the development of rational behavioral and pharmacological treatment and management of AD.

ACKNOWLEDGEMENT

J.T.B. is the recipient of a Research Scientist Development Award (Level II) from the National Institute of Mental Health (MH03177). The authors are grateful to R.D. Nebes for discussion about semantic memory in AD, and to S. Bell McGinty for comments on an earlier version of this manuscript.

REFERENCES

American Psychiatric Association (APA). (1987). *Diagnostic and Statistical Manual of Mental Disorders—Revised (DSM-III-R)*, 3rd (revised) edn. Washington, DC: American Psychiatric Press.

Ashburner, J. & Friston, K.J. (1997). Spatial transformation of images. In R.S.J. Frackowiak, K.J. Friston, C.D. Frith et al. (eds), *Human Brain Function* (pp. 43–58). San Diego, CA: Academic Press.

Atkinson, R.C. & Shiffrin, R.M. (1968). Human memory: a proposed system and its control processes. In K.W. Spence & J.T. Spence (eds), *The Psychology of Learning and Motivation: Advances in Research and Theory*, Vol. 2 (pp. 89–195). New York: Academic Press.

Baddeley, A. (2000). The episodic buffer: a new component of working memory? *Trends in Cognitive Science*, **4**(11), 417–423.

Baddeley, A., Cocchini, G., Della Sala, S. et al. (1999). Working memory and vigilance: evidence from normal aging and Alzheimer's disease. *Brain and Cognition*, **41**(1), 87–108.

Baddeley, A.D. (1986). *Working Memory*. Oxford: Clarendon.

Baddeley, A.D., Bressi, S., Della Salla, S. et al. (1986). Senile dementia and working memory. *Quarterly Journal of Experimental Psychology*, **38A**, 603–618.

Baddeley, A.D., Della Salla, S. & Spinnler, H. (1991). The two-component hypothesis of memory deficit in Alzheimer's disease. *Journal of Clinical and Experimental Neuropsychology*, **13**, 372–380.

Baddeley, A.D. & Hitch, G. (1974). Working memory. In G.H. Bower (ed.), *The Psychology of Learning and Motivation*, Vol. 8 (pp. 47–90). San Diego, CA: Academic Press.

Baddeley, A.D. & Wilson, B.A. (1988). Frontal amnesia and dysexecutive syndrome. *Brain and Cognition*, **1**, 212–230.

Barker, M.G. & Lawson, J.S. (1968). Nominal aphasia in dementia. *British Journal of Psychiatry*, **114**, 1351–1356.

Bayles, K.A. & Tomoeda, C.K. (1983). Confrontation naming in dementia. *Brain and Language*, **19**, 98–114.

Bayles, K.A., Tomoeda, C.K., Kaszniak, A.W. & Trosset, M.W. (1991). Alzheimer's disease effects on semantic memory: loss of structure or impaired processing. *Journal of Cognitive Neurosciences*, **3**, 166–182.

Becker, J.T. (1988). Working memory and secondary memory deficits in Alzheimer's disease. *Journal of Clinical and Experimental Neuropsychology*, **10**, 739–753.

Becker, J.T., Bajulaiye, O. & Smith, C. (1992a). Longitudinal analysis of a two-component model of the memory deficits in Alzheimer's disease. *Psychological Medicine*, **22**, 437–446.

Becker, J.T., Boller, F., Lopez, O.L. et al. (1994a). The natural history of Alzheimer's disease: description of study cohort and accuracy of diagnosis. *Archives of Neurology*, **51**, 585–594.

Becker, J.T., Boller, F., Saxton, J. & McGonigle-Gibson, K. (1987). Normal rates of forgetting of verbal and non-verbal material in Alzheimer's disease. *Cortex*, **23**, 59–72.

Becker, J.T., Caldararo, R., Lopez, O.L. et al. (1995). Qualitative features of the memory deficit associated with HIV infection and AIDS: cross-validation of a discriminant function classification scheme. *Journal of Clinical and Experimental Neuropsychology*, **17**, 134–142.

Becker, J.T., Huff, F.J., Nebes, R.D. et al. (1988). Neuropsychological functioning in Alzheimer's disease: pattern of impairment and rates of progression. *Archives of Neurology*, **45**, 263–268.

Becker, J.T. & Lopez, O.L. (1992). Episodic memory in Alzheimer's disease: breakdown of multiple memory processes. In L. Backman (ed.), *Memory Functioning in Dementia* (pp. 27–44). Amsterdam: North Holland.

Becker, J.T., Lopez, O.L. & Wess, J. (1992b). Material specific memory loss in probable Alzheimer's disease. *Journal of Neurology Neurosurgery & Psychiatry*, **55**, 1177–1181.

Becker, J.T., Mintun, M.A., Aleva, K. et al. (1996). Compensatory reallocation of brain resources supporting verbal episodic memory in Alzheimer's disease. *Neurology*, **46**, 692–700.

Becker, J.T., Mintun, M.A., Diehl, D.J. et al. (1994b). Functional neuroanatomy of verbal free recall: a replication study. *Human Brain Mapping*, **1**, 284–292.

Benton, A.L. (1968). Differential behavioral effects in frontal lobe disease. *Neuropsychologia*, **6**, 53–60.

Benton, A.L., Hamsher, K., Varney, N.R. & Spreen, O. (1983). *Contributions to Neuropsychological Assessment. A Clinical Manual*. New York: Oxford University Press.

Braak, H. & Braak, E. (1991). Neuropathological staging of Alzheimer-related changes. *Acta Neuropathologica*, **82**, 239–259.

Buschke, H. & Fuld, P.A. (1974). Evaluating storage, retention, and retrieval in disoriented memory and learning. *Neurology*, **24**, 1019–1025.

Butters, M.A., Lopez, O.L. & Becker, J.T. (1996). Focal temporal lobe dysfunction in probable Alzheimer's disease predicts a slow rate of cognitive decline. *Neurology*, **46**, 692–700.

Butters, N., Granholm, E.L., Salmon, D.P. et al. (1986a). Episodic and semantic memory: a comparison of amnesic and demented patients. *Journal of Clinical and Experimental Neuropsychology*, **9**, 479–497.

Butters, N., Salmon, D.P., Heindel, W. & Granholm, E. (1988). Episodic, semantic and procedural memory: some comparisons of Alzheimer's and Huntington's disease patients. In R. D. Terry (ed.), *Aging and the Brain* (pp. 63–87). New York: Raven.

Butters, N., Wolfe, J., Granholm, E. & Martone, M. (1986b). An assessment of verbal recall, recognition and fluency abilities in patients with Huntington's disease. *Cortex*, **22**, 11–32.

Chan, A.S., Butters, N., Paulsen, J.S. et al. (1993a). An assessment of the semantic network in patients with Alzheimer's disease. *Journal of Cognitive Neuroscience*, **5**, 254–261.

Chan, A.S., Butters, N., Salmon, D.P. & Johnson, S.A. (1995a). Semantic network abnormality predicts rate of cognitive decline in patients with probable Alzheimer's disease. *Journal of the International Neuropsychological Society*, **1**, 297–303.

Chan, A.S., Butters, N., Salmon, D.P. et al. (1995b). Comparison of the semantic networks in patients with dementia and amnesia. *Neuropsychology*, **9**, 177–186.

Chan, A.S., Butters, N., Salmon, D.P. & McGuire, K.A. (1993b). Dimensionality and clustering in the semantic network of patients with Alzheimer's disease. *Psychology and Aging*, **8**, 411–419.

Chertkow, H. & Bub, D. (1990). Semantic memory loss in dementia of Alzheimer's type. What do various measures measure? *Brain*, **113**(2), 397–417.

Chertkow, H., Bub, D. & Seidenberg, M. (1989). Priming and semantic memory loss in Alzheimer's disease. *Brain and Language*, **36**, 420–446.

Christensen, H., Kopelman, M.D., Stanhope, N. et al. (1998). Rates of forgetting in Alzheimer dementia. *Neuropsychologia*, **36**(6), 546–557.

Delis, D.C., Massman, P.J., Butters, N. et al. (1991). Profiles of demented and amnesic patients on the California Verbal Learning Test: implications for the assessment of memory disorders. *Psychological Assessment: A Journal of Consulting and Clinical Psychology*, **3**, 19–26.

Diller, L., Ben-Yishay, Y., Gerstman, L.J. et al. (1979). *Studies in Cognition and Rehabilitation in Hemiplegia (Rehabilitation Monograph No. 50)*. New York: New York University.

Ericsson, K.A. & Kintsch, W. (1995). Long-term working memory. *Psychological Review*, **102**(2), 211–245.

Farah, M.J., Gazzaniga, M.S., Holtzman, J.D. & Kosslyn, S.M. (1985). A left-hemisphere basis for visual imagery. *Neuropsychologia*, **23**, 115–118.

Flicker, C., Ferris, S.H. & Reisberg, B. (1991). Mild cognitive impairment in the elderly: predictors of dementia. *Neurology*, **41**(7), 1006–1009.

Friston, K.J. (1997). Characterizing distributed functional systems. In R.S.J. Frackowiak, K.J. Friston, C.D. Frith et al. (eds), *Human Brain Function* (pp. 107–126). San Diego, CA: Academic Press.

Friston, K.J. & Frith, C.D. (1995). Schizophrenia: a disconnection syndrome? *Clinical Neuroscience*, **3**, 89–97.

Friston, K.J., Frith, C.D., Liddle, P.F. & Frackowiak, R.S.J. (1993). Functional connectivity: the principal-component analysis of large (PET) data sets. *Journal of Cerebral Blood Flow and Metabolism*, **13**, 5–14.

Fuld, P.A., Katzman, R., Davies, P. & Terry, R.D. (1982). Intrusions as a sign of Alzheimer's dementia: Chemical and pathological verification. *Annals of Neurology*, **11**, 155–159.

Geula, C. (1998). Abnormalities of neural circuitry in Alzheimer's disease: hippocampus and cortical cholinergic innervation. *Neurology*, **51**(suppl 1), S18–S29.

Graham, K.S., Becker, J.T. & Hodges, J.R. (1997a). On the relationship between knowledge and memory for pictures: evidence from the study of patients with semantic dementia and Alzheimer's disease. *Journal of the International Neuropsychological Society*, **3**(6), 534–544.

Graham, K.S., Becker, J.T., Patterson, K. & Hodges, J.R. (1997b). Lost for words: a case of primary progressive aphasia. In A. Parkin (ed.), *Case Studies in the Neuropsychology of Memory* (pp. 83–110). Hove.

Granholm, E. & Butters, N. (1988). Associative encoding and retrieval in Alzheimer's and Huntington's disease. *Brain and Cognition*, **7**, 335–347.

Greene, J.D., Baddeley, A.D. & Hodges, J.R. (1996). Analysis of the episodic memory deficit in early Alzheimer's disease: evidence from the Doors and People Test. *Neuropsychologia*, **34**(6), 537–551.

Grober, E., Buschke, H., Kawas, C. & Fuld, P. (1985). Impaired ranking of semantic attributes in dementia. *Brain and Language*, **26**, 276–286.

Grossi, D., Lopez, O.L. & Martinez, A.J. (1989). The mammillary bodies in Alzheimer's disease. *Acta Neurological Scandinavica*, **80**, 41–45.

Herbster, A.N., Nichols, T., Wiseman, M.B. et al. (1996). Functional connectivity in auditory verbal short-term memory in Alzheimer's disease. *NeuroImage*, **4**, 67–77.

Hirono, N., Mori, E., Ishii, K. et al. (2001). Neuronal substrates for semantic memory: a positron emission tomography study in Alzheimer's disease. *Dementia and Geriatric Cognitive Disorders*, **12**(1), 15–21.

Hodges, J.R. & Patterson, K. (1995). Is semantic memory consistently impaired early in the course of Alzheimer's disease? Neuroanatomical and diagnostic implications. *Neuropsychologia*, **33**, 441–460.

Hodges, J.R., Patterson, K., Garrard, P. (1999). The differentiation of semantic dementia and frontal lobe dementia (temporal and frontal variants of frontotemporal dementia) from early Alzheimer's disease: a comparative neuropsychological study. *Neuropsychology*, **13**, 31–40.

Hodges, J.R., Patterson, K., Graham, N. & Dawson, K. (1996). Naming and knowing in dementia of Alzheimer's type. *Brain and Language*, **54**, 302–325.

Hodges, J.R., Patterson, K., Oxbury, S. & Funnell, E. (1992). Semantic dementia: progressive fluent aphasia with temporal lobe atrophy. *Brain*, **115**, 1783–1806.

Hodges, J. R., Salmon, D.P. & Butters, N. (1990). Differential impairment of semantic and episodic memory in Alzheimer's and Huntington's disease: a controlled prosepective study. *Journal of Neurology Neurosurgery and Psychiatry*, **53**, 1089–1095.

Howard, D. & Patterson, K. (1992). *The Pyramid and Palm Trees Test: A Test of Semantic Access from Words and Pictures*. Bury St Edmunds: Thames Valley Test Company.

Huff, F.J., Becker, J.T., Belle, S. et al. (1987). Cognitive deficits and clinical diagnosis of Alzheimer's. *Neurology*, **37**, 1119–1124.

Huff, J.F., Corkin, S. & Growdon, J.H. (1986). Semantic impairment and anomia in Alzheimer's disease. *Brain and Language*, **28**, 235–249.

Hyman, B.T., Van Hoesen, G.W. & Damasio, A.R. (1984). Alzheimer's disease: cell-specific pathology isolates the hippocampal formation. *Science*, **225**, 1168–1170.

Hyman, B.T., Van Hoesen, G.W. & Damasio, A.R. (1990). Memory-related neural systems in Alzheimer's disease: an anatomic study. *Neurology*, **40**, 1721–1730.

Hyman, B.T., Van Hoesen, G.W., Kromer, L.J. & Damasio, A.R. (1986). Perforant pathway changes and the memory impairment of Alzheimer's disease. *Annals of Neurology*, **20**, 472–481.

Jack, C.R., Petersen, R.C., Xu, Y.C. et al. (1999). Prediction of AD aith MRI-based hippocampal volume in mild cognitive impairment. *Neurology*, **52**(7), 1397–1403.

Jack, C.R., Petersen, R.C., Xu, Y.C. et al. (1997). Medial temporal atrophy on MRI in normal aging and very mild Alzheimer's disease. *Neurology*, **49**, 786–794.

Jernigan, T.L., Salmon, D.P., Butters, N. & Hesselink, J.R. (1991). Cerebral structure on MRI: II. specific changes in Alzheimer's and Huntington's diseases. *Biological Psychiatry*, **29**, 68–81.

Johnson, K.A., Jones, K., Holman, B.L. et al. (1998). Preclinical prediction of Alzheimer's disease using SPECT. *Neurology*, **50**, 1563–1571.

Jorm, A.F. (1985). Subtypes of Alzheimer's dementia: a conceptual analysis and critical review. *Psychological Medicine*, **15**, 543–553.

Kaszniak, A.W. (1988). Cognition in Alzheimer's disease: theoretic models and clinical implications. *Neurobiology of Aging*, **9**(1), 92–94.

Kaszniak, A.W., Poon, L.W. & Riege, W. (1986). Assessing memory deficits: an information-processing approach. In L.W. Poon (ed.), *Handbook for Clinical Memory Assessment of Older Adults*. Washington: American Psychological Association.

Kay, J., Lesser, R. & Coltheart, M. (1992). *PALPA: Psycholinguistic Assessments of Language Processing in Aphasia*. Hove: Erlbaum.

Kessler, J., Ghaemi, M., Mielke, R. et al. (1996). Visual vs. auditory memory stimulation in patients with probable Alzheimer's disease: a PET study with 18 FDG. *Annals of the New York Academy of Science*, **777**, 233–238.

Kessler, J., Herholz, K., Grond, M. & Heiss, W.-D. (1991). Impaired metabolic activation in Alzheimer's disease: a PET study during continuous visual recognition. *Neuropsychologia*, **29**(3), 229–243.

Killiany, R.J., Moss, M.B., Albert, M.S. et al. (1993). Temporal lobe regions on magnetic resonance imaging identify patients with early Alzheimer's disease. *Archives of Neurology*, **50**, 949–954.

Kirshner, H.S., Webb, W.G. & Kelly, M.P. (1984). The naming disorder of dementia. *Neuropsychologia*, **22**, 23–30.

Kopelman, M.D. (1985a). Multiple memory deficits in Alzheimer-type dementia: implications for pharmacotherapy. *Psychological Medicine*, **15**, 527–541.

Kopelman, M.D. (1985b). Rates of forgetting in Alzheimer-type dementia and Korsakoff's syndrome. *Neuropsychologia*, **23**, 623–638.

Kopelman, M.D. (1989). Remote and autobiographical memory, temporal context memory and frontal atrophy in Korsakoff and Alzheimer patients. *Neuropsychologia*, **27**, 437–460.

Kramer, J.H., Delis, D.C., Blusewitz, M.J. et al. (1988). Verbal memory errors in Alzheimer's and Huntington's dementias. *Developmental Neuropsychology*, **4**, 1–15.

Kramer, J.H., Levin, B.E., Brandt, J. & Delis, D.C. (1989). Differentiation of Alzheimer's, Huntington's, and Parkinson's disease patients on the basis of verbal learning characteristics. *Neuropsychology*, **3**, 111–120.

Lambon-Ralph, M.A., Patterson, K. & Hodges, J.R. (1997). The relationship between naming and semantic knowledge for different categories in dementia of Alzheimer's type. *Neuropsychologia*, **35**(9), 1251–1260.

Mair, W.P., Warrington, E.K. & Weiskrantz, L. (1979). Memory disorders in Korsakoff's psychosis: a neuropathological and neuropsychological investigation of two cases. *Brain*, **102**, 749–783.

Martin, A. (1987). Representation of semantic and spatial knowledge in Alzheimer's patients: implication for models of preserved learning in amnesia. *Journal of Clinical and Experimental Neuropsychology*, **9**, 191–224.

Martin, A. (1990). Neuropsychology of Alzheimer's disease: the case for subgroups. In M. F. Schwartz (ed.), *Modular Deficits in Alzheimer's-type Dementia* (pp. 143–176). Cambridge, MA: Bradford/MIT.

Martin, A., Brouwers, P., Lalonde, F. et al. (1986). Towards a behavioral typology of Alzheimer's patients. *Journal of Clinical and Experimental Neuropsychology*, **8**, 594–610.

Martin, A. & Chao, L.L. (2001). Semantic memory and the brain: structure and processes. *Current Opinions in Neurobiology*, **11**, 194–201.

Martin, A., Cox, C., Brouwers, P. & Fedio, P. (1985). A note on the different patterns of impaired and preserved cognitive abilities and their relation to episodic memory deficits in Alzheimer's patients. *Brain and Language*, **25**, 323–341.

Martin, A. & Fedio, P. (1983). Word production and comprehension in Alzheimer's disease: the breakdown of semantic knowledge. *Brain and Language*, **19**, 124–141.

Martin, A., Wiggs, C.L., Ungerleider, L.G. & Haxby, J.V. (1996). Neural correlates of category-specific knowledge. *Nature*, **379**, 649–652.

Mattis, S. (1976). Mental status examination for organic mental syndrome in the elderly patient. In L. Bellak & T.B. Karuso (eds), *Geriatric Psychiatry*. New York: Grune & Stratton.

Mazziotta, J.C., Toga, A., Evans, A. et al. (1997). Brain maps: linking the present to the future. In R.S.J. Frackowiak, K.J. Friston, C.D. Frith et al. (eds), *Human Brain Function* (pp. 429–466). San Diego, CA: Academic Press.

McClelland, J.L. (1998). Complementary learning systems in the brain: a connectionist approach to explicit and implicit cognition and memory. *Annals of the New York Academy of Science*, **843**, 153–169.

McKhann, G., Drachman, D.A., Folstein, M.F. (1984). Clinical diagnosis of Alzheimer's disease: report of the NINCDS–ADRDA Work Group under the auspices of the Department of Health and Human Services Task Force on Alzheimer's disease. *Neurology*, **34**, 939–944.

Miller, E. (1971). On the nature of the memory disorder in presenile dementia. *Neuropsychologia*, **9**, 75–81.

Morris, J.C., McKeel, D.W., Storandt, M. et al. (1991). Very mild Alzheimer's disease: informant-based clinical psychometric and pathological distinction from normal aging. *Neurology*, **41**, 469–478.

Morris, J.C., Storandt, M., Miller, J.P. et al. (2001). Mild cognitive impairment represents early-stage Alzheimer disease. *Archives of Neurology*, **58**, 397–405.

Morris, R.G. (1986). Short-term forgetting in senile dementia of the Alzheimer type. *Cognitive Neuropsychology*, **3**, 77–97.

Morris, R.G. & Baddeley, A. D. (1988). A review of primary and working memory functioning in Alzheimer-type dementia. *Journal of Clinical and Experimental Neuropsychology*, **10**, 279–296.

Morris, R.G. & Kopelman, M.D. (1986). The memory deficits in Alzheimer-type dementia: a review. *Quarterly Journal of Experimental Psychology*, **38**, 575–602.

Moss, M.B., Albert, M.S., Butters, N. & Payne, M. (1986). Differential patterns of memory loss among patients with Alzheimer's disease, Huntington's disease, and alcoholic Korsakoff's syndrome. *Archives of Neurology*, **43**, 239–246.

Mummery, C.J., Patterson, K., Price, C.J. et al. (2000). A voxel-based morphometry study of semantic dementia: relationship between temporal lobe atrophy and semantic memory. *Annals of Neurology*, **47**(1), 36–45.

Mummery, C.J., Patterson, K., Wise, R.J.S. et al. (1999). Disrupted temporal lobe connections in semantic dementia. *Brain*, **122**, 61–73.

Neary, D., Snowden, J.S. & Mann, D.M.A. (1993). Familial progressive aphasia: its relationship to other forms of lobar atrophy. *Journal of Neurology Neurosurgery and Psychiatry*, **56**, 1122–1125.

Nebes, R.D. (1992). Semantic memory dysfunction in Alzheimer's disease: disruption of semantic knowledge or information-processing limitation? In L.R. Squire & N. Butters (eds), *Neuropsychology of Memory*, 2nd edn. New York: Guilford.

Nebes, R.D. & Brady, C.B. (1988). Integrity of semantic fields in Alzheimer's disease. *Cortex*, **24**, 291–300.

Nebes, R.D. & Brady, C. B. (1989). Focused and divided attention in Alzheimer's disease. *Cortex*, **25**, 305–315.

Norman, D.A. & Shallice, T. (1980). *Attention to Action: Willed and Automatic Control of Behavior.* CHIP Report No. 99. San Diego, CA: University of California.

Ouchi, Y., Nobezawa, S., Okada, B.A. et al. (1998). Altered glucose metabolism in the hippocampal head in memory impairment. *Neurology*, **51**, 136–142.

Pepin, E.P. & Eslinger, P.J. (1989). Verbal memory decline in Alzheimer's disease: a multiple-process deficit. *Neurology*, **39**(1477–1482).

Perry, R.J. & Hodges, J.R. (1996). Spectrum of memory dysfunction in degenerative disease. *Current Opinion in Neurology*, **9**, 281–285.

Petersen, R.C., Smith, G.E., Waring, S.C. et al. (1999). Mild cognitive impairment: clinical characterization and outcome. *Archives of Neurology*, **56**, 303–308.

Posner, M.I. & Petersen, S.E. (1990). The attention system of the human brain. *Annual Review of Neuroscience*, **13**, 25–42.

Rombouts, S.A., Barkhof, F., Veltman, D.J. et al. (2000). Functional MR imaging in Alzheimer's disease during memory encoding. *American Journal of Neuroradiology*, **21**(10), 1869–1875.

Salmon, D.P., Galasko, D., Hansen, L.A. et al. (1996). Neuropsychological deficits associated with diffuse Lewy body disease. *Brain and Cognition*, **31**(2), 148–165.

Salthouse, T.A. & Becker, J.T. (1998). Independent effects of Alzheimer's disease on neuropsychological functioning. *Neuropsychology*, **12**(2), 242–252.

Saykin, A.J., Flashman, L.A., Frutiger, S.A. et al. (1999a). Neuroanatomic substrates of semantic memory impairment in Alzheimer's disease: patterns of functional fMRI activation. *Journal of the International Neuropsychological Society*, **5**, 377–392.

Saykin, A.J., Johnson, S.C., Flashman, L.A. et al. (1999b). Functional differentiation of medial temporal and frontal regions involved in processing novel and familiar words: an fMRI study. *Brain*, **122**, 1963–1971.

Schacter, D.L., Curran, T., Reiman, E.M. et al. (1999). Medial temporal lobe activation during episodic encoding and retrieval: a PET study. *Hippocampus*, **9**(5), 575–581.

Shallice, T. & Warrington, E.K. (1970). Independent functioning of verbal memory stores: a neuropsychological study. *Quarterly Journal of Experimental Psychology*, **22**, 261–273.

Snowden, J.S., Neary, D., Mann, D.M.A. et al. (1992). Progressive language disorder due to lobar atrophy. *Annals of Neurology*, **31**, 174–183.

Sowell, E.R., Thompson, P.M., Holmes, C.J. et al. (1999). *In vivo* evidence for post-adolescent brain maturation in frontal and striatal regions. *Nature Neuroscience*, **2**(10), 859–861.

Squire, L.R. (1992). Memory and the hippocampus: a synthesis from findings with rats, monkeys, and humans. *Psychological Review*, **99**, 195–231.

Squire, L.R. & Zola-Morgan, S. (1991). The medial temporal lobe system. *Science*, **253**, 1380–1386.

Stout, J.C., Bondi, M.W., Jernigan, T.L. et al. (1999). Regional cerebral volume loss associated with verbal learning and memory in dementia of the Alzheimer type. *Neuropsychology*, **13**(2), 188–197.

Thomas, G., Hostetter, G. & Barker, D.J. (1968). Behavioral function of the limbic system. In E. Stellar & J.M. Sprague (eds), *Progress in Physiological Psychology*, Vol. 2. New York: Academic Press.

Troster, A.I., Butters, N., Salmon, D.P. et al. (1993). The diagnostic utility of savings scores: differentiating Alzheimer's and Huntington's diseases with the Logical Memory and Visual Reproduction tests. *Journal of Clinical and Experimental Neuropsychology*, **15**(5), 773–788.

Troster, A.L., Salmon, D.P., McCullough, D. & Butters, N. (1989). A comparison of category fluency deficits associated with Alzheimer's and Huntington's disease. *Brain and Language*, **37**, 500–513.

Tulving, E. (1972). Episodic and semantic memory. In E. Tulving & W. Donaldson (eds), *Organization of Memory*. New York: Academic Press.

Tulving, E. (1984). Relations among components and processes of memory. *Behavior and Brain Science*, **1**, 257–268.

Tulving, E. (1987). Multiple memory systems and consciousness. *Human Neurobiology*, **6**, 67–80.

Vallar, G. & Baddeley, A.D. (1984). Fractionation of working memory: neuropsychological evidence for a phonological short-term store. *Journal of Verbal Learning and Verbal Behavior*, **23**, 151–161.

Vandenberghe, R., Price, C., Wise, R. et al. (1996). Functional anatomy of a common semantic system for words and pictures. *Nature*, **383**, 254–256.

Victor, M., Adams, R. D. & Collins, G. H. (1971). *The Wernicke–Korsakoff Syndrome*. Philadelphia, PA: Davis.

Wagner, A.D., Schacter, D.L., Rotte, M. et al. (1998). Building memories: remembering and forgetting of verbal experiences as predicted by brain activity. *Science*, **281**(5380), 1188–1191.

Wechsler, D. (1945). A standardized memory scale for memory use. *Journal of Psychology*, **19**, 87–95.

Weigl, E. (1927). On the psychology of so-called process of abstraction. *Journal of Abnormal Social Psychology*, **36**, 3–33.

Welsh, K., Butters, N., Hughes, J. (1991). Detection of abnormal memory decline in mild cases of Alzheimer's disease using CERAD neuropsychological measures. *Archives of Neurology*, **48**, 278–281.

Welsh, K.A., Butters, N., Hughes, J.P. (1992). Detection and staging of dementia in Alzheimer's disease: use of neuropsychological measures developed for the consortium to establish a registry for Alzheimer's disease. *Archives of Neurology*, **49**, 448–452.

Whitehouse, P.J. (1986). The concept of subcortical and cortical dementia: another look. *Annals of Neurology*, **19**, 1–6.

Williams, R.N., MacIntosh, D.E., Eells, G.T. (1996). Neuropsychological subgroups of dementia of the Alzheimer's type. *International Journal of Neuroscience*, **87**(1–2), 79–90.

Wilson, R.S., Bacon, L.D. & Fox, J.H. (1983a). Primary memory and secondary memory in dementia of the Alzheimer type. *Journal of Clinical and Experimental Neuropsychology*, **5**(4), 337–344.

Wilson, R.S., Bacon, L.D. & Fox, S.H. & Kaszniak, A.W. (1983b). Word frequency effect and recognition memory in dementia of the Alzheimer type. *Journal of Clinical and Experimental Neuropsychology*, **5**, 97–104.

Wilson, R.S., Kaszniak, A.W., Bacon, L.D. et al. (1982). Facial recognition memory in dementia. *Cortex*, **18**, 329–336.

Zelkowicz, B.J., Herbster, A.N., Nebes, R.D. et al. (1997). An examination of regional cerebral blood flow during object naming tasks. *Journal of the International Neuropsychological Society*, **4**, 160–166.

CHAPTER 7

Memory Disorders in Subcortical Dementia

Jason Brandt

and

Cynthia A. Munro

Johns Hopkins University School of Medicine, Baltimore, MD, USA

Contemporary discussions of "subcortical dementia" often cite the work of Albert et al. (1974) on progressive supranuclear palsy and/or McHugh & Folstein (1975) on Huntington's disease as the origin of the concept. However, descriptions of what would come to be known as *subcortical dementia* actually appeared in the medical literature at least as early as the mid-nineteenth century (Mandell & Albert, 1990). The term itself was not coined until 1932, when "subcorticale demenz" was used to describe the cognitive impairments associated with encephalitis (von Stockert, 1932). Thus, research on subcortical dementia may have a short history, but the concept has a long past.

Subcortical dementia is a neuropsychological/neuropsychiatric syndrome. It consists of slowed mentation (bradyphrenia), sustained attention and working memory deficits, forgetfulness, impaired planning and judgment, and changes in drive and/or mood states (with apathy, irritability and depression being most common). Because subcortical dementia is usually seen in diseases that also feature prominent movement disorders, dysarthric speech and psychomotor slowing, and problems with motor set acquisition and switching are typically seen as well. In contrast to the clinical presentation of cortical dementia (the prototype of which is seen in Alzheimer's disease), frank aphasia, apraxia, agnosia and amnesia are rare (Lovell & Smith, 1997; Darvesh & Freedman, 1996; Cummings & Benson, 1984).

Almost since its reintroduction a quarter-century ago, the term "subcortical dementia" has been the subject of controversy. In fact, criticisms of the concept are so widespread that virtually every time the term appears in the literature, its authors seem almost apologetic and justify using the term by appealing to its history and its clinical usefulness. Opponents of the concept argue that describing some dementia syndromes as "cortical" and others as "subcortical" ignores the fact that subcortical nuclei and pathways are affected in diseases like Alzheimer's disease (AD) and, conversely, that cortical changes are seen in conditions like Huntington's disease (HD) and Parkinson's disease (PD) (Whitehouse, 1986). Furthermore, even if the neuropathology of so-called subcortical dementias were confined

The Essential *Handbook of Memory Disorders for Clinicians*. Edited by A.D. Baddeley, M.D. Kopelman and B.A. Wilson.
© 2004 John Wiley & Sons, Ltd. ISBN 0-470-09141-X.

to specific striatal, thalamic, cerebellar or brainstem nuclei, the cognitive impairments may be a manifestation of impaired cortical activity via the disruption of corticostriatothalamocortical circuits (Crosson, 1992; Domesick, 1990). Accordingly, the term "subcortical dementia", as used in this chapter, should not be interpreted literally. It should be construed as a clinical entity found most prominently in diseases with severe subcortical neuropathology, and not as a precisely specified, anatomically delimited entity (Cohen & Freedman, 1995; Cummings, 1993).

CONCEPTUAL AND METHODOLOGICAL ISSUES IN STUDYING MEMORY IN SUBCORTICAL DEMENTIA

Definition of Dementia

To appreciate what the existing literature does and does not reveal about memory impairments in subcortical dementia, a number of conceptual issues need to be considered. The first of these is the very definition of "dementia". The *Diagnostic and Statistical Manual of Mental Disorders* (DSM-IV) criteria for dementia require impairment in memory and at least one other cognitive domain, as well as impairment in social or occupational functioning (American Psychiatric Association, 1994). Whereas the requirement of disordered memory is quite appropriate for the dementia of AD, it may not be appropriate for diseases of subcortical brain structures. Much neuropsychological evidence (discussed later in this chapter) suggests that impaired performance on tests of new learning and episodic recall in subcortical dementia are not due to failures in memory encoding and storage, but rather are attributable to deficits in attention or central executive functions. Thus, one might argue that memory *per se* is less clearly affected in these conditions, and therefore the diagnosis of "dementia" might not be appropriate.

Another problem with the DSM-IV definition of *dementia* concerns the criterion of impaired social or occupational functioning. If a disease affecting subcortical structures causes impairment in everyday functioning, but this impairment is due to a movement disorder rather than cognitive deficits, is the diagnosis of dementia appropriate? For example, PD, by virtue of its motor features, causes clear impairment in social and/or occupational functioning. Although there may be pervasive cognitive deficits in PD, these are often mild and, in and of themselves, might not impair social/occupational functioning. Is it legitimate to diagnose very mild dementia in such patients, even if daily functioning is not yet affected or is impaired only by bradykinesia? Finally, requiring that social role functioning be impaired for the diagnosis of dementia complicates empirical investigation of the differential impact of various dementias on individuals, families, organizations and society.

Severity of Dementia and Group Matching

A second conceptual and methodological issue that needs to be addressed when studying memory (or any other cognitive) impairment across dementia syndromes is that of matching individuals or groups for overall severity of dementia. In order to conclude that a particular aspect of memory is differentially impaired in one patient population compared to another (i.e. that there is a *selective* deficit), one must eliminate the possibility that one patient group is simply more impaired overall (i.e. that there is a *generalized* deficit). How one accomplishes this is not a simple matter. Matching study groups for mean score and variance on the Mini-Mental State Exam (MMSE) (Folstein et al., 1975) is problematic because the test has a heavy language loading and is known to be relatively insensitive to the subcortical dementias (Rothlind & Brandt, 1993; Brandt, 1994). As a result, it is difficult to construct groups with AD and HD, for example, matched for MMSE score. Any such groups will consist of very early AD patients and very advanced HD patients (e.g. Brandt et al., 1992). The Dementia Rating Scale (DRS) (Mattis, 1988) has also been used for this purpose (e.g. Heindel et al., 1989; Paulsen et al., 1995) and is subject to the same limitations. Matching groups on functional disability is an alternative strategy but is likely to yield very mildly impaired subcortical dementia patients, since movement disorders are typically a major source of their disability.

Rather than attempt group matching, many studies have dealt with differences between groups by using statistical procedures (e.g. analysis of covariance) to "correct" for nuisance variables. These approaches are also problematic for a variety of technical reasons (Adams et al., 1985). In addition, they have the potential to create groups that simply do not exist in nature.

Disease Heterogeneity

A third issue to consider in discussions of subcortical dementia is disease heterogeneity. Although the bulk of research on subcortical dementia has been in HD and PD, more than a dozen disorders, each with a unique morbid anatomy and physiology, have been described as causing this syndrome. Grouping all these disorders under the single category "subcortical dementia" is likely to obfuscate important differences among them (Pillon et al., 1991). In addition, there is significant heterogeneity *within* clinically defined disease entities. For example, among patients with Wilson's disease there may be at least two distinct subtypes—those who have neurological deficits and dementia and those who do not—that may reflect genuine biological subtypes (i.e. different genotypes). Among the spinocerebellar ataxias, at least 12 genetically distinct subtypes have been identified. Several of these have neuropathology extending beyond the cerebellum, and almost all of them produce some cognitive changes of the subcortical type. Identifying the sources of such heterogeneity is a major task for the clinical neurosciences in the twenty-first century.

SPECIFIC DISORDERS CAUSING SUBCORTICAL DEMENTIA

Disorders of the Basal Ganglia

The basal ganglia consist of the striatum (caudate nucleus and putamen) and globus pallidus. Since these forebrain nuclei have intricately-patterned connections to many other brain regions, many authors include highly interrelated structures, especially the subthalamic nucleus and substantia nigra, in discussions of the basal ganglia.

Through their interconnections with thalamic, cerebellar and cortical motor areas, the basal ganglia are thought to modulate movement (Benecke et al., 1987; Middleton & Strick, 2000). As such, diseases of the basal ganglia, including HD, basal ganglia calcification, neuroacanthocytosis and Wilson's disease, typically present with movement disorders. Only more recently have the interconnections of basal ganglia with association cortices, and their implications for memory and cognition, been appreciated.

Huntington's Disease

This inherited neurodegenerative disease is characterized by the full "subcortical triad" of movement disorder, dementia and emotional disorder (McHugh, 1989). The onset of HD is insidious, with symptoms typically emerging between ages 35 and 45 (Folstein, 1989). Involuntary movements of the upper limbs and face are often early signs, progressing to more generalized choreic and athetoid movements. Neuropathologically, the disease is characterized by neuronal death in the head of the caudate nucleus and putamen, progressing in later stages to the cerebral cortex (Vonsattel et al., 1985).

Memory functioning in HD has been the focus of numerous investigations, and several consistent findings have emerged. First, at any given level of dementia (defined by MMSE or DRS), episodic memory appears to be less severely impaired in HD than in AD (Brandt et al., 1988; Salmon et al., 1989). Second, HD patients typically have impairments in retrieval (i.e. the organization and execution of effortful memory search) that are manifest most clearly on tests of free recall. This contrasts with their normal, or near-normal, performance on tests of yes/no or multiple-choice recognition (Butters et al., 1978; Caine et al., 1978; Pillon et al., 1993; Rohrer et al., 1999; Weingartner et al., 1979). A comparison of 23 patients with HD and 23 with AD, equated for total score on the DRS, found performance on the Memory subtest of the DRS to be worse in AD and performance on the Initiation/Perseveration subtest to be worse in HD (Salmon et al., 1989). This was later found to be the case even for patients with advanced dementia (Paulsen et al., 1995). Pillon et al. (1993) found that the memory performance of HD patients was more highly correlated with performance on tests of executive function (including the Initiation subtest of the DRS, Wisconsin Card Sorting Test, and initial letter fluency) than was the case in AD. Pillon and associates concluded that the learning and memory deficit of HD patients may be more apparent than real.

Another consistent finding in HD is a deficit in particular types of perceptual and motor learning. In one of the first studies exploring these phenomena, Martone et al. (1984) administered a task requiring the rapid reading of mirror-reversed words to patients with HD and amnesic patients with alcoholic Korsakoff syndrome. Subjects were administered this task three times, one day apart, with a recognition trial administered following the last trial. The Korsakoff amnesics demonstrated normal ability to learn the skill of mirror reading, but were severely impaired on the recognition portion of the task. In contrast, HD patients exhibited normal word recognition, but had much slower rates of perceptual skill acquisition. Defects in perceptual adaptation have also been demonstrated in HD (Heindel et al., 1991; Paulsen et al., 1993).

Heindel et al. (1988) compared procedural learning (using the pursuit rotor task) and declarative learning (using the Verbal Recognition Span Test; Moss et al., 1986) in HD and AD. The HD patients were severely impaired on the pursuit rotor task, improving much less over learning trials than did the AD patients. In contrast, the HD group's performance was superior to that of the AD group on the verbal recognition span test. These findings support a role for the striatum in motor skill learning, a system dissociable from the temporal–limbic explicit memory system impaired in AD.

Gabrieli et al. (1997) examined procedural learning in HD using two psychomotor tasks. HD patients performed worse than a normal control group on the pursuit rotor task; however, they performed as well as the normal subjects on a mirror-tracing task. The authors concluded that the basal ganglia, affected in HD, are involved in the learning of repetitive motor sequences (as on the rotary pursuit task) but not with the learning of new mappings between visual cues and motor responses (as on the mirror-tracing task). Several studies further specify the motor learning deficit in HD as involving impaired ability to benefit from the predictability of movement sequences (Bylsma et al., 1990; Brandt, 1994; Knopman & Nissen, 1991; Willingham et al., 1996).

Basal Ganglia Calcification

This syndrome, first described in the mid-nineteenth century (Delacour, 1850; cited in Klein & Vieregge, 1998), is characterized by parkinsonian symptoms as well as seizures, ataxia and dementia. Basal ganglia calcification (BGC) can be caused by a number of conditions, including anoxia, radiation, infections and metabolic disturbances (Lopez-Villegas et al., 1996). Idiopathic BGC, also known as Fahr's disease, is usually familial and is associated with dementia and schizophreniform psychosis (Cummings et al., 1983). Neuropathologically, BGC is characterized by mineral deposits in the putamen, globus pallidus, thalamus, corona radiata, cerebellar dentate nuclei and cerebellar white matter (Hier & Cummings, 1990).

In the few studies on cognition in BGC, deficits are usually found on tests of memory, visuospatial processing and aspects of executive function (Lopez-Villegas et al., 1996; Cummings et al., 1983). In the most comprehensive studies to date, Lopez-Villegas et al. (1996) compared the performance of 18 BGC patients to that of 16 normal control subjects matched for age, education, sex and estimated premorbid IQ on a battery of neuropsychological tests. The BGC patients performed worse than the control subjects on several tests of motor skills and executive functions. Memory was assessed with the Visual Reproduction subtest of the Wechsler Memory Scale, the multiple-choice version of the Benton Visual Retention Test, the Rey Auditory Verbal Learning Test (RAVLT), the Digit Span subtest from the Wechsler Adult Intelligence Scale, the Corsi span test, and 30-min recall of the Rey Complex Figure Test. Only degree of improvement over the five learning trials of the RAVLT differed between the patient and control groups. Lopez-Villegas et al. (1996) concluded that the memory impairment of BGC is characterized by poor free recall with relative preservation of recognition. Furthermore, they conceptualized this memory deficit as based on dysfunction of the frontal-subcortical circuits that impair retrieval, and noted that this pattern is similar to that observed among patients with other basal ganglia diseases. To explore the possibility of subtypes of BCG, the researchers stratified the patients by presence/absence of neurological signs (seizures, parkinsonism, dysarthria, and orthostatic hypotension), presumed etiology, and extent of calcification (i.e. limited to the putamen and globus pallidus, or more widespread). There were few meaningful differences in cognition between these subgroups of BCG and the sample as a whole.

Neuroacanthocytosis

This rare, presumably autosomal-recessive degenerative disorder is clinically and pathologically similar to HD. The disease usually first presents at ages 30–50 years. It is characterized
by choreiform movements but can often be distinguished from HD by its prominent orofacial
dyskinesia, including involuntary vocalizations and biting of the lips and tongue (Quinn &
Schrag, 1998; Kutcher et al., 1999). Pathologically, neuroacanthocytosis (NA) is associated
with neuronal loss in the caudate, putamen, pallidum and substantia nigra, without involvement of the locus coeruleus, cerebral cortex, brainstem or cerebellum (Hardie et al., 1991;
Brooks et al, 1991; Rinne et al., 1994).

Only a single study could be found that attempted to identify the cognitive profile of
patients with NA. In a chart review of 10 NA patients who received neuropsychological
assessments, Kartsounis & Hardie (1996) found that all 10 had evidence of executive dysfunction (measured by various tests considered to be sensitive to frontal lobe dysfunction),
whereas only half demonstrated memory impairment. The latter was assessed using the
Recognition Memory Test (Warrington, 1984) and a three-choice test of recognition memory (Warrington, 1995, unpublished data). Because patients' memories were tested only
with recognition procedures, it cannot be determined whether NA patients, like those with
other subcortical dementias, would have greater impairments in free recall.

Wilson's Disease

Also known as progressive hepatolenticular degeneration, Wilson's disease (WD) is inherited as an autosomal recessive trait. It is caused by a mutated gene on chromosome 13 that
results in the absence of a copper-carrying protein, resulting in copper deposits in the liver,
cornea and basal ganglia (Scheinberg & Sternlieb, 1984; Wilson, 1912). Clinically, WD
patients may be neurologically asymptomatic. When they do display symptoms, dysarthria,
flapping tremor, rigidity, drooling, gait disturbance and bradykinesia are common (Hefter
et al., 1993; Lang et al., 1990).

Brain-imaging studies in WD often reveal focal abnormalities in the brainstem, white
matter and subcortical nuclei. Bilaterally symmetrical changes in the basal ganglia, particularly the putamen, are common, as is some degree of cortical atrophy (Hefter et al.,
1993; Chen et al., 1983; Williams & Walshe, 1981). Neuropathological studies have found
accumulations of copper in the striatum and globus pallidus (Scheinberg & Sternlieb, 1984).
Vascular changes, including perivascular thickening in the basal ganglia, have also been
found (Scheinberg & Sternlieb, 1984).

Whether the cognitive deficits that accompany WD constitute a full-blown dementia is
a matter of some debate (cf. Lang, 1989; Medalia, 1991). In his original description of
the condition, Wilson (1912) noted mental status changes and a "narrowing of the mental
horizons", but did not believe that his patients were "demented" (Hier & Cummings, 1990).
In a report on 31 WD patients, Starosta-Rubenstein et al. (1987) commented that dementia
was "rare", although neither the exact prevalence nor the way in which dementia was
assessed was reported. Lang (1989) reported no memory impairment in his sample of 15 WD
patients, whereas Medalia (1991) maintains that memory impairment is common, at least
among those with other signs of neurologic involvement. The cognitive impairments in WD

have been shown to lessen following treatment with penicillamine, a copper-chelating agent (Hach & Hartung, 1979; Lang et al., 1990).

Because cognitive impairment seems to occur only among those who have other neurological signs of the illness (Lang, 1989; Medalia, 1991), most studies categorize patients into those with and without such signs (Medalia et al., 1988; Isaacs-Glaberman et al., 1989). In spite of this, there appears to be little correlation between the severity of neurological deficits and cognitive impairments, except for the effect of motor performance on neuropsychological test performance (Medalia, 1991). Performance on tests of memory, for example, is generally not correlated with the extent of neurological impairment (Medalia, 1991).

Medalia et al. (1992) administered a battery of neuropsychological tests to 31 patients with WD and reported the number of patients who fell below established cutoffs on the tests. Among the 12 neurologically asymptomatic WD patients, two (16%) had performances below the cutoff for impairment on the DRS and the Rey Auditory Verbal Learning Test, and three (25%) were impaired on the Trail Making Test. Roughly 30% of the 19 neurologically symptomatic patients were impaired on every test in the battery (Medalia et al., 1992).

Among neurologically symptomatic WD patients, motor slowing and memory deficits are the most common findings (Isaacs-Glaberman et al., 1989). Memory impairment has been demonstrated on tests of free recall for short stories, list of words and geometric designs (Rosselli, 1987). Isaacs-Glaberman et al. (1989) administered the RAVLT to 19 neurologically symptomatic WD patients and 15 normal control subjects. The patients recalled fewer words than the control group on the RAVLT, but performed as well as the control group on the recognition trial. On other memory tests, the WD patients demonstrated normal rates of learning and forgetting and were aided by recognition cues. These findings, combined with the patients' impaired performance on a word list generation task, led the authors to conclude that the memory deficit in WD is due to a retrieval deficit. The qualitative similarities in memory characteristics between patients with WD and those with HD are obvious.

Disorders of Brainstem Nuclei

Parkinson's Disease

First described by James Parkinson in 1817, PD is one of the earliest characterized neurodegenerative diseases affecting primarily subcortical brain areas. Despite its long recognition by the medical and scientific communities, its etiology remains incompletely understood. Abnormalities of movement, primarily resting tremor, stooped and unstable posture, rigidity and slowness, are the most common, and typically the earliest, manifestations of PD. Onset of PD is typically at age 40–70, with average age of onset in the 50s (Freedman, 1990). Neuropathologic studies reveal loss of dopamine-producing neurons and the presence of Lewy bodies in the substantia nigra and locus coeruleus. Dopamine depletions in the head of the caudate nucleus and the frontal cortex are common (Kish et al., 1986; Kish et al., 1988a). Neuronal loss is also frequently seen in the nucleus basalis of Meynert, a major source of cholinergic innervation to the forebrain (Adams & Victor, 1985; Whitehouse et al., 1982).

A relatively consistent finding in early studies comparing memory in PD to that in HD is that PD patients are less severely impaired on tests of word list recall and recognition (Drebing et al., 1993; Caine et al., 1977; Fisher et al., 1983; Kramer et al., 1989). Several of these studies could be criticized, however, for neglecting to match patient groups for age, sex, presumed premorbid intelligence and other factors that influence verbal memory performance. To remedy this, Massman et al. (1990) compared well-matched groups of PD patients, HD patients and normal control subjects on the California Verbal Learning Test (CVLT). Immediate recall (Trial 1 of List A) did not differ between the HD and PD groups, but both were worse than the control group. However, rate of learning over trials was significantly higher in PD than in HD. Performance of the PD group was also better than that of the HD group on the delayed recall trials. The yes/no recognition performance of both groups was mildly impaired. These results led Massman et al. to conclude that verbal memory in PD is characterized by a retrieval deficit that is less severe than that seen in HD, but not qualitatively different.

As in HD, there are selective impairments in procedural learning and implicit memory in PD (Saint-Cyr et al., 1988; Harrington et al., 1990; Heindel et al., 1989). Harrington et al. (1990) found PD patients to be impaired in learning the pursuit rotor task, but normal on a more perceptually-based implicit memory task (reading mirror-reversed text). Bondi & Kazniak (1991) also found PD patients to perform normally in reading mirror-reversed text, but their patients, carefully screened for the absence of frank dementia, also improved at a normal rate over trials on the pursuit rotor task. A selective impairment on a perceptual learning task (fragmented pictures) was the only implicit memory deficit that could be discerned.

In an attempt to further characterize the motor-learning deficit in PD, Haaland et al. (1997) compared the performance of 40 patients with PD to 30 normal control subjects on the pursuit rotor task. Patients were assigned to one of two conditions. In one condition, the speed of the rotating target varied randomly across trials. In the other condition, speed was fixed within blocks of trials and varied across blocks. The PD patients were impaired only in the variable speed condition of this task. The authors concluded that PD patients display their procedural learning deficit only when required to rapidly adjust their motor programming to changing environmental demands.

Progressive Supranuclear Palsy

Progressive supranuclear palsy (PSP) is a rare degenerative disorder of unknown etiology. Also known as Steele–Richardson–Olszewski syndrome, PSP was first described as a distinct disorder in the mid-1960s (Steele et al., 1964). The disease is characterized by parkinsonism, including axial rigidity, gait disturbance, bradykinesia and profound ophthalmoplegia, but absent a resting tremor. Neuropathological changes associated with PSP include neurofibrillary tangles in the basal ganglia, brainstem and cerebellar nuclei (Steele et al., 1964). PSP is perhaps the prototypical subcortical dementia, as the cerebral cortex appears to remain intact even late in the course of the disease (Jellinger & Bancher, 1992). Structural brain imaging studies are often normal (Grafman et al., 1990; Zakzanis et al., 1998), but sometimes reveal midbrain atrophy (Soliveri et al., 1999). PET imaging often shows hypometabolism in the frontal lobes, presumably due to disrupted subcortical projections (Blin et al., 1992).

Whether PSP is invariably associated with memory impairment has not been firmly established. A review of early clinical descriptions led Albert and colleagues (1974) to conclude that there is indeed a "dementia" in this illness, but also that "memory as such may not be truly impaired" (p. 126). Grafman et al. (1990) found that scores on the Wechsler Memory Scale (WMS; Wechsler, 1945) were lower among 12 PSP patients than among 12 normal control subjects. The authors attributed the deficits to deficient subcortical input to the frontal lobes. In this study, however, the memory scores of both the patient and control groups were consistent with their IQ scores. Thus, it is difficult to make the case for a selective memory impairment in the PSP group.

Milberg & Albert (1989) studied nine PSP patients and compared them to 16 patients with AD and 23 normal control subjects. They found no impairment in the PSP group on tests of new learning and memory (Logical Memory and Visual Reproduction subtests of the WMS) or semantic memory (Boston Naming Test; Kaplan et al., 1983). Van der Hurk & Hodges (1995) also found that episodic memory, measured by the Logical Memory subtest of the WMS and the word list learning task from the CERAD battery (Welsh et al., 1994), was preserved in PSP. However, they found that semantic memory, assessed with the Synonym Judgment subtest of the Action for Dysphasic Adults Battery (Franklin et al., 1992) and the Pyramids and Palm Trees Test (Howard & Patterson, 1982), was as impaired in PSP as it was in AD. The authors attempted to reconcile their findings with those of Milberg & Albert (1989) by suggesting that their patients were more cognitively impaired overall. A comparison of total DRS scores between the two studies, however, reveals that is not the case. Patient heterogeneity and/or differences in the sensitivity of the semantic memory tests used are likely sources of the discrepant findings. Nevertheless, van der Hurk & Hodges (1995) suggested that the difficulty with semantic memory among those with PSP is not due to a loss of stored information as it is in AD. Rather, they posited faulty retrieval due to a functional deactivation of the prefrontal cortex caused by subcortical pathology.

In a truly comparative neuropsychological study of subcortical dementia, Pillon et al. (1994) compared 15 patients with PSP to equal numbers of PD, HD and AD patients as well as 19 normal control subjects. Although a few minor differences among the three subcortical groups were found on the CVLT and the Grober–Buschke category-cued recall test (Grober et al., 1988), the authors concluded that, "their [the groups'] similarities . . . are more impressive than their differences . . . ".

After conducting a meta-analysis of 23 studies of PSP published between 1984 and 1997, Zakzanis et al. (1998) concluded that memory impairment is not a "core" feature of PSP. Rather, they maintained, the disease is characterized primarily by impaired ability to manipulate acquired knowledge and to process information rapidly, resulting in a sluggish and inefficient memory system.

Disorders of Thalamic Nuclei

Thalamic Degeneration

Selective thalamic degeneration is a rapidly progressing disorder, which can be inherited as an autosomal dominant trait (Lugaresi et al., 1986). It appears to be an extremely rare condition, with fewer than 50 cases reported worldwide. Neuropathological studies reveal degeneration almost exclusively in the anterior and dorsomedial nuclei of the thalamus (Lugaresi et al., 1986), with up to 90% reduction in cell counts.

Because of its rarity, thalamic degeneration has been the focus of very few neuropsychological or neuropsychiatric studies. The few that exist describe profound apathy, psychomotor retardation, deficits in attention and concentration, and forgetfulness, without aphasia, apraxia or agnosia (McDaniel, 1990). In other words, the picture appears to be one of classic subcortical dementia.

The rapidity with which the thalamic degeneration progresses, coupled with its attendant profound deficits in arousal and attention, render formal neuropsychological study of these patients difficult. A single report of three patients with familial thalamic degeneration is perhaps the most comprehensive attempt to date to characterize the cognitive abilities in this disorder (Gallassi et al., 1992). In this study, repeated cognitive assessments were conducted on each patient, but the tests administered varied among them. In general, immediate and short-term memory were less impaired than was memory after a delay. Verbal memory was deficient relatively early in the course of the disease, whereas spatial memory did not become impaired until later. Finally, tests of semantic memory and procedural memory were performed normally. The authors attributed the memory impairment of these patients to deficits in the encoding and manipulation of information and in the ordering of events. They concluded that the primary neuropsychological deficits in thalamic degeneration are in attention, working memory and planning, with preservation of memory stores.

Disorders of Cerebral White Matter

Ischemic Vascular Disease

Small vessel disease in the periventricular and deep white matter can produce cognitive impairment (Libon et al., 1993; Rao, 1996). Ischemic vascular disease (IVD) is a subtype of vascular dementia (VaD), a category that also includes multi-infarct dementia and strategic single-infarct dementia (Román et al., 1993). Included under the classification of IVD is Binswanger's disease, a disorder characterized by numerous areas of demyelination and infarction in the cerebral white matter.

In one of the early neuropsychological studies of IVD, Kertesz et al. (1990) compared the MRI findings and cognitive functioning of 11 VaD patients, 27 AD patients and 15 control subjects. The patient groups were matched for DRS scores. Fewer than half (11 of 27) of the AD patients had white matter changes, compared to eight of the 11 VaD patients. Scores on the Logical Memory, Visual Reproduction and Paired Associates subtests of the WMS were all higher among patients with white matter changes than in those without, regardless of diagnosis. In contrast, scores on attention and comprehension tests were worse in those with periventricular hyperintensities. This general finding, that subcortical hyperintensities are associated with better memory performance but poorer executive control, has since been replicated (Libon et al., 1997). A similar study by Bernard et al. (1990) found that patients with Binswanger's disease performed better than DRS-matched AD patients on a verbal recognition memory test, but worse on a conceptual reasoning task.

Lafosse et al. (1997) compared 32 IVD patients to an equal number of AD patients, matched for dementia severity by MMSE scores, on performance on the Memory Assessment Scale (MAS) (Williams, 1991). The IVD group performed better on delayed free recall, produced fewer intrusions on the cued recall trial, and had better recognition discrimination than the AD patients. The authors highlighted the much better score of the IVD group on recognition compared to free recall, and attributed this to retrieval difficulties. Among the IVD patients, greater white matter abnormalities were associated with poorer free recall, whereas ventricular enlargement was related to poorer delayed cued recall. In a very similar investigation, Libon et al. (1997) compared CVLT performance of 33 AD and 27 IVD patients, matched on MMSE score. Although the groups did not differ in immediate free recall (measured by trials 1–5 of list A and list B), differences were found on delayed free recall, cued recall and recognition, with the IVD group faring better in all cases. Libon et al. concluded that the memory performance in IVD could be distinguished from that of AD, and is qualitatively similar to that seen in PD and HD.

Reed et al. (2000) compared regional glucose metabolism using PET in IVD and AD during a continuous recognition memory task. Fifteen AD patients and 15 IVD patients, matched for MMSE score, identified visually-presented words as "old" or "new", depending whether they had seen the words before. Performance on the task was worse in both patient groups than in normal subjects but the IVD and AD groups did not differ from each other. Lower metabolism in the prefrontal cortex was associated with the memory impairment in IVD but not AD, whereas lower metabolism in the left hippocampus and left medial temporal gyrus was associated with memory impairment in AD but not IVD. Because the continuous recognition task requires both working and episodic memory, the authors concluded that the frontal dysfunction observed in IVD impairs the task via its effects on attention, working memory or other executive abilities.

To determine whether a double dissociation between IVD and AD could be elicited from a comparison of declarative and procedural memory performance, Libon et al. (1998) used methodology borrowed from Butters et al. (1990). They compared 16 AD patients to 14 IVD patients, matched for disease severity by MMSE score, on the CVLT and the pursuit rotor learning task. There was no difference between groups on CVLT free recall (trials 1–5 on list A), but the IVD group made fewer intrusion errors and had better recognition discrimination. In contrast, the AD group outperformed the IVD group on the pursuit rotor task, as measured by both total time on target and slope of the learning curve over trials. Furthermore, severity of white matter pathology was associated with greater pursuit rotor learning impairment. Like HD patients, patients with IVD demonstrated impaired procedural learning on the pursuit rotor task, with preserved recognition (relative to free recall) on the CVLT (Libon et al., 1998).

Multiple Sclerosis

The cognitive characteristics of multiple sclerosis (MS) have been described since the nineteenth century (Peyser & Poser, 1986; Rao, 1990). While the cause of MS remains unknown, the neuropathology is well described. The disease consists of patchy areas of de-myelination in the cerebrum, brainstem, cerebellum and spinal cord (Rao, 1990). Selective degeneration of the corpus callosum has also been recognized (Brownell & Hughes, 1962). Extreme variability in clinical course distinguishes MS from most other subcortical diseases; symptoms can exacerbate and remit at unpredictable times and for unpredictable durations. Whereas some investigators have found more severe cognitive impairment in chronic-progressive MS than in relapsing–remitting MS (Heaton et al., 1985), this is not always the case (e.g. Beatty et al., 1990). In addition, no consistent relationship has been found between duration of illness and cognitive test performance (Ivnik, 1978; Rao et al., 1984).

Some type of memory impairment is often reported in patients with MS (Ruchkin et al., 1994). There is some debate, however, as to whether the memory impairment in MS is due to an encoding or a retrieval deficit (DeLuca et al., 1994; Arnett et al., 1997). Ruchkin et al. (1994) compared 10 patients with MS to 10 normal control subjects with the goal of identifying the neurophysiological substrate of working memory deficits. Although the groups did not differ significantly on most tests of episodic memory (Logical Memory, Visual Paired Associates, Visual Reproduction, and Digit Span from the WMS-R), the MS patients performed more poorly than the control group on the WAIS-R Digit Symbol subtest and articulation of irregular words. The authors interpreted these performance deficits as reflecting a defect in the phonological loop of the working memory system (Baddeley, 1986), though the sparing of digit span seems to contradict this. Furthermore, the authors suggested that this defect is related to the often-observed pathology in the corpus callosum in MS.

Wishart & Sharpe (1997) conducted a meta-analysis of 37 studies comparing the neuropsychological functioning of MS patients to that of normal control subjects conducted between 1974 and 1994. They found that no cognitive domains were spared in MS. Within the domain of memory, the effect sizes for visual and verbal learning were greater than for delayed visual recall and recognition. Additionally, the effect size for immediate recall of verbal information was larger than that for delayed recall of visual information. Taken together, these results suggest that recognition memory does appear to be affected in MS, although less so than free recall. Wishart & Sharpe also opined that the contribution of both processing speed and working memory must be considered in understanding the recognition failures in MS.

HIV-related Dementia

The neuropsychology of acquired immune deficiency syndrome (AIDS) is distinguished from that of other diseases associated with subcortical pathology by virtue of its youth; the first cases of AIDS were reported just two decades ago (Navia, 1990). In spite of this (or perhaps because of it), several different terms have been used to refer to cognitive impairment associated with the human immunodeficiency virus (HIV) and the resulting illness (AIDS). *AIDS dementia complex* (ADC) requires cognitive, motor and behavioral dysfunction (Navia et al., 1986b; Price, 1996), whereas a more recent term, *AIDS-related dementia* (ARD) refers to AIDS dementia without motor impairment (Price, 1996). Since there may be neurocognitive and neuromotor abnormalities in patients infected with the virus who do not meet clinical criteria for AIDS, the terms "HIV-related dementia" and "HIV-related cognitive impairment" may be preferred terms. Neuropathological studies of HIV-related dementia have found lesions in the basal ganglia, thalamus, brainstem and central periventricular white matter (Navia et al., 1986a; Lang et al., 1989). However, investigations of the effects of the HIV virus itself are complicated by the presence of opportunistic infections in AIDS.

Early in its course, HIV-related dementia produces impairments in sequential problem solving, fine manual dexterity and motor speed (summarized by Navia, 1990). Other studies find impairment on tests of executive function (Wisconsin Card Sorting Test), memory (Selective Reminding Test recall, but not recognition) and complex attention (Trail Making Test, Symbol Digit Modalities Test, Digit Span backwards) (Maruff et al., 1994). With disease progression, additional impairments are seen in word-list generation and constructional praxis, as well as more pervasive verbal and spatial memory deficits. Because HIV-related cognitive impairment has been shown to be more similar to that found in HD than AD, many consider it a subcortical dementia (Van Gorp et al., 1992). White et al. (1995) critically reviewed the literature on cognitive impairment in asymptomatic, HIV-seropositive persons, and concluded that these individuals have a rate of cognitive impairment three times that of seronegative control subjects.

Systemic Lupus Erythematosus

Systemic lupus erythematosus (SLE), or lupus, is an autoimmune disorder that affects multiple organ systems. First described by the French dermatologist Laurent Biett in 1833, the term "lupus erythemateux" was not introduced until almost 20 years later (Benedek, 1997). SLE can sometimes produce frank neurological and/or psychiatric signs, including stroke, seizures, sensory and motor neuropathies and psychosis, clearly indicating central nervous system involvement (Denburg & Denburg, 1999; Kozora et al., 1996; West, 1996). The presence of such neuropsychiatric signs reliably predicts cognitive impairment in SLE (Carlomagno et al., 2000; Kozora et al., 1998). However, even patients without such signs (i.e. "non-CNS" SLE) often complain of, and can have, significant cognitive impairment (Leritz et al., 2000; Denburg & Denburg, 1999).

Structural imaging studies of non-CNS SLE are often inconclusive, but some have revealed white matter lesions as well as increased ventricle:brain ratios (Chinn et al., 1997; Kozora et al., 1996). Functional imaging studies have proven more sensitive in detecting abnormalities associated with SLE, but their findings have been inconsistent with regard to the specific regions involved. SPECT studies, for example, have revealed hypometabolism in the basal ganglia and thalamus, but also in multiple regions of the neocortex (Kao et al., 1999; Falcini et al., 1998).

While some investigators have suggested that memory is particularly vulnerable in non-CNS SLE (Denburg & Denburg, 1999), others have found no memory impairment (Ginsburg et al., 1992; Skeel et al., 2000). Kozora et al. (1996) compared 51 patients with non-CNS SLE to 29 patients with rheumatoid arthritis (RA) and 27 healthy control subjects. RA is a well-suited clinical control group for SLE because it is rarely associated with CNS abnormalities. A comparable proportion of both patient groups (approximately 30%) demonstrated overall cognitive impairment, defined as scoring 2 SDs below the mean in at least two of eight cognitive domains. However, the proportion of patients who were impaired in the learning domain, assessed by the Story and Figure Memory Tests (Heaton et al., 1991) and the CVLT (Delis et al., 1987), was greater in SLE than in RA.

In one of the largest studies of its type, Denburg et al. (1997) investigated the relationship of antiphospholipid antibodies to cognitive function in 118 SLE patients with and without CNS signs and symptoms. Antiphospholipid antibodies are immunoglobulins in the bloodstream that react with specific fat molecules and predispose the patient to thromboembolic events. The authors found that roughly half of SLE patients testing positive for these antibodies demonstrated cognitive impairment (defined as having at least 3/18 cognitive summary scores below the 5th percentile), whereas only 25% of the antibody-negative patients were cognitively impaired. Presence of antibodies predicted cognitive impairment, even in non-CNS patients. Verbal memory, assessed with WMS Logical Memory and Paired-Associate Learning, and trials 1–5 of the RAVLT, was one of three domains in which the antibody-positive patients performed worse than antibody-negative patients (the others being cognitive flexibility and psychomotor speed). Leritz et al. (2002) also found that antibody-positive SLE patients performed worse than antibody-negative patients on tests of attention, working memory, visuospatial search, and psychomotor speed.

Although the cognitive impairment associated with SLE is suggestive of a subcortical dementia, the variability of cognitive deficits makes the identification of a "typical" pattern of impairments difficult. Leritz et al. (2000) used the algorithm developed by Brandt et al. (1988) to classify the performance of non-CNS SLE patients on the MMSE as suggestive of "cortical" or "subcortical" dysfunction. Of the 93 patients, 95% were categorized as having "subcortical" deficits, whereas 5% were categorized as having "cortical" deficits. The authors concluded that even among a group of SLE patients without gross neurological impairment, the pattern of cognitive performance reflects subtle disturbances in attention, working memory and mental tracking.

Dementia of Depression

Neuroimaging and neuropathological studies have suggested that patients with major depressive disorder often have localized metabolic abnormalities or structural lesions in subcortical nuclei (including the striatum and locus coeruleus) and/or cerebral white matter (Baxter et al., 1985; O'Connell et al., 1989; Coffey et al., 1989).

It has long been recognized that the cognitive deficits observed among patients with major depression can be differentiated from those seen in AD. Whitehead (1973) reported that their new learning and memory is less variable and less prone to false-positive errors than is the case in AD. Since that time, a consistent finding is that of mild anterograde amnesia, typically not as severe as in early-stage AD and without semantic deficits (Weingartner, 1986; Hart et al., 1987). King & Caine (1990) were among the first to note the similarity of the dementia of depression to the dementia of HD and other subcortical dementias.

Clinical and neuroradiological variability among patients with depression has led to the suggestion that there are subtypes of depression, some of which are associated with dementia and others which are not. Massman et al. (1992) used discriminant function analysis to classify 49 patients with major depression into like-HD, like-AD, and normal groups, based on their performance on the CVLT and other neuropsychological tests. Whereas 29% were classified as like HD, none were classified as like AD, suggesting that at least a subset of depressed patients have a subcortical dementia profile.

Disorders of the Cerebellum

Although the cerebellum is most clearly implicated in the coordination of movement, its role in cognition is becoming more widely recognized (Rapoport et al., 2000; Schmahmann, 1997). Cerebellar lesions can arise acutely, as in stroke, or as part of a neurodegenerative process, as in the inherited spinocerebellar ataxias. A functional disconnection of the cerebellum from the cerebrum, especially the prefrontal cortex (via the basal ganglia and thalamus), is often implicated in these higher cognitive impairments (Botez et al., 1991a). Neurochemical abnormalities of the cholinergic system (Kish et al., 1987) and of the dopaminergic system (Botez et al., 1991b) have also been suggested as contributing to the cognitive disorder of some cerebellar patients.

Patients with cerebellar disease may suffer from a variety of cognitive and affective impairments (Schmahmann & Sherman, 1998), with particularly prominent disorders of executive functioning (Grafman et al., 1992). Schmahmann & Sherman (1998) studied a heterogeneous group of 20 patients with isolated cerebellar pathology. Most prominent among the cognitive deficits and emotional disturbances found were impairments in executive functioning, including deficits in working memory (assessed with backward digit span).

Spinocerebellar Ataxias

The autosomal dominant cerebellar ataxias (ADCAs), also known as the spinocerebellar ataxias (SCAs), are a group of inherited movement disorders, several of which, like HD, are caused by triplet repeat (*CAG*) mutations coding for glutamine. This group of disorders overlaps with the entity known as olivopontocerebellar atrophy (OPCA), a disease that occurs sporadically as well as familially and is caused by progressive degeneration of the cerebellar cortex, pons and inferior olives. Kish et al. (1988) studied 11 OPCA patients with standardized cognitive tests and found prominent impairments in the recall of stories (WMS Logical Memory subtest), as well as deficits in verbal and nonverbal intelligence and executive functions. Because these patients were not aphasic, apractic or agnosic, the authors described their mental state as a mildly disabling subcortical dementia. In contrast, Berent et al. (1990) reported no cognitive performance differences between 39 OPCA patients (ill for an average of 6 years) and education-matched control subjects. In a follow-up study of 43 patients with a variety of SCAs, ill for an average of 11 years, Kish et al. (1994) found mildly ataxic patients to perform near-normally on a battery of neuropsychological tests. Moderately ataxic patients in this study displayed executive functioning deficits and mild memory deficits (WMS Mental Control and Logical Memory subtests, and Memory Quotient) that could not be explained by depression, whereas severely ataxic patients had more pervasive deficits but were nonetheless nonaphasic.

On verbal list-learning tasks, deficient immediate and delayed free recall with preservation of yes/no or forced-choice recognition is often taken as the *sine qua non* of subcortical dementia. This is generally what has been found among patients with spinocerebellar degeneration (Hirono et al., 1991).

In one of the most comprehensive memory studies of cerebellar patients to date, Appollonio et al. (1993) studied both effortful and automatic aspects of explicit memory performance in 11 patients with isolated cerebellar degeneration. The patients performed worse than normal control subjects on the DRS (Mattis, 1988) and word-list generation tasks, as well as free recall of word lists (Hasher frequency monitoring task; Hasher & Zacks, 1984) and a paired-associate learning task using both word and picture stimuli. Importantly, the patients were not impaired on the cued recall or recognition portion of either task. Neither were they impaired in their incidental monitoring of frequency of occurrence or modality of stimuli, two measures of automatic processing. Implicit memory was also investigated by Appollonio et al. (1993). Cerebellar patients and normal control subjects displayed equivalent improvement over trials on both a word fragment completion test and an identification of incomplete pictures test. The results led the authors to conclude that only attention-demanding cognitive processes are impaired in patients with pure cerebellar pathology, and these contribute to their "frontal-like" executive dysfunction.

The cognitive processing deficit(s) underlying the dysexecutive syndrome and mild subcortical dementia seen in cerebellar patients has also been the subject of several other investigations. In many cases, a defect in some aspect of sequencing or timing has been implicated (Ivry & Keele, 1989; Botez-Marquard & Routhier, 1995). Possibly related to this, it is well established that cerebellar lesions severely impair classical conditioning of the eyeblink response (Daum & Schugens, 1996; Woodruff-Pak et al., 1996), known to depend on precise timing of conditioned and unconditioned stimuli.

CONCLUSIONS

"Subcortical dementia" is simultaneously a frequently invoked and much maligned concept in neuropsychology and behavioral neurology. It is a syndrome that is clearly more difficult to define than it is to apply. It implies anatomical delineations that fall apart on close scrutiny and a clinical phenotype that is broad and imprecise. Nonetheless, several relatively consistent themes emerge from the literature reviewed here:

1. Impairments in anterograde learning and memory, to the extent that they exist in diseases affecting primarily subcortical nuclei and pathways, are relatively milder than those seen in AD.
2. Tests of free recall are more sensitive to the new learning deficits of these patients than are tests of recognition. While this is likely true for most, if not all, conditions, the relative difference between recognition and recall is greater in the subcortical dementias than, for example, in AD.
3. Fluency/generativity and working memory are typically more impaired than memory storage, and may contribute to performance deficits on episodic memory tests.
4. There are probably subtypes of many subcortical diseases; some of them are associated with memory impairment and others not.
5. Memory impairments are usually most significant in patients with clear signs and symptoms of neurological disease (e.g. sensory or motor deficits).

Methodological advances in brain imaging and neuropathology have increased our understanding of the differences in pathological anatomy and chemistry underlying specific diseases affecting primarily the brainstem nuclei, cerebellum, thalamus, basal ganglia and subcortical white matter. Unfortunately, the same level of detail is often lacking when discussing the mental states of these patients. Most clinicians and scientists will agree that the term "subcortical dementia" is too coarse for further progress to be made in this field. The term will almost certainly give way eventually to the more precise delineation of specific cognitive syndromes linked to specific neurobiological entities.

ACKNOWLEDGEMENTS

Preparation of this chapter was supported, in part, by grants AG05146 and NS16375 from the National Institutes of Health, USA.

REFERENCES

Adams, R.D. & Victor, M. (1985). *Principles of Neurology*, 3rd edn. New York: McGraw-Hill.
Adams, K.M., Grant, I. & Brown, G.G. (1985). The use of analysis of co-variance as a remedy for demographic group mismatch: some sobering simulations. *Journal of Clinical and Experimental Neuropsychology*, **7**, 445–462.

Albert, M.L., Feldman, R.G. & Willis, A.L. (1974). The "subcortical dementia" of progressive supranuclear palsy. *Journal of Neurology, Neurosurgery, and Psychiatry*, **37**, 121–130.

American Psychiatric Association. (1994). *Diagnostic and Statistical Manual of Mental Disorders*, 4th edn. Washington, DC: American Psychiatric Association.

Appollonio, I.M., Grafman, J., Schwartz, V. et al. (1993). Memory in patients with cerebellar degeneration. *Neurology*, **43**, 1536–1544.

Arnett, P.A., Higginson, C.I., Voss, W.D. et al. (1997). Working memory span and long-term memory in multiple sclerosis [Abstract]. *Journal of the International Neuropsychological Society*, **2**, 19.

Baddeley, A. (1986). *Working Memory*. Oxford: Clarendon.

Baxter, L.R., Phelps, M.E., Mazziotta, J.C. et al. (1985). Cerebral metabolic rates for glucose in mood disorders: studies with positron emission tomography and fluorodeoxyglucose F18. *Archives of General Psychiatry*, **46**, 243–250.

Beatty, W.W., Goodkin, D.E., Hertsgaard, D. & Monson, N. (1990). Clinical and demographic predictors of cognitive performance in multiple sclerosis. Do diagnostic type, disease duration, and disability matter? *Archives of Neurology*, **47**, 305–308.

Benecke, R., Rothwell, J.C. & Dick, J.P. (1987). Disturbance of sequential movements in patients with Parkinson's disease. *Brain*, **110**, 361–379.

Benedek, T. (1997). Historical background of discoid and systemic lupus erythematosus. In D.J. Wallace & B.H. Hahn (eds), *Dubois' Lupus Erythematosus* (pp. 3–16). Baltimore, MD: Williams & Wilkins.

Berent, S., Giordani, B., Gilman, S. et al. (1990). Neuropsychological changes in olivopontocerebellar atrophy. *Archives of Neurology*, **47**, 997–1001.

Bernard, B.A., Wilson, R.S., Gilley, D.W. et al. (1990). Performance of patients with BD and AD on the Mattis Dementia Rating Scale [Abstract]. *Journal of Clinical and Experimental Neuropsychology*, **12**, 22.

Blin, J., Ruberg, M. & Baron, J.C. (1992). Positron emission tomography studies. *Progressive Supranuclear Palsy: Clinical and Research Approaches* (pp. 155–168). New York: Oxford University Press.

Bondi, M.W. & Kazniak, A.W. (1991). Implicit and explicit memory in Alzheimer's disease and Parkinson's disease. *Journal of Clinical and Experimental Neuropsychology*, **13**, 339–358.

Botez, M.I., Léveillé, J., Lambert, R. & Botez-Marquard, T. (1991a). Single photon emission computed tomography (SPECT) in cerebellar disease: cerebello-cerebral diaschisis. *European Neurology*, **31**, 405–412.

Botez, M.I., Young, N.S., Botez-Marquard, T. & Pedraza, O.L. (1991b). Treatment of heredodegenerative ataxias with amantadine hydrochloride. *Canadian Journal of Neurological Sciences*, **18**, 307–311.

Botez-Marquard, T. & Routhier, I. (1995). Reaction time and intelligence in patients with olivopontocerebellar atrophy. *Neuropsychiatry, Neuropsychology, and Behavioral Neurology*, **8**, 168–175.

Brandt, J., Folstein, S.E. & Folstein, M.F. (1988). Differential cognitive impairment in Alzheimer's disease and Huntington's disease. *Annals of Neurology*, **23**, 555–561.

Brandt, J. (1994). Cognitive investigations in Huntington's disease. In L. Cermak (ed.), *Neuropsychological Explorations of Memory and Cognition: Essays in Honor of Nelson Butters* (pp. 135–146). New York: Plenum.

Brandt, J., Corwin, J. & Krafft, L. (1992). Is verbal recognition memory really different in Alzheimer's and Huntington's disease? *Journal of Clinical and Experimental Neuropsychology*, **14**, 773–784.

Brooks, D.J., Ibanez, V., Playford, E.D. et al. (1991). Presynaptic and postsynaptic striatal dopaminergic function in neuroacanthocytosis: a positron emission tomographic study. *Annals of Neurology*, **30**, 166–171.

Brownell, B. & Hughes, J.F. (1962). The distribution of plaques in the cerebrum in multiple sclerosis. *Journal of Neurology, Neurosurgery, and Psychiatry*, **25**, 315–320.

Butters, N., Sax, D., Montgomery, K. & Tarlow, S. (1978). Comparison of the neuropsychological deficits associated with early and advanced Huntington's disease. *Archives of Neurology*, **35**, 585–589.

Butters, N., Heindel, W.C., & Salmon, D.P. (1990). Dissociation of implicit memory in dementia: neurological implications. *Bulletin of the Psychonomic Society*, **28**, 359–366.

Bylsma, F.W., Brandt, J. & Strauss, M.E. (1990). Aspects of procedural memory are differentially impaired in Huntington's disease. *Archives of Clinical Neuropsychology*, **5**, 287–297.

Caine, E.D., Hunt, R.D., Weingartner, H. & Ebert, M.H. (1978). Huntington's dementia: clinical and neuropsychological features. *Archives of General Psychiatry*, **35**, 377–384.

Caine, E.D., Ebert, M.H. & Weingartner, H. (1977). An outline for the analysis of dementia. The memory disorder of Huntington's disease. *Neurology*, **27**, 1087–1092.

Carlomagno, S., Migliaresi, S., Ambrosone, L. et al. (2000). Cognitive impairment in systemic lupus erythematosus: a follow-up study. *Journal of Neurology*, **247**, 273–279.

Chinn, R.J.S., Wilkinson, I.D., Hall-Craggs, M.A. et al. (1997). Magnetic resonance imaging of the brain and cerebral proton spectroscopy in patients with systemic lupus erythematosus. *Arthritis and Rheumatism*, **40**, 36–46.

Chen, X.R., Shen, T.Z., Li, N.Z. & Liu, D.K. (1983). Computed tomography in hepatolenticular degeneration (Wilson's disease). *Computed Radiology*, **7**, 361–364.

Coffey, C.E., Figiel, G.S., Djang, W.T. et al. (1989). White matter hyperintensity on magnetic resonance imaging: clinical and neuroanatomic correlates in the depressed elderly. *Journal of Neuropsychiatry and Clinical Neurosciences*, **3**, 18–22.

Cohen, S. & Freedman, M. (1995). Cognitive and behavioural changes in Parkinson-plus syndromes. In W.J. Weiner & A.E. Lang (eds), *Advances in Neurology: Behavioral Neurology of Movement Disorders*, Vol. 65 (pp.139–157). New York: Raven.

Crosson, B. (1992). *Subcortical Functions in Language and Memory*. New York: Guilford.

Cummings, J.L., Gosenfeld, L.F., Houlihan, J.P. & McCaffrey, T. (1983). Neuropsychiatric disturbances associated with idiopathic calcification of the basal ganglia. *Biological Psychiatry*, **18**, 591–601.

Cummings, J.L. (1993). Frontal-subcortical circuits and human behavior. *Archives of Neurology*, **50**, 873–880.

Cummings, J.L. & Benson, D.F. (1984). Subcortical dementia. Review of an emerging concept. *Archives of Neurology*, **41**, 874–879.

Darvesh, S. & Freedman, M. (1996). Subcortical dementia: a neurobehavioral approach. *Brain and Cognition*, **31**, 230–249.

Daum, I. & Schugens, M.M. (1996). On the cerebellum and classical conditioning. *Current Directions in Psychological Science*, **5**, 58–61.

Delis, D.C., Kramer, J.H., Kaplan, E. & Ober, B.A. (1987). *California Verbal Learning Test*. New York: Psychological Corporation.

DeLuca, J., Barbieri-Berger, S. & Johnson, S.K. (1994). The nature of memory impairments in multiple sclerosis: acquisition vs. retrieval. *Journal of Clinical and Experimental Neuropsychology*, **16**, 183–189.

Denberg, S.D., Carbotte, R.M. & Denberg, J.A. (1987). Cognitive impairment in systemic lupus erythematosus: a neuropsychological study of individual and group deficits. *Journal of Clinical and Experimental Neuropsychology*, **9**, 323–339.

Denburg, S.D., Carbotte, R.M., Ginsberg, J.S. & Denburg, J.A. (1997). The relationship of antiphospholipid antibodies to cognitive function in patients with systemic lupus erythematosus. *Journal of the International Neuropsychological Society*, **3**, 377–386.

Denburg, S.D. & Denburg, J.A. (1999). Cognitive dysfunction in systemic lupus erythematosus. In D.J. Walace & B.H. Hahn (eds), *Dubois' Lupus Erthematosus* (pp. 611–629). Philadelphia, PA: Lea & Febiger.

Domesick, V.B. (1990). Subcortical anatomy: the circuitry of the striatum. In J.L. Cummings (ed.), *Subcortical Dementia* (pp. 31–43). New York: Oxford University Press.

Drebing, C.E., Moore, L.H., Cummings, J.L. et al. (1993). Patterns of neuropsychological performance among forms of subcortical dementia: a case study approach. *Neuropsychiatry, Neuropsychology, and Behavioral Neurology*, **7**, 57–66.

Falcini, F., DeCristofaro, M.T., Ermini, M. et al. (1998). Regional cerebral blood flow in juvenile systemic lupus erythematosus: a prospective SPECT study. *Journal of Rheumatology*, **25**, 583–588.

Fisher, J.M., Kennedy, J.L., Caine, E.D. & Shoulson, I. (1983). Dementia in Huntington's disease: a cross-sectional analysis of intellectual decline. *Advances in Neurology*, **38**, 229–238.

Folstein, S.E. (1989). *Huntington's Disease: A Disorders of Families*. Baltimore, MD: Johns Hopkins University Press.

Folstein, M.F., Folstein, S.E. & McHugh, P.R. (1975). Mini-Mental State: a practical method of grading the cognitive state of patients for the clinician. *Journal of Psychiatric Research*, **12**, 189–198.

Franklin, S., Turner, J.E. & Ellis, A.W. (1992). *The ADA Comprehension Battery*. University of York: Human Neuropsychology Laboratory.

Freedman, M. (1990). Parkinson's Disease. In J.L. Cummings (ed.), *Subcortical Dementia* (pp. 71–86). New York: Oxford University Press.

Gabrieli, J.D.E., Stebbins, G.T., Jaswinder, S. et al. (1997). Intact mirror-tracing and impaired rotary-pursuit skill learning in patients with Huntington's disease: evidence for dissociable memory systems in skill learning. *Neuropsychology*, **11**, 272–281.

Gallassi, R., Morreale, A., Montagna, P. et al. (1992). Fatal familial insomnia: neuropsychological study of a disease with thalamic degeneration. *Cortex*, **28**, 175–187.

Ginsburg, K.S., Wright, E.A., Larson, M.G. et al. (1992). A controlled study of the prevalence of cognitive dysfunction in randomly selected patients with systemic lupus erythematosus. *Arthritis and Rheumatism*, **35**, 776–782.

Grafman, J., Litvan, I., Massaquoi, S. et al. (1992). Cognitive planning deficit in patients with cerebellar atrophy. *Neurology*, **42**, 1493–1496.

Grafman, J., Litvan, I., Gomez, C. & Chase, T.N. (1990). Frontal lobe function in progressive supranuclear palsy. *Archives of Neurology*, **47**, 553–558.

Grober, E., Buschke, H., Crystal, H. et al. (1988). Screening for dementia by memory testing. *Neurology*, **38**, 900–903.

Haaland, K.Y., Harrington, D.L., O'Brien, S. & Hermanowicz, N. (1997). Cognitive-motor learning in Parkinson's disease. *Neuropsychology*, **11**, 180–186.

Hach, B. & Hartung, M.L. (1979). The effect of penicillamine on the mental disorders associated with Wilson's disease (in German). *Nervenarzi*, **50**, 115–120.

Hardie, R.J., Pullon, H.W.H., Harding, A.E. et al. (1991). Neuroacanthocytosis: a clinical, haematological and pathological study of 19 cases. *Brain*, **114**, 13–49.

Harrington, D.L., Haaland, K.Y., Yeo, R.A. & Marder, E. (1990). Procedural memory in Parkinson's disease: impaired motor but not visuoperceptual learning. *Journal of Clinical and Experimental Neuropsychology*, **12**, 323–339.

Hart, R.P., Kwentus, J.A., Taylor, J.R. & Harkins, S.W. (1987). Rate of forgetting in dementia and depression. *Journal of Consulting and Clinical Psychology*, **55**, 101–105.

Hasher, L. & Zacks, R. (1984). Automatic processing of fundamental information: the case of frequency of occurrence. *American Psychologist*, **39**, 1372–1388.

Heaton, R.K., Grant, I. & Matthews, C.G. (1991). *Comprehensive Norms for an Extended Halstead Reitan Battery*. Odessa, FL: Psychological Assessment Resources.

Heaton, R.K., Nelson, L.M., Thompson, D.S. et al. (1985). Neuropsychological findings in relapsing-remitting and chronic-progressive multiple sclerosis. *Journal of Consulting and Clinical Psychology*, **53**, 103–110.

Hefter, H., Arendt, G., Stremmel, W. & Freund, H.-J. (1993). Motor impairment in Wilson's disease: slowness of voluntary limb movements. *Acta Neurologica Scandinavia*, **87**, 133–147.

Heindel, W.C., Salmon, D.P. & Butters, N. (1991). The biasing of weight judgments in Alzheimer's and Huntington's disease: a priming or programming phenomenon? *Journal of Clinical and Experimental Neuropsychology*, **13**, 189–203.

Heindel, W.C., Butters, N. & Salmon, D.P. (1988). Impaired learning of a motor skill in patients with Huntington's disease. *Behavioral Neuroscience*, **102**, 141–147.

Heindel, W.C., Salmon, D.P., Shults, C.W. et al. (1989). Neuropsychological evidence for multiple implicit memory systems: a comparison of Alzheimer's, Huntington's, and Parkinson's disease patients. *Journal of Neuroscience*, **9**, 582–587.

Hier, D.B. & Cummings, J.L. (1990). Rare acquired and degenerative subcoirtical dementias. In J.L. Cummings (ed.), *Subcortical Dementia* (pp. 199–217). New York: Oxford University Press.

Hirono, N., Yamadori, A., Kameyama, M. et al. (1991). Spinocerebellar degeneration (SCD): cognitive disturbances. *Acta Neurologica Scandinavica*, **84**, 226–230.

Howard, D. & Patterson, K. (1992). *The Pyramids and Palm Trees Test*. Bury St. Edmunds: Thames Valley Test Co.

Isaacs-Glaberman, K., Medalia, A. & Scheinberg, H. (1988). Verbal recall and recognition abilities in patients with Wilson's disease. Paper read at the 16th annual meeting of the International Neuropsychological Society, New Orleans, January.

Ivnik, R.J. (1978). Neuropsychological test performance as a function of the duration of MS-related symptomatology. *Journal of Clinical Psychiatry*, **39**, 304–307.

Ivry, R.B. & Keele, S.W. (1989). Timing functions of the cerebellum. *Journal of Cognitive Neurosciences*, **1**, 136–152.

Jellinger, K.A. & Bancher, C. (1992). Neuropathology. In *Progressive Supranuclear Palsy: Clinical and Research Approaches* (pp. 44–88). New York: Oxford University Press.

Kao, C-H., Ho, Y-J., Lan, J-L. et al. (1999). Discrepancy between regional cerebral blood flow and glucose metabolism of the brain in systemic lupus erythematosus patients with normal brain magnetic resonance imaging findings. *Arthritis and Rheumatism*, **42**, 61–68.

Kaplan, E.F., Goodglass, H. & Weintraub, S. (1983). *The Boston Naming Test*. Philadelphia, PA: Lea & Febinger.

Kartsounis, L.D. & Hardie, R.J. (1996). The pattern of cognitive impairments in neuroacanthocytosis: a frontosubcortical dementia. *Archives of Neurology*, **53**(1), 77–80.

Kertesz, A., Polk, M. & Carr, T. (1990). Cognition and white matter changes on magnetic resonance imaging in dementia. *Archives of Neurology*, **47**, 387–391.

King, D.A. & Caine E.D. (1990). Depression. In J.L. Cummings (ed.), *Subcortical Dementia* (pp. 218–230). New York: Oxford University Press.

Kish, S.J., Rajput, A., Gilbert, J. et al. (1996). Elevated GABA level in striatal but not extrastriatal brain regions in Parkinson's disease: correlation with striatal dopamine loss. *Annals of Neurology*, **20**, 26–31.

Kish, S.J., Shannak, K. & Hornykiewicz, O. (1988a). Uneven pattern of dopamine loss in the striatum of patients with idiopathic Parkinson's disease: pathophysiologic and clinical implications. *New England Journal of Medicine*, **318**, 876–880.

Kish, S.J., El-Awar, M., Stuss, D. et al. (1994). Neuropsychological test performance in patients with dominantly inherited spinocerebellar ataxia: Relationship to ataxia severity. *Neurology*, **44**, 1738–1746.

Kish, S.J., Currier, R.D., Schut, L. et al. (1987). Brain choline acetyltransferase reduction in dominantly inherited olivopontocerellar atrophy. *Annals of Neurology*, **22**, 272–275.

Kish, S.J., El-Awar, M., Schut, L. et al. (1988b). Cognitive deficits in olivopontocerebellar atrophy: Implications for the cholinergic hypothesis of Alzheimer's disease. *Annals of Neurology*, **24**, 200–206.

Klein, C. & Vieregge, P. (1998). Fahr's disease—far from a disease. *Movement Disorders*, **13**, 620–621.

Knopman, D.S. & Nissen, M.J. (1991). Procedural learning is impaired in Huntington's disease: evidence from the serial reaction time task. *Neuropsychologia*, **29**, 245–254.

Kozora, E., Thompson, L., West, S.G. & Kotzin, B.L. et al. (1996). Analysis of cognitive and psychological deficits in systemic lupus erythematosus patients without overt central nervous system disease. *Arthritis & Rheumatism*, **39**, 2035–2045.

Kozora, E., West, S.G., Kotzin, B.L. et al. (1998). Magnetic resonance imaging abnormalities and cognitive deficits in systemic lupus erythematosus patients without overt central nervous system disease. *Arthritis and Rheumatism*, **41**, 41–47.

Kramer, J.H., Levin, B.E., Brandt, J. & Delis, D.C. (1989). Differentiation of Alzheimer's, Huntington's, and Parkinson's disease patients on the basis of verbal learning characteristics. *Neuropsychology*, **3**, 111–120.

Kutcher, J.S., Kahn, M.J., Andersson, H.D. & Foundas, A.L. (1999). Neuroacanthocytosis masquerading as Huntington's disease: CT/MRI findings. *Journal of Neuroimaging*, **9**, 187–189.

Lafosse, J.M., Reed, B.R., Mungas, D. et al. (1997). Fluency and memory differences between ischemic vascular dementia and Alzheimer's disease. *Neuropsychology*, **11**, 514–522.

Lang, C., Müller, D., Claus, D. & Druschky, K.F. (1990). Neuropsychological findings in treated Wilson's Disease. *Acta Neurologica Scandinavica*, **81**, 75–81.

Lang, C. (1989). Is Wilson's disease a dementing condition? *Journal of Clinical and Experimental Neuropsychology*, **14**, 569–570.

Lang, W., Miklossy, J., Deruaz, J.P. et al. (1989). Neuropathology of the acquired immune deficiency syndrome (AIDS): a report of 135 consecutive autopsy cases from Switzerland. *Acta Neuropathologica*, **77**, 379–390.

Leritz, E., Brandt, J., Minor, M. et al. (2000). "Subcortical" cognitive impairment in patients with systemic lupus erythematosus. *Journal of the International Neuropsychological Society*, **6**, 821–825.

Leritz, E., Brandt, J., Minor, M. et al. (2002). Neuropsychological functioning and its relationship to antiphospholipid antibodies in patients with systemic lupus erythematosus. *Journal of Clinical and Experimental Neuropsychology*, **24**, 527–533.

Libon, D.J., Bogdanoff, B., Bonavitak, J. et al. (1997). Dementia associated with periventricular and deep white matter alterations: a subtype of subcortical dementia. *Archives of Clinical Neuropsychology*, **12**, 239–250.

Libon, D.J., Bogdanoff, B., Cloud, B.S. et al. (1998). Declarative and procedural learning, quantitative measures of the hippocampus, and subcortical white alterations in Alzheimer's disease and ischaemic vascular dementia. *Journal of Clinical and Experimental Neuropsychology*, **20**, 30–41.

Libon, D.J., Swenson, R., Malamut, B.L. et al. (1993). Periventricular white matter alterations, Binswanger's disease, and dementia. *Developmental Neuropsychology*, **9**, 87–102.

Lopez-Villegas, D., Kulisevsky, J., Deus, J. et al. (1996). Neuropsychological alterations in patients with computed tomography-detected basal ganglia calcification. *Archives of Neurology*, **53**, 251–256.

Lovell, M.R. & Smith, S.S. (1997). Neuropsychological evaluation of subcortical dementia. In P. David (ed.), *Handbook of Neuropsychology and Aging. Critical Issues in Neuropsychology* (pp. 189–200). New York: Plenum.

Lugaressi, E., Medori, R., Montagna, P. et al. (1986). Fatal familial insomnia and dysautonimia with selective degeneration of thalamic nuclei. *New England Journal of Medicine*, **315**, 997–1003.

Mandell, A.M. & Albert, M.L. (1990). History of subcortical dementia. In J.L. Cummings (ed.), *Subcortical Dementia* (pp. 17–30). New York: Oxford University Press.

Martone, M., Butters, N., Payne, J. et al. (1984). Dissociations between skill learning and verbal recognition in amnesia and dementia. *Archives of Neurology*, **41**, 965–970.

Maruff, P., Currie, J., Malone, V. et al. (1994). Neuropsychological characterization of the AIDS dementia complex and rationalization of a test battery. *Archives of Neurology*, **51**, 689–695.

Massman, P.J., Delis, D.C., Butters, N. et al. (1990). Are all subcortical dementias alike? Verbal learning and memory in Parkinson's and Huntington's disease patients. *Journal of Clinical and Experimental Neuropsychology*, **12**, 729–744.

Massman, P.J., Delis, D.C., Butters, N. et al. (1992). The subcortical dysfunction hypothesis of memory deficits in depression: neuropsychological validation in a subgroup of patients. *Journal of Clinical and Experimental Neuropsychology*, **14**, 687–706.

Mattis, S. (1988). *Dementia Rating Scale: Professional Manual*. Odessa, FL: Psychological Assessment Resources.

McDaniel, K.D. (1990). Thalamic degeneration. In J.L. Cummings (ed.), *Subcortical Dementia* (pp. 132–144). New York: Oxford University Press.

McHugh, P.R. (1989). The neuropsychiatry of basal ganglia disorders: a triadic syndrome and its explanation. *Neuropsychiatry, Neuropsychology, and Behavioral Neurology*, **2**, 239–246.

McHugh, P.R. & Folstein, M.F. (1975). Psychiatric syndrome of Huntington's chorea: a clinical and pharmacologic study. In D.F. Benson & D. Blumer (eds), *Psychiatric Aspects of Neurologic Disease*. New York: Grune & Stratton.

Medalia, A., Isaacs-Glaberman, K. & Scheinberg, I.H. (1988). Neuropsychological impairment in Wilson's disease. *Archives of Neurology*, **45**, 502–504.

Medalia, A., Galynker, I. & Scheinberg, H. (1992). The interaction of motor, memory, and emotional dysfunction in Wilson's disease. *Biological Psychiatry*, **31**, 823–826.

Medalia, A. (1991). Memory deficit in Wilson's disease: a response to Lang. *Journal of Clinical and Experimental Neuropsychology*, **13**(2), 359–360.

Middleton, F.A. & Strick, P.L. (2000). Basal ganglia and cerebellar loops: motor and cognitive circuits. *Brain Research Reviews*, **31**, 236–250.

Milberg, W. & Albert, M. (1989). Cognitive differences between patients with progressive supranuclear palsy and Alzheimer's disease. *Journal of Clinical and Experimental Neuropsychology*, **11**(5), 605–614.

Moss, M.D., Albert, M.S., Butters, N. & Payne, M. (1986). Differential patterns of memory loss among patients with Alzheimer's disease, Huntington's disease, and alcoholic Korsakoff's syndrome. *Archives of Neurology*, **43**, 239–246.

Navia, B.A., Cho, E.S., Petito, C.K. & Price, R.W. (1986a). The AIDS dementia complex: II. Neuropathology. *Annals of Neurology*, **19**(6), 525–535.

Navia, B.A., Jordan, B.D. & Price, R.W. (1986b). The AIDS dementia complex. I. Clinical features. *Annals of Neurology*, **19**, 517–524.

Navia, B.A. (1990). The AIDS dementia complex. In J.L. Cummings (ed.), *Subcortical Dementia* (pp. 181–198). New York: Oxford University Press.

O'Connell, R.A., Van Heertum, R.L., Billick, S.B. et al. (1989). Single photon emission computed tomography (SPECT) with [123I] IMP in the differential diagnosis of psychiatric disorders. *Journal of Neuropsychiatry and Clinical Neurosciences*, **1**, 145–152.

Paulsen, J.S., Butters, N., Salmon, D.P. et al. (1993). Prism adaptation in Alzheimer's and Huntington's disease. *Neuropsychology*, **1**, 73–81.

Paulsen, J.S., Butters, N., Sadek, J.R. et al. (1995). Distinct cognitive profiles of cortical and subcortical dementia in advanced illness. *Neurology*, **45**, 951–956.

Peyser, J.M. & Poser, C.M. (1986). Neuropsychological correlates of multiple sclerosis. In S.B. Filskov & T.J. Boll (eds), *Handbook of Clinical Neuropsychology*, Vol. 2 (pp. 364–397). New York: Wiley.

Pillon, B., Deweer, B., Michon, A. et al. (1994). Are explicit memory disorders of progressive supranuclear palsy related to damage to striatofrontal circuits? *Neurology*, **44**, 1264–1270.

Pillon, B., Deweer, B., Agid, Y. & Dubois, B. (1993). Explicit memory in Alzheimer's, Huntington's, and Parkinson's diseases. *Archives of Neurology*, **50**, 374–379.

Pillon, B., Dubois, B., Ploska, A. & Agid, Y. (1991). Severity and specificity of cognitive impairment in Alzheimer's, Huntington's, and Parkinson's diseases and progressive supranuclear palsy. *Neurology*, **41**, 634–643.

Price, R.W. (1996). AIDS dementia complex: a complex, slow virus "model" of acquired genetic neurodegenerative disease. *Cold Spring Harbor Symposium on Quantitative Biology*, **61**, 759–770.

Quinn, N. & Schrag, A. (1998). Huntington's disease and other choreas. *Journal of Neurology*, **245**, 709–715.

Rao, S.M. (1996). White matter disease and dementia. *Brain and Cognition*, **31**, 250–268.

Rao, S.M., Hammeke, T.A., McQuillen, M.P. et al. (1984). Memory disturbance in chronic progressive multiple sclerosis. *Archives of Neurology*, **41**, 625–631.

Rao, S.M. (1986). Neuropsychology of multiple sclerosis: a critical review. *Journal of Clinical and Experimental Neuropsychology*, **8**, 503–542.

Rapoport, M., van Reekum, R. & Mayberg, H. (2000). The role of the cerebellum in cognition and behavior: a selective review. *Journal of Neuropsychiatry and Clinical Neurosciences*, **12**, 193–198.

Reed, B.R., Eberling, J.L., Mungas, D. et al. (2000). Memory failure has different mechanisms in subcortical stroke and Alzheimer's disease. *Annals of Neurology*, **48**, 275–284.

Rinne, J.O., Daniel, S.E., Scaravilli, F. et al. (1994). The neuropathological features of neuroacanthocytosis. *Movement Disorders*, **9**, 297–304.

Rohrer, D., Salmon, D.P., Wixted, J.T. & Paulsen, J.S. (1999). The disparate effects of Alzheimer's disease and Huntington's disease on semantic memory. *Neuropsychology*, **13**, 381–388.

Román, G.C., Tatemichi, T.K., Erkinjuntti, T. et al. (1993). Vascular dementia: diagnostic criteria for research studies. Report of the NINDS–AIREN International Workshop. *Neurology*, **43**, 250–260.

Rosselli, M. (1987). Wilson's disease, a reversible dementia: case report. *Journal of Clinical and Experimental Neuropsychology*, **9**, 399–406.

Rothlind, J. & Brandt, J. (1993). Validation of a brief assessment of frontal and subcortical functions in dementia. *Journal of Neuropsychiatry and Clinical Neurosciences*, **5**, 73–77.

Ruchkin, D.S., Grafman, J., Krauss, G.L. et al. (1994). Event-related brain potential evidence for a
    verbal working memory deficit in multiple sclerosis. *Brain*, **117**, 289–305.
Saint-Cyr, J.A., Taylor, A.E. & Lang, A.E. (1988). Procedural learning and neostriatal dysfunction in
    man. *Brain*, **111**, 941–959.
Salmon, D.P., Kwo-on-Yuen, P.F., Heindel, W.C. et al. (1989). Differentiation of Alzheimer's disease
    and Huntington's disease with the Dementia Rating Scale. *Archives of Neurology*, **46**, 1204–1208.
Scheinberg, I.H. & Sternlieb, I. (1984). *Wilson's Disease*. Philadelphia, PA: Saunders.
Schmahmann, J.D. (ed.) (1997). *The Cerebellum and Cognition*. New York: Academic Press.
Schmahmann, J.D. & Sherman, J.C. (1998). The cerebellar cognitive affective syndrome. *Brain*, **121**,
    561–576.
Skeel, R.J., Johnstone, B., Yangco, D.T. et al. (2000). Neuropsychological deficit profiles in systemic
    lupus erythematosus. *Applied Neuropsychology*, **7**, 96–101.
Soliveri, P., Monza, D., Paridi, D. et al. (1999). Cognitive and magnetic resonance imaging aspects
    of corticobasal degeneration and progressive supranuclear palsy. *Neurology*, **53**, 502–507.
Starosta-Rubinstein, S., Young, A.B., Kluin, K. et al. (1987). Clinical assessment of 31 patients with
    Wilson's disease. *Archives of Neurology*, **4**, 365–370.
Steele, J.C., Richardson, J.C. & Olszewski, J. (1964). Progressive supranuclear palsy: a hetero-
    geneous degeneration involving the brain stem, basal ganglia, and cerebellum, with verti-
    cal gaze and pseudobulbar palsy, nuclear dystonia, and dementia. *Archives of Neurology*, **10**,
    339–359.
van der Hurk, P.R. & Hodges, J.R. (1995). Episodic and semantic memory in Alzheimer's disease
    and progressive supranuclear palsy: a comparative study. *Journal of Clinical and Experimental
    Neuropsychology*, **17**, 459–471.
Van Gorp, W.G., Mandelkern, M.A., Gee, M. et al. (1992). Cerebral metabolic dysfunction in AIDS:
    Findings in a sample with and without dementia. *Journal of Neuropsychiatry and Clinical Neuro-
    science*, **4**, 280–287.
Von Stockert, F.G. (1932). Subcorticale demenz. *Archives of Psychiatry*, **97**, 77–100.
Vonsattel, J.P., Myers, R.H., Stevens, T.J. et al. (1985). Neuropathological classification of Hunting-
    ton's disease. *Journal of Neuropathology and Experimental Neurology*, **44**, 559–577.
Warrington, E.K. (1984). *Recognition Memory Test*. Windsor: NFER-Nelson.
Wechsler, D. (1945). A standardized memory scale for clinical use. *Journal of Psychology*, **19**, 87–95.
Weingartner, H. (1987). Automatic and effort-demanding cognitive processes in depression. In J.W.
    Poon & T. Crook (eds), *Handbook of Clinical Memory Assessment of Older Adults* (pp. 218–225).
    Washington, DC: American Psychological Association.
Weingartner, H., Caine, E.D. & Ebert, M.H. (1979). Imagery, encoding, and retrieval of informa-
    tion form memory: some specific encoding-retrieval changes in Huntington's disease. *Journal of
    Abnormal Psychology*, **88**, 52–58.
Welsh, K.A., Butters, N., Mohs, R.C. et al. (1994). The Consortium to Establish a Registry for
    Alzheimer's Disease (CERAD). Part V. A normative study of the neuropsychological battery.
    Neurology, **44**, 609–614.
West, S.G. (1996). Lupus and the central nervous system. *Current Opinion in Rheumatology*, **8**,
    408–414.
White, D.A., Heaton, R.K., Monsch, A.U. & the HNRC Group. (1995). Neuropsychological studies
    of asymptomatic Human Immunodeficiency Virus Type-1 infected individuals. *Journal of the
    International Neuropsychological Society*, **1**, 304–315.
Whitehead, A. (1973). Verbal learning and memory in elderly depressives. *British Journal of Psychi-
    atry*, **123**, 203–208.
Whitehouse, P.J., Price, D.L., Struble, R.G. et al. (1982). Alzheimer's disease and senile dementia:
    loss of neurons in the basal forebrain. *Science*, **215**, 237–239.
Whitehouse, P.J. (1986). The concept of subcortical and cortical dementia: another look. *Annals of
    Neurology*, **19**, 1–6.
Williams, J.M. (1991). *Memory Assessment Scales Manual*. Odessa, FL: Psychological Assessment
    Resources.
Williams, F.J.B. & Walshe, J.M. (1981). Wilson's disease—an analysis of the cranial computerized
    tomography appearances found in 60 patients and the changes in response to treatment with
    chelating agents. *Brain*, **104**, 735–752.

Willingham, D.B., Koroshetz, W.J. & Peterson, E.W. (1996). Motor skills have diverse neural bases: Spared and impaired skill acquisition in Huntington's disease. *Neuropsychology*, **10**, 315–321.

Wilson, S.A.K. (1912). Progressive lenticular degeneration: a familiar nervous disease associated with cirrhosis of the liver. *Brain*, **34**, 294–507.

Wishart, H. & Sharp, D. (1997). Neuropsychological aspects of multiple sclerosis: a quantitative review. *Journal of Clinical and Experimental Neuropsychology*, **19**, 810–824.

Woodruff-Pak, D.S., Papka, M. & Ivry, R.B. (1996). Cerebellar involvement in classical eyeblink conditioning in humans. *Neuropsychology*, **10**, 443–458.

Zakzanis, K.K., Leach, L. & Freedman, L. (1998). Structural and functional meta-analytic evidence for fronto-subcortical system deficit in progressive supranuclear palsy. *Brain and Cognition*, **38**, 283–296.

CHAPTER 8

Assessment of Memory Disorders

Barbara A. Wilson

MRC Cognition and Brain Sciences Unit, Cambridge, and Oliver Zangwill Centre for Cognitive Rehabilitation, Ely, UK

This chapter is concerned with the assessment of memory disorders in people whose problems follow an injury or insult to the brain. Assessment can be taken to mean the systematic collection, organisation and interpretation of information about a person and his/her situation. It is also concerned with the prediction of future behaviour in new situations (Sundberg & Tyler, 1962).

Ways in which information is collected, organized and interpreted will depend on reasons why the information is needed. Assessments carried out for research purposes may require a different approach from assessments carried out for clinical purposes. Both research and clinically-orientated assessments will differ further, depending on the nature of the question or questions each is asking. So, for example, someone interested in the underlying processes involved in memory would carry out a different assessment procedure from someone interested in whether or not a memory impaired patient can return to work. An example of the former might be to find out whether or not part of a theoretical model is true, for example Baddeley et al. (1986) wanted to support or refute the hypothesis that patients with Alzheimer's disease had a deficit in the central executive component of the working memory model (Baddeley & Hitch, 1974). An example of the latter might be to identify the tasks involved in a particular job and observe whether or not a memory-impaired person could do those tasks in various situations, at different times of day and with increasing amounts of distraction. Mayes (1986, 1995) discusses the different concerns of researchers and clinicians.

This chapter focuses on clinical assessments and how clinically-orientated questions can be answered. Some can be answered using standardized tests, while others require a more functional or behavioural approach. Standardized tests are appropriate for certain questions and answer these reasonably well. As assessment of memory is typically part of a broader cognitive assessment, important questions might include the following:

- What is this person's general level of intellectual functioning?
- What was the probable level of premorbid functioning?

The Essential *Handbook of Memory Disorders for Clinicians.* Edited by A.D. Baddeley, M.D. Kopelman and B.A. Wilson.
© 2004 John Wiley & Sons, Ltd. ISBN 0-470-09141-X.

- Does this person have an organic memory deficit?
- Is there a difference in ability between recognition and recall tasks?
- Is there a difference between verbal and visual memory ability?
- To what extent are the memory problems due to language, perceptual or attention deficits?
- How do these scores compare with people of the same age in the general population?

These and similar questions can, on the whole, be answered by the administration of standardized tests; for example, there are adequately normed, reliable and valid tests available to answer each of the above questions. It is when we turn to treatment or rehabilitation issues that standardized tests are perhaps less satisfactory. They are less effective in telling us how memory deficits identified on tests affect everyday life. Standardized tests tend to be more concerned with the structure of memory, rather than the manifestations of memory difficulties in real life. Furthermore, they do not take into account factors such as premorbid lifestyle, personality, motivation, family support and so forth.

The kind of questions people in rehabilitation want answered include the following:

- What problems are causing the greatest difficulty for this person and the family?
- What coping strategies are used?
- Are the problems exacerbated by anxiety or depression?
- Can this person return home/to school/to work?
- Should we try to restore lost functioning or teach compensatory strategies?

Although results from standardized tests can throw light on some of these questions (e.g. someone with widespread cognitive deficits plus a severe memory impairment is unlikely to return to work), they do not directly answer them. Instead, a more behavioural or functional approach is required, such as that provided by direct observation, self-report measures (usually from relatives or therapists) or interviews.

In concluding this introduction, it needs to be pointed out that the two methodologies are not in opposition to each other. In fact, they are complementary and can be combined in order to plan treatment strategies (see Chapter 10).

MODELS OF ASSESSMENT

Current assessment procedures in neuropsychology have been influenced by several theoretical models or approaches. Perhaps the most widely known is the psychometric approach, based on statistical analysis. Test development typically involves establishing a procedure for administration, collecting norms from a representative population, developing a scoring procedure, and determining the reliability and validity of the test. Although other models of assessment may include many of these features, the rationale behind them is not based solely on statistical analysis. Anastasi (1982), Lezak (1995) and Evans et al. (1996) provide accounts of the characteristics of psychometric tests. The revised Wechsler Memory Scales (Wechsler, 1987, 1997) are examples of psychometrically-influenced memory tests.

Another approach to assessment is the localisation model, whereby the examiner attempts to assess damage to a particular part of the brain, such as the frontal lobes or the hippocampus. Until about 20 years ago, one of the main purposes of a neuropsychological assessment was to identify damage of this kind in order to help neurologists or neurosurgeons obtain a diagnosis. With the advent of scanners, this is no longer the case. Less often used in clinical memory assessments, localisation models have been traditionally associated with the detection of frontal lobe damage rather than other areas of the brain. The Halstead–Reitan battery (Halstead, 1947; Reitan & Davison, 1974) is a classic example of this approach, and was originally used to discriminate between patients with frontal lobe damage and controls.

Researchers interested in the anatomy of memory are, perhaps, more concerned with localisation than clinicians. Markowitsch (1998) discusses different types of memory problems associated with particular anatomical sites. Some believe that the left frontal lobe is particularly involved with encoding of information, while the right is more concerned with retrieval of information (see for example Shallice et al., 1994; Tulving et al., 1994). In short, people with typical episodic anterograde amnesia are likely to have lesions in and around the hippocampal area (i.e. the medial temporal lobes). Those with confabulation, poor attention or encoding, poor retrieval and prospective memory difficulties are likely to have frontal lobe damage.

Working memory deficits are associated with frontal lobe lesions (Goldman-Rakic & Friedman, 1991), although they may also be associated with other areas. One component of working memory, the phonological loop, appears to involve several sites, such as the left basal frontal, the parietal and the superior temporal areas (Vallar & Papagno, 1995). Another working memory component, the visuospatial sketchpad, appears to involve the right occipital, parietal and prefrontal areas (Baddeley, 1999). Semantic memory deficits are associated with damage to the lateral temporal neocortex, with the hippocampal areas being relatively unaffected (Graham et al., 1997). Procedural memory appears to depend on the basal ganglia and cerebellar regions (Markowitsch, 1998; Tranel & Damasio, 1995). Recall and recognition deficits may follow both hippocampal and frontal lobe damage, although recognition may be less impaired in frontal patients. This is because such patients are likely to have poor retrieval skills and recognition tasks avoid the need for retrieval strategies.

Retrograde amnesia is believed to result from lesions in different areas of the brain from those causing anterograde amnesia. Medial temporal lobe structures are responsible for anterograde memory, and anterolateral temporal lobe areas, especially on the right, are thought to be critical for the retrieval of anterograde factual knowledge (Calabrese et al., 1996; Jones et al., 1998). Another paper, by Eslinger (1998), argues for both left and right temporal lobe involvement in one component of retrograde memory, namely autobiographical memory, with more severe impairment following bilateral damage.

Although researchers are interested in the anatomy of memory, assessments are not always administered to identify location of lesion. Instead, lesions are used to confirm the functional distinctions of memory. In clinical memory assessments, the localisation approach is perhaps mostly associated with: (a) whether or not a client has a pure amnesic syndrome (associated with hippocampal damage) or more widespread damage, in which case there will be additional cognitive deficits; and (b) whether the memory deficit is due to hippocampal or frontal lobe damage. Hippocampal damage results in a different pattern of memory deficits than frontal lobe damage. Within the frontal lobes there are several systems involved in memory. Some argue that they have an indirect rather than a direct role in memory, and exert their influences through processes such as attention, encoding and problem solving (see Tranel & Damasio, 2002). What is clear is that memory disorders associated with damage to the frontal lobes are different from those that occur with medial temporal lobe damage.

Frontal lobe memory deficits include poor prospective memory, problems in judging how recently or how frequently something has happened, confabulation, poor retrieval problems, and difficulty in linking various components of a memory together, so that mismatching may occur (i.e. components from different memories may be incorrectly linked together).

A third approach to the assessment of memory derives from theoretical models from cognitive psychology and cognitive neuropsychology. Models of language, reading, perception and attention have provided a rich source of ideas for assessment procedures. In memory, the working memory model of Baddeley & Hitch (1974) has had a big influence on the assessment of people with organic memory impairment. At one time, memory was assessed either as if it were one skill or function or as if the subdivisions were gross; for example, the first Wechsler Scale (Wechsler, 1945) did not include delayed recall. Since the working memory and other memory models appeared, clinicians have become increasingly likely to separate assessments into visual and verbal, semantic and episodic, and short- and long-term memory. Furthermore, it is now routine to examine phonological loop, visual spatial sketchpad and central executive deficits, although it was unheard of to do this when I first entered neuropsychology in the mid-1970s. These models enable us to predict patterns of functioning and explain phenomena that on the surface might appear improbable (for example that someone should have an excellent digit span but fail to recall anything of a story after 20 s). Wilson & Patterson (1990) discuss this in more detail.

One of the latest memory assessments to appear, based on the visual–verbal and recall–recognition distinctions within memory, is "Doors and People: a test of visual and verbal recall and recognition" (Baddeley et al., 1994), which is described in more detail below. Other recent, theoretically-driven assessments include the Camden Memory Test (Warrington, 1996) and the Visual Patterns Test (Della Sala et al., 1997).

One of the earliest approaches to neuropsychological assessment involves defining a condition through the exclusion of other possible explanations. Thus, to determine whether someone has visual agnosia, it is necessary to exclude poor eyesight and anomia as explanations for the problem. Although such definition by exclusion is not directly relevant to the assessment of memory, as we typically determine memory impairment through test scores, the exclusion approach is used indirectly. For example, when assessing a memory-impaired person, we need to know whether the problems observed can be explained wholly or in part by poor attention, perception or language. We therefore assess these functions and, if necessary, exclude them as explanations for the results. Howieson & Lezak (Chapter 9, this volume) address this issue when they discuss "separating memory from other cognitive disorders".

The final model of assessment described in this section involves an ecological approach whereby the main focus of interest is in predicting the problems that are likely to occur in everyday life. If someone scores in the impaired range on a standardized memory test, we do not necessarily learn that he/she will have problems coping in real life; for example, one of my ex-patients, J.C., is a densely amnesic young man who is able to live alone, hold down a job and fill in his own tax forms, despite scoring zero on all tests of delayed, episodic memory (see Wilson & Hughes, 1997). V.K., on the other hand, achieves scores in the normal or mild range on the same delayed, episodic memory tests, yet she cannot live alone, is unemployed and needs help with many of her activities. The main reason for the difference between these two clients is that J.C. has a pure amnesia, his other cognitive functions are intact, he is of above average intelligence and he can compensate well for his memory problems. V.K., on the other hand, has diffuse brain damage and widespread cognitive impairments.

In many assessments, particularly if one is concerned with rehabilitation or helping people manage their memory difficulties, one needs to predict the nature, frequency and severity of everyday problems. This is often best done through a more functional assessment (discussed in the following section). However, there are tests specifically designed to predict everyday problems. The first memory test designed to do this was probably the Rivermead Behavioural Memory Test (RBMT: Wilson et al., 1985).

The RBMT grew out of the need to provide professionals working in rehabilitation with functionally relevant information. When I first began working in rehabilitation in 1979 I would carry out assessments I had been taught and report the findings at the weekly ward rounds, using such terminology as, "She is two standard deviations below the mean on the Rey–Osterreith figure", or "He is below the fifth percentile on the story recall". The response from the other staff was often, "But can she return to work?" or "Is he safe to go home?". I could not answer such questions because the tests I gave were not representative of the problems faced in real life. The priorities of patients, family and other rehabilitation staff were different from mine. I set about designing a test that would predict everyday memory problems, based partly on observations of the real-life memory problems exhibited by patients and partly on some earlier work by Sunderland et al. (1983), in which they had found that, although some standardized tests were good at distinguishing between head injured patients and controls, they were not good at predicting the kinds of everyday problems reported by patients or their relatives. In collaboration with Alan Baddeley and Janet Cockburn, we carried out 5 years of research to produce the RBMT, which proved useful in predicting independence and employability (Schwartz & McMillan, 1989; Wilson, 1991) as well as correlating very well with observed memory failures (Wilson et al., 1989b). A more difficult version, the RBMT-E (extended), appeared in 1999 to assess people with more subtle memory deficits (Wilson et al., 1999b).

The RBMT was not the first ecologically valid test. In 1980, Holland published the Test of Functional Communication for Aphasic Adults (Holland, 1980), based on the principle that scores from conventional tests do not give sufficient information about real-life competencies or difficulties faced by people who have sustained an insult to the brain. Several other ecologically valid tests have appeared in recent years including the Behavioural Inattention Test for unilateral neglect (Wilson et al., 1988), the Test of Everyday Attention (Robertson et al., 1994), the Behavioural Assessment of the Dysexecutive Syndrome (Wilson et al., 1996a) and the Wessex Head Injury Matrix (Shiel et al., 2000).

Ecologically valid tests may never provide sufficient information on their own but they can provide complementary information to other tests in our "toolbox". We need a complete range of neuropsychological assessments to provide the clearest picture of a person's strengths and weaknesses. It is unhelpful for neuropsychologists who ask a particular set of questions to attack other neuropsychologists who ask a different set of questions. Some questions are answered best by theoretically-driven assessment procedures and others by more practically orientated procedures. To return to my earlier statement, much depends upon reasons why information is needed.

Standardized and Behavioural (Functional) Assessment Procedures

In order to obtain the broadest picture of deficit and impairment we need to collate information from all sources. If we want to plan, implement and evaluate a rehabilitation programme (see Chapter 10, this volume) we must include information from all forms of assessment available to us. Ecological tests may be relatively good at predicting whether or not everyday problems are likely to occur, but they may not provide sufficient detail about an individual's specific problems requiring isolation for treatment. For example, one problem that frequently arises and causes great irritation to families is repetition on the part of the patient of previously told stories or statements. People with severe memory problems are likely to repeat a question, story or joke over and over again. Although this may sound trivial, it can drive staff and relatives to breaking point. Standardized tests will neither identify this problem nor measure its frequency. Furthermore, standardized tests cannot detect whether certain situations or people make the repetition better or worse, neither can they detect the level of distress caused to family members.

Standardized tests can build up a picture of an individual's cognitive profile and this is important in planning treatment. We need to know that we are not asking the cognitively impossible, that instructions or requests are understood, that material can be perceived or read and so forth. However, they are insufficient on their own for all questions needing to be answered about a memory-impaired individual. A behavioural assessment involves an analysis of the relationship between a person's behaviour, its antecedents and its consequences. There are several ways this can be carried out, including direct observations, self-report measures and interviews.

Direct observations of everyday memory failures may be carried out in real-life settings or in analogue situations. In the example of repetition given above, one could observe the client during therapy sessions, on the ward, at home or at work, whatever is appropriate. It may be possible to follow the client around for several hours a day for a period of time or it may only be practical to see him/her for half an hour a day for several days or weeks. The crucial thing is to ensure there is a stable baseline. It is also helpful to recruit a colleague or student to do the same recording for some of the time to check for inter-rater reliability.

If the person conducting the observation (e.g. a relative, therapist or work colleague) is present, when the observations are taking place, then the observer is said to be dependent. The advantage of a dependent observer is that the person being observed is with a familiar person and less likely to change his/her natural behaviour. The disadvantage here is that certain targeted behaviours may be missed because the relative, therapist or colleague is engaged in his/her own activities. If the observer is specially recruited to carry out the observations, and is not there for any other purpose, then he/she is said to be an independent observer. The advantage of an independent observer is that all attention can be focused on the client. The disadvantage is that the client may be aware of being observed and may consequently change or modify behaviour under observation.

Given the fact that direct observations are time consuming, it is not always possible for busy clinicians to engage in them. An alternative is to set up an analogue situation, either through role-play or through simulating a particular setting (for example, role-play could be employed to find out information about how the memory-impaired person copes with passing on messages). A therapist could be recruited to play the person giving the message and the memory-impaired client could be asked to role-play how he/she would deal with the situation. The assessor might want to find out whether the client wrote down or tape-recorded the information, or repeated it back. A simulated setting might be employed to see how a person copes at work. A mock office or shop could be set up and certain tasks given to the client to see what kinds of problem occur. With all direct observations the assessor should carry out the observations several times to check for consistency.

Another approach to collecting information about everyday memory failures is to use self-report measures, such as questionnaires, checklists, rating scales and diaries. It has been known for a number of years that there is poor agreement between self-report measures and traditional or laboratory memory tasks (for example, Sunderland et al. (1984) designed a study to look at the relationship between laboratory tests of memory and subjective reports of memory difficulties by brain-injured people and their relatives). Questionnaires were used to investigate the type and frequency of memory lapses noted in everyday life after a severe brain injury. Correlations with objective tests were low. However, relatives' responses had a greater relationship to the test than responses by the brain-injured people themselves. This was explained as a result of the fact that people with memory problems cannot remember their own memory failures. A related study (Sunderland et al., 1983) found that daily checklists kept by the patients related better to objective test results than did responses to questionnaires, possibly because filling in a checklist provides a more immediate evaluation of problems.

Although self-report measures are a quick way to identify everyday problems and can target relevant issues, it is important to remember that filling in the measures is, in itself, a memory task, so one should not expect accuracy from the memory-impaired person. Nevertheless, such measures are useful because they give us insight into the patients' perceptions and understanding of their problems. Perhaps more importantly, however, one can give the measures to relatives and members of staff to complete on behalf of the memory-impaired person in order to get a more accurate picture. Thus, it is usual, at least in the settings where I work, to administer measures to the client and to an independent other who knows the memory-impaired person well. Examples of self-report measures can be found in Wilson (1999).

The main differences between standardized and the more functional or behavioural assessments include the following. First, standardized tests tend to tell us what a person *has*; for example, a person might have a severe memory impairment or a visuospatial memory deficit. Behavioural assessments, on the other hand, tend to tell us what a person *does*. Thus, a person might forget to put her wheelchair brakes on when transferring to the toilet, or asks the same question 50 times each hour.

Second, in standardized tests, behaviours observed are typically *signs* of a disorder, so for example, if someone fails to recall a prose passage after a delay, this can be taken as a sign of memory impairment. In behavioural assessments, however, the behaviours observed are seen as *samples* of performance, so we might sample a person's remembering or forgetting performance.

Third, standardized tests are usually carried out in *one situation*, typically the neuropsychologist's office; whereas behavioural assessments are more likely to be carried out in a *number of situations*, such as the hospital ward, occupational therapy, at home or at work.

Fourth, standardized tests are carried out as part of a *diagnosis*: we want to find out whether there is organic memory impairment or whether there are additional cognitive problems. In contrast, behavioural assessments are usually implemented to *help select or plan treatment*; for example, we need to know whether the problems are particularly likely to occur in certain situations or at certain times of day.

Fifth, the standardized tests have an *indirect relationship to treatment*. We need to know as much as possible about the nature of the memory deficit and of other cognitive functions but we do not (or should not) treat the inability to do well on a memory test. Behavioural assessments, on the other hand, have a *direct relationship to treatment*.

Finally, standardized tests are typically carried out prior to treatment (or perhaps post-treatment) but they are *not part of the treatment process itself*. In contrast, behavioural assessments may well be carried out during treatment and are therefore *part of the treatment process*. If we are trying to ensure, for example, that wheelchair brakes are applied by a patient, or the repetition of a question decreases, we need to measure these behaviours during treatment. Although there are fundamental differences between standardized test and behavioural assessments, both are important and provide complementary information. We need standardized test results to build up a cognitive map of strengths and weaknesses; we need behavioural assessments to clarify everyday problems, set goals for and evaluate treatment.

ASPECTS OF MEMORY TO BE ASSESSED

Leaving aside behavioural assessments of memory problems (see Chapter 10 for more on this), what should be included in a clinical memory assessment? Not every person referred for memory assessment will need to be assessed in great detail. Again, the nature of the question(s) one is trying to answer will determine this. Sometimes a quick screening test might suffice. If, for example, one is looking for signs of organic memory impairment, then one of the existing tests, such as WMS-R/WMS III, might provide evidence of this. If the pattern of results is consistent with organic memory impairment (e.g. normal forward digit span, poor delayed memory and problems with paired-associate learning particularly hard verbal pairs), then one could conclude there is evidence of organic memory impairment.

Frequently, however, testers will need a more thorough and fine-grained assessment, particularly for people who are referred for rehabilitation. In such cases, one may want to look at a wide range of memory functions, together with other cognitive functions In these cases, as far as memory is concerned, one will probably need to look at:

1. Orientation for time, place and person.
2. Immediate memory, including verbal, visual and spatial short-term/immediate memory.
3. Delayed episodic memory, including visual recall, visual recognition, verbal recall and verbal recognition.
4. New episodic learning, including verbal, visual and spatial.
5. Implicit memory, including, perhaps, motor, verbal and visual aspects of implicit memory.
6. Remote memory, to look at retrograde amnesia—one may want to subdivide this into personal/autobiographical memory and memory for public information.
7. Prospective memory, perhaps subdivided into remembering to do things (a) at a given time, (b) within a certain time interval, and (c) when a certain event happens.
8. Semantic memory, for both verbal and visual material.

How should these aspects of memory be assessed?

Most of the subtypes of memory functioning above will be able to be measured by one or more of the many published memory tests. A number of the published tests are described in Lezak (1995) and Spreen & Strauss (1998). Orientation should be included in all memory assessments (Erickson & Scott, 1977) and it is easy to find tests containing orientation questions (e.g. The Wechsler Scales, the RBMT and the Randt et al. (1980) test). People with organic memory impairment are almost always orientated for person and most will be able to give their date of birth. Problems may arise with orientation for time and place. If someone does not know what year it is, it is difficult to work out how old one is, so it is not uncommon to find memory-impaired patients who do not know their current age unless they are given the date and can thus work it out. Immediate memory for verbal material is almost always assessed clinically with forward digit span. Test items, age-related norms and percentiles can be found in the Wechsler Memory Scales and in the Wechsler Adult Intelligence Scales. It is less clear what is being measured by backward digit span, although it is often used to assess attention. Immediate visuospatial span can be measured by the visual memory span tasks in the Wechsler Memory Scales and a purer measure of visual memory by the Visual Patterns Test (Della Sala et al., 1997). Some studies have shown double dissociations between the visual and spatial aspects of immediate memory. Thus, there may be differences between the Visual Patterns Test, which reduces the spatial component, and the Wechsler Memory Scales visual tapping tasks (Della Sala et al., 1999; Wilson et al., 1999a).

Other ways of testing immediate memory can be employed. These include:

- The recency effect in free recall. The testee is requested to recall a list of words in any order. If the last word(s) are consistently recalled (i.e. a recency effect is found), one can conclude that there is normal short-term/immediate memory.
- Other pattern recognition tasks, such as those used by Phillips (1974).
- The Token Test (De Renzi, 1982). Although this is normally used as a test of comprehension, it is also sensitive to deficits of immediate memory span.

Delayed/long-term episodic memory can be subdivided into (a) verbal recall, (b) verbal recognition, (c) visual recall and (d) visual recognition. Verbal recall tasks are among the most frequently used of all memory tests and prose recall passages among the most sensitive tests for detecting organic impairment (Sunderland et al., 1984). The stories from the Wechsler Memory Scales, the Adult Memory and Information Processing Battery (AMIPB; Coughlan & Hollows, 1984, 1985) and the Rivermead Behavioural Memory Test all provide prose passages for verbal recall.

One widely used test of recognition, at least in the UK, is the Recognition Memory Test (Warrington, 1984). This is in two parts — Recognition Memory for Words (i.e. verbal recognition) and Recognition Memory for Faces (i.e. visual recognition). The new Camden Memory Tests (Warrington, 1996) include a short recognition memory test for words and faces.

Among the best known visual recall tests are the Rey–Osterreith Complex Figure (Rey, 1958), the Benton Visual Retention Test (BVRT; Benton, 1974) and the Visual Reproduction Tests from the Wechsler Memory Scales. The AMIPB also has a complex figure analogous to the Rey figure. Participants are required to copy the figure first (with the exception of the BVRT) and recall after a delay. Participants with planning, visuospatial or apraxic difficulties may have problems copying these figures and this, in turn, could affect their delayed recall. Another potential disadvantage of these figures is that the scoring is not always straightforward; for example, at least two scoring methods exist for the Rey figure (see Lezak, 1995) and some of the drawings/figures are, at least partly, verbalisable. With the Rey, the overall figure looks rather like a flag, there are vertical, horizontal and diagonal lines with triangles and a component resembling a face.

Recognition memory for faces has already been mentioned. The Camden (Warrington, 1996) also includes a topographical and a pictorial recognition task, as does the RBMT and RBMT-E. Baddeley et al. (1994) produced a test that includes all four components in one battery. This is the Doors and People: a test of visual and verbal recall and recognition. This is a theoretically-derived, broad-based test, using ecologically plausible material which provides a number of scores. Results can be used to derive: (a) a single overall age-scaled score; (b) a verbal memory score; (c) a visual memory score; (d) a recognition memory score; (e) a recall memory score; and (f) a forgetting score. In the visual recall task, participants copy the figures first, so it is possible to ensure there are no problems with the execution of the design. Although the visual material is verbalisable (e.g. "door" or "cross"), in practice this is of little help as all the other material also consists of a "door" or a "cross", so one has to rely on visual detail. Finally, scoring problems are considerably reduced through clear examples and instructions.

New episodic learning can also be subdivided into verbal and visual (or visuospatial learning). The Wechsler Scales include subtests to look at both visual and verbal learning. For verbal learning there is the paired associate learning task. Eight pairs of words are presented, with four pairs having a logical match (e.g. metal–iron) and four pairs having no logical connection (e.g. cabbage–pen). Everyone finds the nonlogical pairs harder to learn but people with organic memory deficits find this task almost impossible, even over several trials. The Wechsler visual paired-associate task involves learning to match a colour with a symbol. Again, this is extremely difficult for memory-impaired people.

A number of other verbal paired-associate learning tasks are available. These include the Camden (Warrington, 1996), the Test for Longitudinal Measurement of Mild to Moderate Deficits (Randt et al., 1980), and the paired-associate learning tests of Inglis (1957) and Walton & Black (1957). Not all new verbal learning tests are paired-associates. The Rey Auditory–Verbal Learning Test (RAVLT; Rey, 1964) and The California Verbal Learning Test (CVLT; Delis et al., 1987) are both readily available and useful tests to include in one's repertoire. In both these tests, the testee is required to listen to a list of 15 or 16 words and repeat back as many as possible in any order. The list is repeated four more times. Each time, free recall is required. There is then a distraction list, followed by recall of the original list. The CVLT (Delis et al., 1987) has some advantages over the RAVLT; for example it includes a short delayed recall and a long (20 min) delayed recall. It also provides category cues to aid recall: "Tell me all the tools that you can recall". Finally, the CVLT enables one to score several different aspects of memory. The Selective Reminding Test (Buschke & Fuld, 1974) is another test of verbal learning and one that is claimed to separate out retention, storage and retrieval (Lezak, 1995); however, as (Lezak, 1995) says, this is a procedure rather than a test and is given in a number of ways, so it is hard to compare different findings.

Apart from the visual paired associates in the WM Scales, tests to assess nonverbal, episodic learning are harder to find. Wilson et al. (1989a) describe a test of new learning in which participants are given three trials to learn a six-step task. The testee is required to put the date and time into an electronic memory aid. All 50 normal control participants learned the task in three trials (and most in one trial), whereas less than 44% of the people with brain injury learned the task in three trials.

Both the RBMT and the RBMT-E include learning a new route (both immediate and delayed recall are required) and a model version of the route in the RBMT-E has recently been published (Clare et al., 2000). The RBMT-E routes combine visuospatial and verbal learning as they attempt to replicate real-life learning of new routes.

A recently published test of visuospatial learning, designed specifically for use with older adults and individuals with dementia or suspected dementia, is the Location Learning Test

(LLT; Bucks et al., 2000). The LLT uses an array on which 10 pictures of everyday items have been placed. The participant is required to learn the location of the pictures over five trials. Rather than using a number correct score for each trial, the LLT is calculated in terms of displacement error, thus allowing for a more sensitive measure of learning.

One final approach to non-verbal learning, which is easy to administer, is a visual-span plus two task. This can be given with the Corsi blocks (described by Milner, 1971), the visual tapping from the WM Scales and the Visual Patterns test. Once span has been established in the usual way, the tester adds two more blocks or squares. Thus if the span is a typical five, the learning sequence of seven is administered and repeated until the participant can reproduce it correctly or until 25 (or even 50) trials have been given. Although norms do not appear to exist, most without brain injury people would learn this within three (and certainly within five) trials, whereas people with a dense amnesia fail to learn the sequence even after 50 trials.

Although implicit memory, or memory without awareness, is of great interest to researchers into theoretical models of memory, implicit memory is not regularly assessed by clinicians. This may be due to the fact that standardized assessments are not available, so each battery or test has to be made separately or obtained from colleagues working in the area. Another reason for the haphazard inclusion of these tasks is that it is not clear how implicit memory relates to everyday problems or rehabilitation goals (although see Chapter 10 for further discussion). As long ago as 1988, Baddeley & Wilson suggested that poor procedural memory (one aspect of implicit memory) in people with organic memory impairment could be a poor prognostic sign (Baddeley & Wilson, 1988). Implicit memory is not a unitary concept, however (Wilson et al., 1996b), and one should probably look at a number of aspects, including implicit memory for motor verbal and visual tasks.

Another way to subdivide implicit memory is to look at tasks involving procedural memory, priming and stem completion. One task for looking at motor implicit or procedural memory is the pursuit rotor task, a visual-motor tracking task. People with organic memory deficits typically improve the percentage of time on target, despite (in some cases) being unable to recognize that they have been tested on the task previously. A variation on pursuit rotor is the mirror tracing task, in which the testee is required to trace a pattern with a light pen. The pattern cannot be seen directly and has to be viewed through a mirror. Woodworth & Schlosberg (1954) report a large practice effect with nonbrain-injured people on this task and improvement has also been shown with people who are amnesic. Wilson et al. (1996b) gave a mirror tracing task to 110 control participants and 12 amnesic participants aged 20–55 years. These results can be seen in Figure 8.1. Thus, it can be seen that although the people with amnesia were slower than controls, the pattern of improvement was similar.

Clinically, the best way to measure motor memory is probably to use a computerized visual tracking task, such as that used by Baddeley et al. (1986) in their study of Alzheimer's disease. The problem with this is that participants would have to be used as their own controls. This would allow one to see whether or not they improved over time, but not how such improvement compared to a normal control group.

One verbal implicit memory task frequently used in theoretical studies is stem completion or verbal priming. This involves the presentation of a list of words and then the presentation of a stem (the first two or three letters). The testee is then required to say the first word that comes to mind when he/she sees the stem. So, for example, if the words CHOKE, TRUST and WHEAT are presented and a few seconds later CH is shown and the testee asked for the first word that comes to mind, the response (even among people with amnesia) is likely

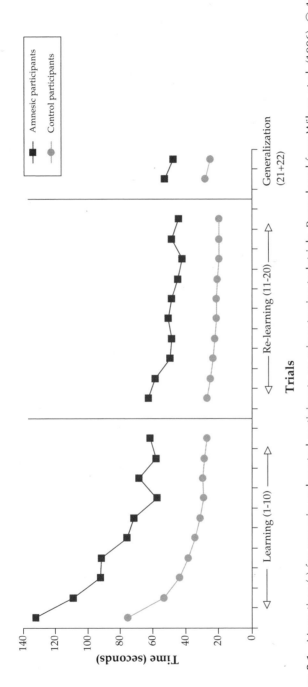

Figure 8.1 Mean time (s) for amnesic and control participants on mirror-tracing task trials. Reproduced from Wilson et al. (1996). © 1996, Swets Zeitlinger

to be CHOKE rather than CHEESE or CHALK (see Davis & Bernstein, 1982; Graf et al., 1984; Chapter 10, this volume, for further discussion). Baddeley & Wilson (1994) used a stem completion task to compare errorful and errorless learning (again, see Chapter 10, this volume).

Perceptual priming involving visual implicit memory is another kind of task employed in a number of studies. Fragmented pictures (degraded from a greater to a lesser degree) are presented until the testee can identify the picture. Originally employed by Warrington & Weiskrantz (1968), it was shown that people with amnesia showed savings, i.e. recognized the pictures earlier in the sequence when these were shown a second time despite having no episodic memory of seeing the pictures earlier. Wilson et al. (1996b), using a computerized method to fragment the pictures based on Snodgrass et al. (1987), administered fragmented pictures to 136 control participants and 16 people with amnesia. The people with amnesia were poorer at recognizing the sequences but showed savings compared to a baseline condition. An auditory priming task was also included in the Wilson et al. (1996b) study. This was a replication of a study by Johnson et al. (1985), whereby melodies heard several times were preferred to melodies heard only once. There was no difference between the controls and the people with amnesia on the preference (implicit memory) task, despite a significant difference on a recognition (explicit memory) task. The Wilson et al. (1996b) study also showed dissociations among people with amnesia in that "normal" performance (compared to controls) on one type of implicit memory task did not guarantee "normal" performance on another. This supported the view that implicit memory is not unitary and can be fractionated like episodic, explicit memory tasks. The time is right for a published standardized test battery to appear for the assessment of several aspects of implicit memory.

Remote memory is another aspect of memory functioning that is rarely assessed routinely in clinical practice, despite having important implications for real life problems. In 1986, Baddeley & Wilson suggested that impaired autobiographical memory can result in anxiety, depression and other problematic behaviours (Baddeley & Wilson, 1986). In order to know who we are, we need a past. People with long periods of retrograde amnesia are frequently angry or bewildered by what seems to them an unexpectedly high cost of living, change in political and geographical circumstances or the loss of several years from their lives. For a description of one man with a very long retrograde amnesia (RA), bewilderment and confusion, see Wilson (1999, Chapter 6).

It is possible to find people whose RA for public events is greater than that for personal events and vice versa (see Hodges & McCarthy, 1993; Kapur, 1993, 1999), although it is more typical to find impairments in both. There is a published semistructured interview to assess autobiographical memory. This is the Autobiographical Memory Interview (AMI; Kopelman et al., 1989b). The AMI encompasses two aspects of autobiographical memory, viz. personal semantic memory, i.e. memory for facts (e.g. names of friends, addresses and schools attended) and memory for specific autobiographical incidents (e.g. something that happened at one's wedding or when one went on holiday). Each of these aspects covers three broad time bands: childhood, early adult life and recent time, i.e. the past year.

Kopelman et al. (1989a) believe that it is useful to assess autobiographical memory for at least three reasons: to understand the nature of the memory deficit, to allow for more adequate counselling and to provide an individual focus for treatment. Baddeley & Wilson (1986) found that subjects who are very similar on intelligence and memory test scores may differ markedly on ability to recall events from their own past life. The AMI has been subject to a number of research studies; for example, Evans et al. (1993) found that a woman assessed during an episode of Transient Global Amnesia (TGA) achieved a reasonable score on the personal semantic sections but scored poorly on the autobiographical incidents. When re-assessed following recovery from the TGA, she scored normally on both personal semantic and autobiographical questions. In contrast, Graham & Hodges (1997) found that patients with semantic dementia (at least in the earlier stages) showed the reverse pattern, i.e. they were poor at the personal semantic sections but relatively unimpaired on the autobiographical incidents.

Famous faces, famous names and famous events from different decades are most often used in assessing remote memory for public events. However, there is not one readily available test for the assessment of public events. Although a number of tools have been developed as research instruments, including a Retrograde Amnesia Battery by Butters & Albert (1982), all such tests need regular updating, so any published RA test is only valid for a couple of years or so. Other problems include: (a) differences in the level of interest, so that people who have always been interested in the news are likely to show a different pattern to those who have shown little interest; (b) cultural specificity, so British politicians or sports stars may have had little exposure in the USA; and (c) differences in exposure, so Charlie Chaplin, dead many years, will still be recognized by many, whereas Lord Mountbatten, who died much more recently, will be recognized by far fewer people. There have been attempts to develop other tests of remote memory, for example the Prices Test (Wilson & Cockburn, 1988), in which people are asked to estimate the cost of some common items; and the Dead-and-Alive Test (referred to in Kapur et al., 1996), in which people have to say whether or not a famous person is dead or alive (and if dead, when and how the death occurred). The aforementioned problems still apply, however, and it will probably always be necessary to produce one's own materials and/or modify material regularly.

Prospective memory involves remembering to perform previously planned actions at the right time (e.g. "at 8 pm tonight telephone your sister") or within the right time interval (e.g. "post a letter before leaving work today") or when a certain event takes place (e.g. "when you next see your colleague pass on a message"). These actions should take place while the person concerned is engaged in other activities. One of the commonest complaints of people with memory problems is forgetting to do things (prospective memory failures), yet once again, this aspect of memory is not always assessed. Mateer et al. (1987) showed that people both with and without brain injury perceive themselves as having more trouble with prospective memory tasks than with other memory tasks, and went on to develop a Prospective Memory Screening tool (PROMS; Sohlberg & Mateer, 1989) to look at the ability to remember to carry out tasks after 60 s, 2 min, 10 min, 20 min, and 24 h. The only other tests to formally include prospective memory items appear to be the RMBT and the RMBT-E. The original RBMT has three (out of 12) items concerned with prospective memory. Participants have to remember to: (a) ask, at the end of the test, for a belonging that was placed out of sight at the beginning of the test; (b) ask about the next appointment when an alarm rings; and (c) deliver a message to a predetermined place during the immediate and delayed recall of a new route. These prospective memory items seem to account for some of the sensitivity of the RBMT; for example, Cockburn & Smith (1989) found that prospective memory items significantly discriminated between two groups of older subjects living in the community: a "young" old group aged 55–70 years and an "old" old group aged 71–90 years.

The RBMT-E has similar prospective memory items but as this test places a greater load on memory, the items are consequently more demanding. Thus two belongings are hidden at the beginning of the test instead of one, two questions are asked when the alarm rings and two messages have to be delivered during the immediate and delayed recall of the route.

As screening tests the RBMT and RBMT-E adequately cover the assessment of prospective memory. However, a more detailed assessment of prospective memory would appear to be clinically useful and work on this is well under way. We are developing a clinical, ecologically valid test of prospective memory in Cambridge, covering time-based prospective memory tasks (e.g. "In 15 min time remind me not to forget my key") and event-based tasks (e.g. "When the alarm rings please open the window").

A pilot study with 36 people with brain injury and 28 people with no known brain injury, showed that: (a) the new test of prospective memory discriminated between those with and without brain injury; (b) time-based tasks were more difficult for both groups than event-based tasks; and (c) people who took notes/wrote down information scored significantly better than those who did not take notes (Groot et al., 2002). We expect the final version of this test to be ready in 2004.

Tulving (1972) first suggested that semantic and episodic memory should be distinguishable. Semantic memory is the system we use to store knowledge about the world. We refer to our semantic store when answering such questions as "Does a rabbit have prick ears?", "What does the word 'happy' mean?" and "What shape is Italy?" We have a huge store of information as to what things mean, look like, sound like, smell like and feel like. Damage to this store or impaired access to this store may follow brain damage; Warrington (1975) suggests that visual object agnosia is a deficit of the visual semantic memory system. Furthermore, some patients lose the ability to recognize living things but are still able to recognize non-living things. They are said to have a category-specific disorder (Warrington & Shallice, 1984). Hillis & Caramazza (1991) and Sacchett & Humphreys (1992) describe the reverse, i.e. people who show greater knowledge of living than of non-living or manufactured objects. Patients with semantic memory deficits are likely to have problems recognizing objects in the real world and problems expressing themselves, and may be considered stupid because of the errors they make.

Semantic memory may be assessed in a variety of ways, including spoken and single-word comprehension, category fluency and general knowledge. Hodges et al. (1992a, 1992b) describe a semantic memory test battery designed to assess semantic knowledge in patients with dementia of the Alzheimer type and patients with progressive semantic dementia. Wilson (1997) also administered the battery, with broadly similar results, to people with non-progressive brain injury. The battery has the major advantage of employing one set of stimulus items designed to assess input to and output from a central store of representational knowledge. Thus, the same group of items is used as stimuli and assessed using different sensory modalities. The battery contains 48 items, representing three categories of manufactured items matched for prototypicality. The three living categories are land animals, water creatures and birds. The three manufactured categories are household items, vehicles and musical instruments. Knowledge of these items is assessed in several ways, namely fluency, naming, picture–word matching, picture sorting and naming to description. Although a considerable amount of work has been carried out on this battery, it has not yet been published as a test. One semantic memory battery that has been published is the Category-Specific Names Test (McKenna, 1998), a test of naming objects and of matching objects with their names in four semantic categories.

In conclusion to this section, it must be pointed out that the above list of potential clinical memory tests is by no means exhaustive. Readers can find details about other tests in Lezak (1995) and Spreen & Strauss (1998).

General Principles in the Assessment of Memory Disorders

Failure to select, administer and interpret tests appropriately can have serious consequences, for example a problem that exists might be missed, incorrect administration can invalidate results, and misinterpretation of results may lead to incorrect conclusions being drawn and, perhaps, inappropriate treatment offered. All people administering tests need to ensure they are competent to do so. Not only is it imperative to know how to administer and score tests, but the tester should also know how to put the person being tested at ease, how to feed back the results to the patient, family member, therapy staff and referring agents. Confidentiality needs to be ensured and the tester needs to know when it is appropriate and inappropriate to disclose information. Guidelines on selecting, administering and interpreting cognitive tests can be found in Evans et al. (1996). Further issues on assessment are dealt with in Lezak (1995) and Spreen & Strauss (1998).

Another factor that may be forgotten in assessment is the effect of practice. If there is an improvement in test scores, does this mean that the person being tested has really improved or that the change reflects the fact that the test is now no longer novel? Similarly, if there is no change in scores, does this mean the patient has stayed at the same level, or that practice effects have masked any decline? These are very real issues in assessment. Practice effects are different for different tests, for example there is virtually no practice effect on forward digit span but a large one on verbal fluency (Wilson et al., 2000). Some tests, such as the RBMT, have several parallel versions, while others, such as the WMS-R, have only one version. This, too, influences results on repeated assessments. Practice effects are also different for people with and without brain injury (Wilson et al., 2000).

Memory assessment, and assessment of other cognitive functions, is not something to be approached in a casual manner. A test is as good as its developers, designers and administrators. All three owe it to the people being tested to do the best job possible. Used responsibly and ethically, good assessments can contribute to the understanding and well-being of memory-impaired people referred to us.

REFERENCES

Anastasi, A. (1982). *Psychological Testing*, 5th edn. New York: Collier/Macmillan.

Baddeley, A.D. (1999). *Essentials of Human Memory*. Hove: Psychology Press.

Baddeley, A.D., Emslie, H. & Nimmo-Smith, I. (1994). *Doors and People: A Test of Visual and Verbal Recall and Recognition*. Bury St Edmunds: Thames Valley Test Company.

Baddeley, A.D. & Hitch, G. (1974). Working memory. In G. H. Bower (ed.), *The Psychology of Learning and Motivation*, Vol. 8 (pp. 47–89). New York: Academic Press.

Baddeley, A.D., Logie, R., Bressi, S. et al. (1986). Dementia and working memory. *Quarterly Journal of Experimental Psychology*, **38**, 603–618.

Baddeley, A.D. & Wilson, B.A. (1986). Amnesia, autobiographical memory and confabulation. In D. Rubin (ed.), *Autobiographical Memory* (pp. 225–252). New York: Cambridge University Press.

Baddeley, A.D. & Wilson, B.A. (1988). Frontal amnesia and the dysexecutive syndrome. *Brain and Cognition*, **7**, 212–230.

Baddeley, A.D. & Wilson, B.A. (1994). When implicit learning fails: amnesia and the problem of error elimination. *Neuropsychologia*, **32**, 53–68.

Benton, A.L. (1974). *The Revised Visual Retention Test: Clinical and Experimental Applications*. New York: Psychological Corporation.

Bucks, R.S., Willison, J.R. & Byrne, L.M.T. (2000). *Location Learning Test*. Bury St Edmunds: Thames Valley Test Company.

Buschke, H. & Fuld, A.P. (1974). Evaluating storage, retention and retrieval in disordered memory and learning. *Neurology*, **24**, 1019–1025.

Butters, N. & Albert, M.L. (1982). Processes underlying failures to recall remote events. In L. Cermak (ed.), *Human Memory and Amnesia* (pp. 257–274). Hillsdale, NJ: Erlbaum.

Calabrese, P., Markowitsch, H.J., Durwen, H.F. et al. (1996). Right temperofrontal cortex as critical locus for the ecphory of old episodie memories. *Journal of Neurology, Neurosurgery and Psychiatry*, **61**, 304–310.

Clare, L., Wilson, B.A., Emslie, H. (2000). Adapting the Rivermead Behavioural Memory Test Extended Version (RBMT-E) for people with restricted mobility. *British Journal of Clinical Psychology*, **39**, 363–369.

Cockburn, J. & Smith, P. (1989). *The Rivermead Behavioural Memory Test. Supplement* 3: *Elderly People*. Bury St Edmunds: Thames Valley Test Company.

Coughlan, A.K. & Hollows, S.E. (1984). Use of memory tests in differentiating organic disorder from depression. *British Journal of Psychiatry*, **145**, 164–167.

Coughlan, A.K. & Hollows, S. (1985). *The Adult Memory and Information Processing Battery (AMIPB)*. Leeds: A. Coughlan, St James University Hospital.

Davis, H.P. & Bernstein, P.A. (1982). Age-related changes in explicit and implicit memory. In L.R. Squire & N. Butters (eds), *Neuropsychology of Memory*, 2nd edn (pp. 249–261). New York: Guilford.

De Renzi, E. (1982). *Disorders of Space Exploration and Cognition*. Chichester: Wiley.

Delis, D., Kaplan, E., Kramer, J. & Ober, B. (1987). *California Verbal Learning Test*. San Antonio, TX: Psychological Corporation.

Della Sala, S., Gray, C., Baddeley, A.D. et al. (1999). Pattern span: a tool of unwelding visuospatial memory. *Neuropsychologia*, **37**, 1189–1199.

Della Sala, S., Gray, C., Baddeley, A.D. & Wilson, L. (1997). *Visual Patterns Test*. Bury St Edmunds: Thames Valley Test Company.

Erickson, R.C. & Scott, M.L. (1977). Clinical memory testing: a review. *Psychological Bulletin*, **84**, 1130–1149.

Eslinger, P.J. (1998). Autobiographical memory after temporal lobe lesions. *Neurocase*, **4**, 481–495.

Evans, J.J., Wilson, B.A. & Emslie, H. (1996). *Selecting, Administering and Interpreting Cognitive Tests: Guidelines for Clinicians and Therapists*. Bury St Edmunds: Thames Valley Test Company.

Evans, J.J., Wilson, B.A., Wraight, E.P. & Hodges, J. (1993). Neuropsychological and SPECT scan findings during and after transient global amnesia: evidence for differential impairment of remote episodic memory. *Journal of Neurology, Neurosurgery and Psychiatry*, **56**, 1227–1230.

Goldman-Rakic, P.S. & Friedman, H.R. (1991). The circuitry of working memory revealed by anatomy and metabolic imaging. In H.S. Levin, H.M. Eisenberg & A.L. Benton (eds), *Frontal Lobe Function and Dysfunction* (pp. 72–91). New York: Oxford University Press.

Graf, P., Squire, L.R. & Mandler, G. (1984). The information that amnesic patients do not forget. *Journal of Experimental Psychology: Learning, Memory, and Cognition*, **10**, 164–178.

Graham, K.S., Becker, J.T. & Hodges, J.R. (1997). On the relationship between knowledge and memory for pictures: evidence from the study of patients with semantic dementia and Alzheimer's disease. *Journal of the International Neuropsychological Society*, **3**, 534–544.

Graham, K.S. & Hodges, J.R. (1997). Differentiating the roles of the hippocampal complex and the neocortex in long-term memory storage: evidence from the study of semantic dementia and Alzheimer's disease. *Neuropsychology*, **11**, 77–89.

Groot, Y.C.T., Wilson, B.A., Evans, J. & Watson, P. (2002). Prospective memory functioning in people with and without brain injury. *Journal of the International Neuropsychological Society*, **8**, 645–654.

Halstead, W.C. (1947). *Brain and Intelligence*. Chicago, IL: University of Chicago Press.

Hillis, A.E. & Caramazza, A. (1991). Category-specific naming and comprehension impairment: a double dissociation. *Brain*, **114**, 2081–2094.

Hodges, J.R. & McCarthy, R.A. (1993). Autobiographical amnesia resulting from bilateral paramedian thalamic infarction. A case study in cognitive neurobiology. *Brain*, **116**, 921–940.

Hodges, J.R., Patterson, K., Oxbury, S. & Funnell, E. (1992b). Semantic dementia: progressive fluent aphasia with temporal lobe atrophy. *Brain*, **115**, 1783–1806.

Hodges, J., Salmon, D.P. & Butters, N. (1992a). Semantic memory impairment in Alzheimer's disease: failure of access or degraded knowledge? *Neuropsychologia*, **30**, 301–314.

Holland, A.L. (1980). *CADL—Communicative Abilities in Daily Living: A Test of Functional Communication for Aphasic Adults*. Baltimore, MD: University Park Press.

Inglis, J. (1957). An experimental study of learning and "memory function" in elderly psychiatric patients. *Journal of Mental Science*, **103**, 796–803.

Johnson, M.K., Kim, J.K. & Risse, G. (1985). Do alcoholic Korsakoff's syndrome patients acquire affective reactions? *Journal of Experimental Psychology: Learning, Memory, and Cognition*, **11**, 22–36.

Jones, R.D., Grabowski, T.J. & Tranel, D. (1998). The neural basis of retrograde memory: evidence from positron emission tomography for the role of non-mesial temporal lobe structures. *Neurocase*, **4**, 471–479.

Kapur, N. (1993). Focal retrograde amnesia in neurological disease: a critical review. *Cortex*, **29**, 217–234.

Kapur, N. (1999). Syndromes of retrograde amnesia: a conceptual and empirical synthesis. *Psychological Bulletin*, **125**, 800–825.

Kapur, N., Thompson, S., Cook, P. et al. (1996). Anterograde but not retrograde memory loss following combined mammillary body and medial thalamic lesions. *Neuropsychologia*, **34**, 1–8.

Kopelman, M., Wilson, B.A. & Baddeley, A.D. (1989a). The Autobiographical Memory Interview: a new assessment of autobiographical and personal semantic memory in amnesic patients. *Journal of Clinical and Experimental Neuropsychology*, **11**, 724–744.

Kopelman, M., Wilson, B.A. & Baddeley, A.D. (1989b). *The Autobiographical Memory Interviews*. Bury St Edmunds: Thames Valley Test Company.

Lezak, M. (1995). *Neuropsychological Assessment*, 3rd edn. New York: Oxford University Press.

Markowitsch, H.J. (1998). Cognitive neuroscience of memory. *Neurocase*, **4**, 429–435.

Mateer, C.A., Sohlberg, M.M. & Crinean, J. (1987). Perceptions of memory functions in individuals with closed head injury. *Journal of Head Trauma Rehabilitation*, **2**, 74–84.

Mayes, A.R. (1986). Learning and memory disorders and their assessment. *Neuropsychologia*, **24**, 25–39.

Mayes, A.R. (1995). *Human Organic Memory Disorders*. Cambridge: Cambridge University Press.

McKenna, P. (1998). *The Category-specific Names Test*. Hove: Psychology Press.

Milner, B. (1971). Interhemispheric differences in the localisation of psychological processes in man. *British Medical Bulletin: Cognitive Psychology*, **27**, 272–277.

Phillips, W.A. (1974). On the distinction between sensory storage and short-term visual memory. *Perception and Psychophysics*, **16**, 283–290.

Randt, C.T., Brown, E.R. & Osborne, D.P. (1980). A memory test for longitudinal measurement of mild to moderate deficits. *Clinical Neuropsychology*, **2**, 184–194.

Reitan, R.M. & Davison, L.A. (1974). *Clinical Neuropsychology: Current Status and Applications*. New York: Hemisphere.

Rey, A. (1958, 1964). *L'Examen Clinique en Psychologie*. Paris: Universitaires de France.

Robertson, I.H., Ward, T., Ridgeway, V. & Nimmo-Smith, I. (1994). *The Test of Everyday Attention*. Bury St Edmunds: Thames Valley Test Company.

Sacchett, C. & Humphreys, G.W. (1992). Calling a squirrel a squirrel but a canoe a wigwam: a category-specific deficit for artifactual objects and body parts. *Cognitive Neuropsychology*, **9**, 73–86.

Schwartz, A.F. & McMillan, T.M. (1989). Assessment of everyday memory after severe head injury. *Cortex*, **25**, 665–671.

Shallice, T., Fletcher, P., Frith, C.D. et al. (1994). Brain regions associated with acquisition and retrieval of verbal episodic memory. *Nature*, **368**, 633–635.

Shiel, A., Wilson, B.A., McLellan, L. et al. (2000). *The Wessex Head Injury Matrix (WHIM)*. Bury St Edmunds: Thames Valley Test Company.

Snodgrass, J.G., Smith, B., Feenan, K. & Corwin, J. (1987). Fragmenting pictures on the Apple Macintosh computer for experimental and clinical applications. *Behavior Research Methods, Instruments, and Computers*, **19**, 270–274.

Sohlberg, M.M. & Mateer, C. (1989). Training use of compensatory memory books: a three-stage behavioural approach. *Journal of Clinical and Experimental Neuropsychology*, **11**, 871–891.

Spreen, O. & Strauss, E. (1998). *A compendium of neuropsychological tests*, 2nd edn. New York: Oxford University Press.

Sundberg, N.S. & Tyler, L.E. (1962). *Clinical Psychology*. New York: Appleton-Century-Crofts.

Sunderland, A., Harris, J.E. & Baddeley, A.D. (1983). Do laboratory tests predict everyday memory? A neuropsychological study. *Journal of Verbal Learning and Verbal Behavior*, **22**, 341–357.

Sunderland, A., Harris, J.E. & Gleave, J. (1984). Memory failures in everyday life after severe head injury. *Journal of Clinical Neuropsychology*, **6**, 127–142.

Tranel, D. & Damasio, A.R. (2002). Neurobiological foundations of human memory. In A.D. Baddeley, M.D. Kopelman & B.A. Wilson (eds), *Handbook of Memory Disorders*, 2nd edn (pp. 17–56). Chichester: Wiley.

Tulving, E. (1972). Episodic and semantic memory. In E. Tulving & W. Donaldson (eds), *Organization of Memory* (pp. 381–403). New York: Academic Press.

Tulving, E., Kapur, S., Craik, F.I.M. et al. (1994). Hemispheric encoding/retrieval asymmetry in episodic memory: positron emission tomography findings. *Proceedings of the National Academy of Sciences of the USA*, **91**, 2016–2020.

Vallar, G. & Papagno, C. (1995). Neuropsychological impairments of short-term memory. In A.D. Baddeley, B.A. Wilson & F.N. Watts (eds), *Handbook of Memory Disorders, 1st edn* (pp. 135–165). Chichester: Wiley.

Walton, D. & Black, D.A. (1957). The validity of a psychological test of brain damage. *British Journal of Medical Psychology*, **30**, 270–279.

Warrington, E.K. (1975). The selective impairment of semantic memory. *Quarterly Journal of Experimental Psychology*, **27**, 635–657.

Warrington, E.K. (1984). *The Recognition Memory Test*. Windsor: NFER-Nelson.

Warrington, E. (1996). *Camden Memory Tests*. Hove: Psychology Press.

Warrington, E.K. & Shallice, T. (1984). Category-specific semantic impairments. *Brain*, **107**, 829–854.

Warrington, E.K. & Weiskrantz, L. (1968). New method of testing long-term retention with special reference to amnesic patients. *Nature*, **217**, 972–974.

Wechsler, D. (1945). A standardized memory scale for clinical use. *Journal of Psychology*, **19**, 87–95.

Wechsler, D. (1987). *The Wechsler Memory Scale—Revised*. San Antonio, TX: Psychological Corporation.

Wechsler, D. (1997). *Wechsler Memory Scale III*. San Antonio, TX: Psychological Corporation.

Wilson, B.A. (1991). Theory, assessment and treatment in neuropsychological rehabilitation. *Neuropsychology*, **5**, 281–291.

Wilson, B.A. (1997). Semantic memory impairments following non-progressive brain damage: a study of four cases. *Brain Injury*, **11**, 259–269.

Wilson, B.A. (1999). *Case Studies in Neuropsychological Rehabilitation*. New York: Oxford University Press.

Wilson, B.A., Alderman, N., Burgess, P. et al. (1996a). *Behavioural Assessment of the Dysexecutive Syndrome*. Bury St Edmunds: Thames Valley Test Company.

Wilson, B.A., Baddeley, A.D. & Cockburn, J. (1989a). How do old dogs learn new tricks? Teaching a technological skill to brain-damaged people. *Cortex*, **25**, 115–119.

Wilson, B.A., Baddeley, A.D. & Young, A.W. (1999a). L.E., a person who lost her "mind's eye". *Neurocase*, **5**, 119–127.

Wilson, B.A., Clare, L., Baddeley, A.D. et al. (1999b). *The Rivermead Behavioural Memory Test— Extended Version*. Bury St Edmunds: Thames Valley Test Company.

Wilson, B.A. & Cockburn, J. (1988). The Prices Test: a simple test of retrograde amnesia. In M.M. Gruneberg, P.E. Morris & R.N. Sykes (eds), *Practical Aspects of Memory: Current Research and Issues*, Vol. 2 (pp. 46–51). Chichester: Wiley.

Wilson, B.A., Cockburn, J. & Baddeley, A.D. (1985). *The Rivermead Behavioural Memory Test*. Bury St Edmunds: Thames Valley Test Company.

Wilson, B.A., Cockburn, J., Baddeley, A.D. & Hiorns, R. (1989b). The development and validation of a test battery for detecting and monitoring everyday memory problems. *Journal of Clinical and Experimental Neuropsychology*, **11**, 855–870.

Wilson, B.A., Cockburn, J. & Halligan, P.W. (1988). *The Behavioural Inattention Test*. Bury St Edmunds: Thames Valley Test Company.

Wilson, B.A., Green, R., Teasdale, T. et al. (1996b). Implicit learning in amnesic subjects: a comparison with a large group of normal control subjects. *Clinical Neuropsychologist*, **10**, 279–292.

Wilson, B.A. & Patterson, K.E. (1990). Rehabilitation and cognitive neuropsychology: does cognitive psychology apply? *Journal of Applied Cognitive Psychology*, **4**, 247–260.

Wilson, B.A., Watson, P.C., Baddeley, A.D. et al. (2000). Improvement or simply practice? The effects of twenty repeated assessments on people with and without brain injury. *Journal of the International Neuropsychological Society*, **6**, 469–479.

Wilson, J.C. & Hughes, E. (1997). Coping with amnesia: the natural history of a compensatory memory system. *Neuropsychological Rehabilitation*, **7**, 43–56.

Woodworth, R.S. & Schlosberg, H. (1954). *Experimental Psychology*, revised edn. London: Methuen.

CHAPTER 9

Separating Memory from Other Cognitive Disorders

Diane B. Howieson

and

Muriel D. Lezak

Oregon Health Sciences University, Portland, OR, USA

The clinician is often asked to evaluate patients' memory or learning problems, even when memory is not the actual problem. It is not uncommon for patients and the people close to them to attribute a variety of cognitive and behavioral problems to failing memory. A spouse brings her husband for evaluation complaining that he does not remember to do anything she has asked. When it turns out that the memory problem is confined to this one category of information, the clinician begins to suspect that the problem lies elsewhere. More often, the complaint is difficulty remembering the names of new acquaintances. In these circumstances the social encounter may provide ample distraction for not properly registering the name at the introduction.

Memory complaints provide fascinating and sometimes amusing insights into the complexities and vagaries of human relationships as well as the human mind, but they can present neuropsychologists with serious diagnostic challenges. In this chapter we will focus on the variety of cognitive problems that (secondarily) produce what patients experience or those dealing with them describe as poor memory. As more is learned about how the brain functions, it becomes increasingly difficult to distinguish between theoretical concepts of memory and other cognitive functions (Damasio et al., 1990; Kosslyn & Thompson, 2000; Lezak, 1995). At the practical level, however, the clinician is able to make distinctions that have important implications for counseling and remediation.

The major sources of the *experience* of memory impairment when new learning and retention actually are spared are *information registration deficits*, which can be due to impaired attention or information processing, and *executive function disorders* (see Figure 9.1). These neuropsychological abnormalities can occur discretely or in combination to affect the efficiency of the learning/memory system. Obviously, the more the problem is compounded, the more impaired will be the patient's memory performance.

The Essential *Handbook of Memory Disorders for Clinicians.* Edited by A.D. Baddeley, M.D. Kopelman and B.A. Wilson.
© 2004 John Wiley & Sons, Ltd. ISBN 0-470-09141-X.

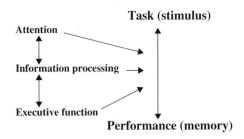

Figure 9.1   Cognitive processes that affect memory as well as other areas of cognition

INFORMATION REGISTRATION

Memory functions are dependent on attention and information processing for proper registration of information to be learned (Curran, 2000; Fischler, 1998; Pashler, 1998). "Attention" refers to the several abilities involved in attending to and grasping all of a specific stimulus (Parasuraman, 1998). "Information processing" refers to the ability to extract the meaning of the stimulus based on past experiences. Some types of information processing are relatively automatic while others require effort and strategies. Reductions in attention and information processing produce marked limitations on memory. The cognitive inefficiencies consequent to attention and information processing deficits are frequently misinterpreted by patients and those close to them as "memory" problems (for example see Di Stefano & Radanov, 1996).

Attention

Many diffusely brain-injured patients have impaired attention (Gasquoine, 1997; Morrow, Robin et al., 1992; Rao, 1996; van Gorp et al., 1989). Their deficit may be obvious only on examination because they appear to attend adequately to tasks. Patients may be limited in attentional capacity, in the ability to direct attention, in the ability to divide attention to more than one stimulus, or in the ability to sustain attention. As attentional tasks increase in complexity, they are often referred to as "tests of concentration" and "mental tracking" or "mental manipulation" (Lezak 1995; Weintraub, 2000). Although many of them involve more complex mental operations as well, attention is a prominent contributing process.

Attentional Capacity

Simple attention span is most frequently examined with a digit repetition task, which tests how many numbers a person can attend to at once and repeat in sequence. The Digit Span tests from the Wechsler Intelligence Scales (WIS) (Wechsler, 1955, 1981, 1997) and the Wechsler Memory Scales (WMS) (Wechsler, 1945, 1987, 1997) assess repetition of digits both forward and backward. The latter task involves a mental tracking component that distinguishes it from the simple span measure. A more subtle disorder may be detected by increasing the demands of the task, such as using a sentence repetition task, which increases the informational load (Benton & Hamsher, 1989; Spreen & Strauss, 1998). A visual measure of attention span may be obtained by the Corsi Cube Test (Milner, 1971) or the WMS Spatial Span Test (Wechsler, 1987, 1997), in which the patient reproduces spatially arranged patterns of increasing length, as demonstrated by the examiner.

These tests of attention require intact short-term memory. Most patients with brain disorders have intact short-term memory when recall follows reception immediately, with neither delay nor interference. When their attention is directed away from tasks by an interpolated activity, retention, even for relatively brief intervals, becomes tenuous. Patients with actual short-term memory impairment do exist but it is relatively rare (Vallar & Shallice, 1990; Warrington & Shallice, 1984), so this possibility should be evaluated. Poor performance on a simple digit span task is more likely to be representative of an attentional impairment rather than a true memory impairment.

Attentional capacity is resistant to the effects of many brain disorders. It may be restricted in the first months following head trauma but it is likely to return to normal during later states (Bazarian et al., 1999; Lezak, 1979; Ponsford & Kinsella, 1992). Most mildly demented Alzheimer's patients have normal capacity for reciting a string of digits (Pachana et al., 1996; Rubin et al., 1998), although not as the dementia progresses (Freed et al., 1989; Storandt et al., 1992). However, when the information becomes more complex, as in sentence span tests, or more information is presented than can normally be grasped at once, as in supraspan tests (Benton et al., 1983; Milner, 1970; see also Lezak, 1995), the reduced attentional capacity of many brain-injured persons becomes evident (Small et al., 2000).

> A 55-year-old advertising executive had his first symptoms of multiple sclerosis 20 years before he was examined for suspected cognitive deficits. At this examination he was confined to a wheelchair, having use of only his left hand. His highest test scores were on a recognition vocabulary test (93rd percentile) and a test of practical reasoning based on well-established information (90th percentile). Working memory, measured by Auditory Consonant Trigrams, was intact. However, he had difficulty repeating sentences of more than 19 syllables accurately (e.g. his recall of "Yesterday he said he would be near the village station before it was time for a train to come" was "Yesterday he said he would be before the station where the train was to come").

Directed Attention

In most settings an individual attending to a task must direct attention to the relevant material and ignore extraneous information, for example that required to read a book while riding a crowded bus. Normally, the clinician examines the patient in an environment relatively free from distractions in order to minimize this factor. Although ideal in one respect and expected when administering standardized tests, this arrangement differs, often radically, from the clatter and clutter of most patients' everyday situations and may mask the problem to be assessed. Therefore, the clinician may wish to interact with the patient in an environment with extraneous noise or activity and observe the patient's ability to be free from distraction. Some tests are designed with distractions included for this reason.

The Stroop Test (Dodrill, 1978; Posner & DiGirolamo, 2000; Stroop, 1935) is a difficult task involving directed attention in addition to other processes. As a baseline measure of speed of responding, the patient is asked to read a page of color names. For the critical condition, the patient is instructed to name the color in which color words are presented, such as saying "green" when the word "red" is printed in green ink. For literate adults, reading the words is prepotent over naming the ink color: therefore, attention must be directed to the color in which the words are printed while inhibiting the prepotent response.

Sustained Attention

Another aspect of attention that may be disrupted by brain injuries frequently involving the frontal lobes, such as that incurred in a moving vehicle accident (Ponsford, 1995; Wrightson & Gronwall, 1999), is the ability to sustain attention (Parasuraman et al., 1998; Swick & Knight, 1998). Many neuropsychological tests require this ability. The WMS Mental Control tests and Subtracting Serial Sevens (Strub & Black, 2000) provide measures of sustained attention as well as other mental operations.

Clinical evaluations of sustained attention often involve vigilance tasks in which stimuli both targets and foils) are presented over an extended period of time and the patient must indicate each target occurrence (Rosvold et al., 1956). Paper and pencil versions are usually in the form of cancellation tests consisting of rows of letters or numbers with instructions to the patient the cross out the target item. The Letter Cancellation Test (Diller et al., 1974) and Vigilance Test (Strub & Black, 2000) are examples of this kind of test. Auditory forms are available in which subjects tap or press a computer key when they hear the designated target letter or word. Complex variations may be devised by asking the patient to indicate when two or more conditions have been fulfilled, such as when two numbers occur in succession on a tape presentation (Licerone, 1997). The Continuous Performance Test (Conners, 1992, 2000) asks the patient to indicate every time a letter other than X appears on a screen. The test measures sustained attention over 14 minutes.

Divided Attention

Divided attention, or the ability to attend to more than one stimulus simultaneously, is yet another aspect of attention that is sensitive to brain injury (Nestor et al., 1991; Raskin & Mateer, 2000; Stuss et al., 1989) or normal aging (Baddeley, 1986; Greenwood & Parasuraman, 1991). Practically, problems in this area show up in inability to follow a recipe while the children are talking or difficulty following a conversation when surrounded by a chattering crowd. However, deficiencies in divided attention may also be at the heart of the "misplaced keys (or wallet, or glasses, etc.)" complaint: upon entering their homes these are patients who become immediately distracted by something (the dog, the mail on the hall table, the children) and lay down their keys without registering where they have put them. Almost inevitably, they attribute this latter problem to "poor memory".

Oral arithmetic stories provide one means of examining this problem, as subjects must perform a second or third set of operations while keeping practical solutions in mind. Take the problem, "Mary has 13 stamps and Jane has five. How many would Mary have to give to Jane for them to have the same number?" To solve this, several sequential calculations must be performed while retaining the question.

Difficulties in doing more than one thing at a time may also show up on list producing tasks, whether they involve learning a series of items or generating items *de novo*. On these tasks patients who may be having no difficulty fulfilling the task requirements, whether they be to learn words or generate line patterns (e.g. Ruff Figural Fluency Test: Ruff et al., 1987), will repeat an abnormally large number of responses just given within the last minute or even the last 10–15 seconds. In these repetitions, the patients demonstrate difficulty in keeping track of their responses while performing an ongoing task. These repetitions are distinguishable from true perseverations, as perseverating patients typically produce very few different responses, and once they begin perseverating, some if not all of the elements of succeeding responses will be perseverations.

The Trail Making Test (Lezak, 1995) is a frequently used test of divided attention or mental tracking. In part A in this timed task, the patient is asked to draw a line connecting in sequence a random display of numbered circles. The level of difficulty is increased in the second part (B) by having the patient again sequence a random display of circles with numbers and letters, going from 1 to A to 2 to B to 3 and so forth. The patient must be able to keep both sequences in mind to perform the task efficiently and quickly. The test also requires visual scanning, flexibility in shifting from set to set, and fine motor coordination and speed. Problems with divided attention show up in abnormally slowed performances on the more complex part B relative to part A.

A working memory test that uses a distractor condition involving divided attention is the "Brown–Peterson technique", the "Peterson task" (Peterson & Peterson, 1959), which is also referred to as "auditory consonant trigrams " (Mitrushina et al., 1999; Spreen & Strauss, 1998). The patient hears three consonants presented at the rate of 1/s, is asked to count backward from a given number until signaled to stop counting, and then to report the stimulus items; for example, the examiner says, "P R L 126" and the subject begins counting, "125, 124" etc., until told "stop" at the end of the predesignated number of seconds and is expected to recall the three letters. Mental tracking problems may also show up, as some patients lose track of numbers as they count backwards (e.g. " . . . 123, 122, 121, 130, 129", etc.).

Everyday Attention

Daily activities place a heavy demand on many aspects of attention. The Test of Everyday Attention is designed to assess attentional demands of common tasks, such as searching maps, looking through telephone directions and listening to lottery number broadcasts (Crawford et al., 1997; Robertson et al., 1996). The eight tasks measure selective attention, sustained attention, attentional switching and divided attention with activities that are meaningful to the patient.

Contributions to Memory

It is often difficult to distinguish between a primary memory disorder and a more general impairment in attention or concentration secondarily disrupting memory. Several theorists (Luria, 1971; Petrides, 1998; Stuss et al., 1997) have described the frontal lobe memory disorder as more a deficit in attention and other control functions than memory *per se*. Some cases sort themselves out, such as when a patient performs well on one class of tests and not on the other. Some amnesic patients appear to have normal attention and several studies have shown that the memory deficit in mild Alzheimer's disease occurs in patients without impaired sustained attention (Lines et al., 1991) or directed attention (Lafleche & Albert, 1995; Nebes & Brady, 1989). Often patients perform poorly on both attentional and memory tasks, thus making the distinction more difficult. Reductions in attentional capacity as well as memory may be seen in patients with diffuse brain dysfunction, such as from severe closed head injury, schizophrenia, metabolic encephalopathy, or dementia of the Alzheimer's type. One method for identifying components of complex cognitive disorders is to examine the correlation between performances on memory tests and other cognitive tests, for example performance on a word-list learning task by a group with mixed neurological disorders was related to performance on tests of attention and mental tracking (Vanderploeg et al., 1994). Using between-group comparisons, rumination in patients with dysphoric mood was associated with deficits in both focused attention and memory not seen in subjects who were not dysphoric (Hertel, 1998). Another method is to alter attention during a memory task. When attention was limited during a recognition memory task, performance was affected by the interaction of attentional resources and study time (Ganor-Stern et al., 1998).

Some standard memory tasks place heavy demands on attention. Lengthy memory tasks require intact sustained attention; for example, in continuous memory recognition tests (Tombaugh, 1996; Trahan & Larrabee, 1988; Warrington, 1984) patients see a long sequence of items out of which they must identify those already seen. Any loss of attention during the early, acquisition phase of the task could affect performance on the remainder of the task. The performance demands of some visuographic memory tasks are substantial and may divide attention. Drawing geometric designs from memory would be expected to produce interference for those patients who labor with the drawing component of the task (Taylor, 1992).

The clinician may choose to minimize the influence of attentional factors by test selection. Some tests are constructed to ensure that the patient overtly attends to material to be learned. The CERAD Word List Task (Morris et al, 1989) requires that the patient read aloud each of the to-be-recalled words, which requires registration of the words. One could argue that the act of reading divides the patient's attention between the performance and memory requirements of the test. However, reading is relatively automatic and the interference would be expected to be small. The examiner may wish to select a memory test with a simple response mode, for example, rather than having patients draw geometric designs, visuospatial memory can be examined by having patients place items in their learned position on a spatial grid. The original 7/24 (Barbizet & Cany, 1968) and modified 7/24 Spatial Recall (Rao et al., 1984) tests, as well as the Visual Spatial Learning Test (Malec et al., 1991) and the Visual Recognition tasks of the Memory Assessment Battery (Williams, 1991), examine memory for the location of stimulus items on a grid.

Information Processing

Many traumatically brain-injured patients, especially those whose damage is diffusely distributed, have reduced ability to process information as rapidly as it is presented to them. They may fail to recall elements of a conversation or the evening's news because they have not been able to assimilate the information as it was presented. Others with more focal and lateralized lesions may no longer be able to process verbal or nonverbalizable information adequately. If not properly examined, these deficits can be misinterpreted as due to memory failures. Hearing loss, common in the elderly, also can interfere with information processing and adversely affect memory performance (van Boxtel et al., 2000).

It is generally accepted that memory deficits that are specific to either verbal or nonverbal material cut across sensory modalities. Most memory tests in clinical use confound the type of material to be learned (verbal and nonverbal) with modality of presentation (aural or visual), i.e. most verbal memory tests consist of having the patient recall material that has been read by the examiner and most nonverbal tasks require the patient to draw from memory or recognize visually presented material. It is possible to dissociate these two factors, such as asking the patient to recall the names of a set of visually presented objects or pictures or to recall a series of familiar sounds, such as a bell, birdsong and paper rustling.

Speed

Information processing speed can be assessed using timed tasks. Timed performances on commonly used mental tracking tasks, such as serial subtraction of sevens, proved to be effective measures of speed of information processing in cardiac transplant patients (Williams et al., 1996). One of the more demanding of these is the Paced Auditory Serial Addition Task (PASAT) (Gronwall, 1977; Gronwall & Sampson, 1974), which has been used extensively to detect subtle disorders in patients with mild brain dysfunction. Although originally developed for patients with mild traumatic brain injury, the PASAT has also been used in other conditions in which brain damage tends to be diffuse, such as AIDS, toxic encephalopathy, and multiple sclerosis. The task requires that the patient report aloud the sum of consecutive pairs of numbers presented at a fixed rate by a tape recorder; for example, if the numbers, "2–7–4–1" are heard in that sequence, the subject should say "9" after hearing the "7", then "11" after hearing the "4", and so on. The task difficulty results from the necessity to inhibit the easier response of adding the last number presented on the tape with the last summation generated by the patient. The level of difficulty can be heightened by speeding up the rate of presentation of numbers. Like most complex tasks, it requires a number of cognitive operations in addition to information processing: sustained as well as divided attention, calculation, and inhibition of a prepotent response.

Verbal Deficits

Patients may have deficits that are specific to the nature of the information to be learned (Fuster, 1995). Many patients with left hemisphere lesions have language impairments and patients with right hemisphere lesions often have visuospatial impairment. Even patients with intact fluent speech who appear to follow a casual conversation may have subtle language-processing deficits. The Token Test (Boller & Vignolo, 1966; Spreen & Strauss, 1998) is sensitive to disrupted language processing that is not readily recognizable (Lezak, 1995; Weintraub, 2000). The test consists of series of oral commands, using "tokens" of varying shapes, sizes and colors. The patient follows commands of increasing length and syntactic complexity. Unlike most information conveyed in social conversations, the commands given during this test lack contextual cuing or redundancy of information, thus bringing to light even fairly subtle comprehension problems. Similarly, reading comprehension tests may identify language-processing deficits that might not be obvious (Greenwald, 2000).

Nonverbal Deficits

Likewise, patients may have deficits that are specific to processing of visuospatial information (Ogden, 1996; Robertson & Rafal, 2000). The WIS subtests include constructional tasks involving reconstructing designs with blocks and assembling puzzle pieces

(Wechsler, 1944, 1955, 1981, 1997). The Complex Figure Test requires more complex visuospatial processing by the drawing from memory of this difficult geometric design (Corwin & Bylsma, 1993; Rey, 1964) or one of the alternative forms (Spreen & Strauss, 1993; Taylor, 1979). Lesions of the posterior cerebral cortex tend to be associated with the greatest difficulty with constructions, with right hemisphere lesions producing greater deficits than left hemisphere lesions. The geometric designs used in some memory tests, such as the Benton Visual Retention Test (Benton, 1974; Sivan, 1991) lend themselves to verbal labels and thus are not useful measures of nonverbal functions.

Contributions to Memory

Speed of information processing influences memory as well as other cognitive abilities. For example, age-related changes in memory are related to changes in speed of processing (Birren et al., 1980; Bryan & Luszcz, 1996; Fastenau et al., 1996; Salthouse, 1996; Verhaeghen & Salthouse, 1997) and memory performance is related to processing speed in patients with Parkinson's disease (Stebbins et al., 1999) and multiple sclerosis (De Luca et al., 1994; Randolph et al., 2001). Slower processing speed can limit the capacity of working memory (Grigsby, et al., 1994; Hinton-Bayre et al., 1997); Salthouse & Babcock, 1991) and reduce the amount of elaboration or formation of associations that are involved in encoding to-be-remembered information (Salthouse, 1994).

The role of slow information processing on memory performance can be examined by comparing performances on tests in which speed is essential and in which speed is relatively irrelevant. Many patients react as though overwhelmed when presented with story recall tasks, such as in the WMS. They experience it as too much information too fast. Presentation rates that are too fast hinder recall in intact persons (Shum et al., 1997) and this effect would be expected to be greatest in the elderly and in patients with brain disorders, whose information processing is slow. To test the limits on such a task, the examiner should slow down the pace, particularly pausing between sentences. Ideally, story recall tests would allow ample information processing by presenting the story more than once, such as with the Heaton Story Recall format (Heaton et al., 1991) or Story B of the WMS-III (Wechsler, 1997). Patients may show better performance on a word-list learning task, in which the pace of presentation is naturally slower and the material is repeated three or more times.

Material-specific processing deficits affect performance on memory tests in which language or visuospatial information is to be learned. Aphasic patients often perform poorly on verbal memory tests, which require both language and memory capacities. Language impairment can affect the patient's comprehension of the material or ability to produce the correct verbal response (Wilshire & Coslett, 2000). Aphasic stroke patients with extensive damage to the left temporal lobe involving both language areas on the convexity and memory structures more anterior and mesial may sustain both memory and language impairments. Both of these areas play important but different roles in the verbal memory impairment. Aphasic patients tend to perform more poorly on word-list learning, paired word associates learning, and prose recall tasks than nonaphasic patients (Fuster, 1995). However, some aphasic patients perform better on the prose tasks because they benefit from contextual information. Others process the grammatical and syntactical information too slowly and perform better on word-list tasks.

For some patients it may be impossible to assess the relative contribution of language impairment on verbal memory performance. One attempt consists of assessing memory with tasks with minimal verbal characteristics, such as memory for complex geometric designs or for faces (Warrington, 1984). Aphasic patients are at a disadvantage even on these tasks because of their disrupted ability to encode material using verbal mediation as well as visual imagery. The difference in performance of a language-impaired patient on a verbal memory task compared with a nonverbal memory task will provide an indication of the material-specificity of the impairment.

Patients with visuospatial disorders who have difficulty in drawing a geometric design will be disadvantaged in recalling the design, because here memory becomes confounded with processing demands. Some examiners have advocated calculating the memory score in relation to the copy score (Brooks, 1972; Kuehn & Snow, 1992), thereby factoring out as much as possible the constructional component from the memory performance. However, if a patient is unable to copy the design within at least the *low average* range, a subsequent recall score is of dubious value. Some frequently used memory tests require the copying of relatively simple geometric designs, thereby minimizing the processing and constructional requirements of the test. The Benton Visual Retention Test and, to a lesser extent, the WMS Visual Reproduction Test fall into this category. However, even the Visual Reproduction Test designs are too difficult for healthy very elderly persons (Howieson et al., 1991). Some memory recognition tests have a spatial as well as pattern or picture component (e.g. Trahan & Larrabee, 1988; Williams, 1991)

EXECUTIVE FUNCTIONS

The distinction between memory and other cognitive functions is perhaps most difficult when describing the motivating, control and regulatory behaviors that are necessary for all goal-directed activities, including memory. In neuropsychological terms, executive functions refer to those abilities necessary to formulate goals and effectively carry them out (Lezak, 1982; Stuss & Benson, 1987). These are difficult tasks for many patients with extensive frontal lobe or diffuse brain injuries (Damasio & Anderson, 1993; Eslinger & Geder, 2000; Luria, 1980). Executive deficits also can be found in patients with disorders involving subcortical structures and connections (Huber & Shuttleworth, 1990) and right hemisphere damage (Cutting, 1990; Pimental & Kingsbury, 1989). The major categories of executive behaviors are: (a) volition; (b) planning; (c) executing activities; and (d) self-monitoring (Lezak, 1995). A deficiency in any of these task-orientating behaviors can interfere with the ability to succeed in all but the simplest of cognitive tasks. Some executive functions have particular bearing on memory performance.

Volition

An individual must be aware of his/her self and surroundings in order to have the capacity to formulate a goal and exercise self-will. The ability to create motives involves an interaction of an appreciation of personal or social needs based on past experiences and self-identity and the capacity to be motivated (Lezak, 1982). Some patients with brain disorders have greatly diminished capacity for self-generating activity, which may be reflected in diminished spontaneous memory retrieval (Markowitsch, 2000). They may have a reasonable plan of action but fail to initiate the plan. These patients typically look their best in a formal evaluation where they can respond to the structure and motivation provided by the examiner (Damasio & Anderson, 1993; Eslinger & Geder, 2000). By their very nature, most examiner-administered tests require little self-generation by the patient (Lezak, 1982). Left on their own, these patients lack the capacity to carry on and appear apathetic (Habib, 2000; Knight & Grabowecky, 2000). Descriptions of patients' self-initiated activities from persons close to them can provide important information.

Planning

Tasks that best assess executive functions are sufficiently complex to require planning or strategies to maximize performance. Examples include mazes, constructional tasks including free drawing (of a bicycle, for example), and complex problem-solving tests, such as the Twenty Questions parlor game, which was modified for neuropsychological use by Laine & Butters (1982). This task requires the subject to identify an object the examiner has in mind by asking questions that can only be answered by "yes" and "no". The object is to identify the task with as few questions as possible. A successful strategy uses questions that include or exclude as many items as possible in one question: the first question might be, "Is it living?" and, if the answer is "No", a follow-up question, "Is it bigger than a car (or whatever comparison nearly equally divides the inanimate objects)?" The tower puzzles, such as the Tower of London task (Shallice, 1982), are solved successfully by planning the movement of rings from one peg to another to achieve a particular display of rings in the fewest moves (Lezak, 1995). Patients who have difficulties on these tests may also fail to use strategies to facilitate their recall during memory testing.

Executing

Carrying out activities requires the capacities to initiate behavior and modify that behavior through switching, maintaining or stopping behavior in an integrated manner, according to an analysis of appropriate actions (Lezak, 1982). The Brixton Spatial Anticipation Test (Burgess & Shallice, 1996a), the Category Test (Halstead, 1947) and the Wisconsin Card Sorting Test (Berg, 1948; Grant & Berg, 1948; Heaton et al., 1993) are designed to measure rule attainment, flexibility of thinking and appropriate switching of behavior. They present patterns of stimuli and require the patients to select a response based on a principle or concept learned through feedback about the correctness of previous responses. The patients must realize when a shift in principles occurs and act accordingly. These tasks also assess capacity for concept formation. Deficits in modulation of behavior may result in inconsistent responses, perseverations and impersistence. Using six tests that are more exemplary of everyday tasks, the Behavioural Assessment of the Dysexecutive Syndrome (BADS) examines cognitive flexibility, novel problem solving, planning, judgment and estimation, and behavioural regulation (Wilson et al., 1996). It is designed to predict patients' abilities to handle problems that are likely to be encountered in daily activities.

Some brain-injured patients lack the ability to persist with lengthy or complex tasks. There are few open-ended tests that measure persistence directly. However, a fluency task can be used to measure persistence (Lezak, 1995; Spreen & Strauss, 1998). Patients may be asked to name all the words they can think of beginning with a designated letter of the alphabet. Impaired patients will think of a few that come to mind and stop generating items prematurely. These patients often will perform adequately if frequently prompted by the examiner. The Tinkertoy Test (Bayless et al., 1989; Lezak, 1982, 1995) was designed to measure planning and persistence. Patients are simply instructed to make what they want with these simple construction materials and thus must decide what to build and how to design it. Severely impaired patients begin the task without a plan and their final product may be the result of serendipity.

Self-monitoring

Another executive function necessary for successful performance on cognitive tasks is the capacity to monitor and self-correct spontaneously and reliably. The person who is able to regulate the relevance and accuracy of their responses on tests will have an advantage over those who make careless errors or contaminate their performance with perseverative or extraneous responses. Some patients with brain disorders, particularly those with frontal lobe damage, are impulsive and may trade accuracy of performance for speed (Knight & Grabowecky, 2000; Ogden, 1996).

Impulsivity occurs when inhibiting an undesirable, often easy, behavior fails. It can be seen on the Trail Making Test, Part B, when a patient fails to shift set and gives the easier, same-set response. Maze-tracing tests may also elicit impulsivity as the patient charges into turns that lead to blind alleys. The Stroop Test requires inhibiting an easy response, as the patient is asked to state the color of ink in which a conflicting color word is printed. After asking the patient to supply a reasonable word for the missing last word in a series of sentences, the Hayling Sentence Completion Test then asks the patient to complete each sentence with a word that is unrelated to the sentence in every way (Burgess & Shallice, 1996b). Success requires inhibition of meaningful associations that the sentence activates and use of a strategy to generate unconnected responses. Observations of test-taking behavior differentiate those patients who regularly check their work, such as a reconstructed design on WIS Block Design test or copy of the Complex Figure, from those who do not. Requiring patients to complete a page of arithmetic calculations at their leisure (for example see Lezak, 1995) frequently brings out carelessness tendencies in patients who demonstrate adequate arithmetic skills but make (*and leave*) small computational errors on the page.

Contribution to Memory

When are deficits in volition, planning, persistence or self-monitoring on memory tests a primary feature of the memory disorder, and when are they associated impairments? The executive deficit might be primary, but it can also occur in conjunction with a true memory disorder. The difficulty in making this distinction is illustrated by Baddeley & Wilson (1988) in their analysis of man with a frontal syndrome due to a closed head injury sustained in a traffic accident. They concluded that this patient's memory disorder resembled a classic memory disorder but that it occurred in combination with a frontal syndrome. Trauma patients might be expected to have frontal syndromes because many sustain damage to the frontal lobes as well as to memory areas of the anterior/medial temporal lobes. It has been proposed that memory disorders of frontal patients are related to problems in attention, susceptibility to interference, and problems with planning and organization needed for retrieval, rather than deficits in storage or consolidation as seen in memory-impaired patients with medial temporal lobe and diencephalic areas (Shimamura et al., 1991; Smith et al., 1995; Stuss et al., 1997).

Perhaps the best example of the interaction of executive and memory deficits occurs with Korsakoff's syndrome. The Korsakoff's patient has a severe memory impairment that dramatically interferes with daily activities, but it is the pervasive executive disorders that render them socially dependent and unable to carry out ordinary constructive activities (Lezak, 1995). Memory impairment is presumably related to lesions of primary memory areas, the dorsal-medial nucleus of the thalamus and mammillary bodies, but Korsakoff patients have frontal atrophy as well (Shimamura et al., 1991). Moscovitch (1982) showed that the Korsakoff's patient's poor performance on one memory task, release from proactive interference, is related more to impairment of frontal functions than to the amnesic disorder.

Failure to use strategies to manipulate and organize information will also limit recall on memory tests. These strategies may include chunking information (e.g. digits to recall), making meaningful associations between unrelated items to be recalled (e.g. difficult paired associates), or using semantic attributes to facilitate recall of related bits of information (e.g. words from a list). Several memory tests developed for clinical applications provide useful information about the use of strategies. The California Verbal Learning Test (Delis et al., 1983, 1986, 1987) and the California Verbal Learning Test, 2nd edn (Delis et al., 2000) assess the patient's use of semantic categorizing in the course of memory testing. The items to be learned are 16 words, four from of each of four object categories, such as fruits or clothing. The items are presented in random order with both uncued and category-cued recall trials. The uncued performances can be evaluated for semantic clustering, an effective recall strategy. Thus, patients who cluster according to categories tend to perform better than those who do not. Patients with left hemisphere lesions show impaired semantic clustering and better (although still impaired) recall with category cues (Hildebrandt et at., 1998). Parkinson's patients are impaired when forced to rely on internally generated strategies and function normally when provided with category cues (Knoke et al., 1998). Using similarly constructed word lists, Stuss et al. (1996) found that patients with frontal lesions and adults over the age of 65 perform worse than younger participants on memory measures of strategy, monitoring, and efficiency. Absence of semantic strategy may also reflect a breakdown in semantic knowledge, such as with Alzheimer's disease.

A less structured word list also can provide important information about the use of memory strategies. The commonly used Auditory Verbal Learning Test (Lezak, 1995; Rey, 1964) consists of 15 unrelated words that the patient hears in the same order for each of five trials, with no restriction on order of recall. On first hearing the list, intact subjects show both recency and primacy effects, recalling most often the first few words and the last few words, with perhaps a few in the middle. As trials are repeated, most intact subjects begin to organize the words according to associations and their recall demonstrates these clusters. They also begin to recall first the words they have not given before so they make sure not to forget them. These self-employed strategies assist the patient. We advocate inquiring of the patient who performs poorly on such a task whether they used any particular method for learning the words.

Deficits in self-monitoring can play havoc with memory. Both psychiatric patients and frontal lobe-injured patients may have difficulty distinguishing accurate memories from internal associations (Schacter & Curran, 2000). Some patients elaborate a completely faulty ending to a story they have been asked to remember, or interject associative material here and there. In some instances, if the examiner questions their response, these patients are able to specify the elaborated portion, thereby displaying some capacity to distinguish between external stimuli and their mental contents. Most people have a relatively strong sense of confidence about accuracy of memories, often referred to as the "feeling-of-knowing", and inhibit irrelevant or erroneous associations (Hintzman, 2000).

Impersistence can also result in poor memory performance. Patients may readily recall a few elements of a story to be learned and then stop, sometimes stating and sometimes implying that "that's enough" without attempting to expand the recall.

CONCLUSIONS

Most cognitive tasks involve a composite of mental operations, so that it is often difficult to specify where one ends and the other takes over. Several models have been proposed to relate the cognitive functions discussed in this chapter. The information-processing model proposed by Schneider & Shiffrin (1977) relates attention and information processing by suggesting that divided attention is dependent on adequate speed of information processing. In fact, models of information processing include a stage in which stimuli are compared with memory stores for familiarity. Information processing also is a key element of some theories of memory (Cermak, 1972; Craik & Lockhart, 1972). Shallice (1982) has proposed a model of executive control over attentional resources that regulates the use of attentional resources in a goal-directed fashion, while Baddeley (1986, 1994) has proposed a model of working memory that includes inherent attentional and executive functions.

Memory tasks certainly have multiple demands and it is not always easy to dissociate memory from other cognitive functions (Fuster, 1995; Schacter et al., 2000). Clearly, some patients' cognitive impairments are restricted to memory alone. However, the majority of patients with memory impairment have other cognitive deficits as well; for example, if the patient has difficulty with attention or self-monitoring across a range of tasks, then poor performance on memory tests may be at least partly attributable to these other cognitive problems. Some distinctions are difficult, such as between poor memory retrieval and general impersistence. The clinician is challenged with making the correct distinctions so that necessary counseling and possibly remediation can be accurately directed.

REFERENCES

Baddeley, A.D. (1986). *Working Memory*. Oxford: Oxford University Press.

Baddeley, A.D. (1994). Working memory: the interface between memory and cognition. In D.L. Schacter & E. Tulving (eds), *Memory Systems 1994* (pp. 351–376). Cambridge, MA: MIT Press.

Baddeley, A. & Wilson, B. (1988). Frontal amnesia and the dysexecutive syndrome. *Brain and Cognition*, **7**, 212–230.

Barbizet, J. & Cany, E. (1968). Clinical and psychometrical study of a patient with memory disturbances. *International Journal of Neurology*, **7**, 44–54.

Bayless, J.D., Varney, N.R. & Roberts, R.J. (1989). Tinker Toy Test performance and vocational outcome in patients with closed head injuries. *Journal of Clinical and Experimental Neuropsychology*, **11**, 913–917.

Bazarian, J.J., Wong, T., Harris, M. et al. (1999). Epidemiology and predictors of post-concussive syndrome after minor head injury in an emergency population. *Brain Injury*, **13**, 173–189.

Benton, A.L. (1974). *The Revised Visual Retention Test*. New York: Psychological Corporation.

Benton, A.L. & Hamsher, K. de S. (1989). *Multilingual Aphasia Examination*. Iowa City, IA: AIA Associates.

Benton, A.L., Hamsher K. de S., Varney N.R. & Spreen, O. (1983). *Contributions to Neuropsychological Assessment*. New York: Oxford University Press.

Berg, E.A. (1948). A simple objective test for measuring flexibility in thinking. *Journal of General Psychology*, **39**, 15–22.

Boller, F. & Vignolo, L.A. (1966). Latent sensory aphasia in hemisphere-damaged patients: an experimental study with the Token Test. *Brain*, **89**, 815–831.

Birren, J., Woods, A.M. & Williams, M.V. (1980). Behavioral slowing with age: causes, organization and consequences. In L.W. Poon (ed.), *Aging in the 1980s* (pp. 293–308). Washington, DC: American Psychological Association.

Brooks, D.N. (1972). Memory and head injury. *Journal of Nervous and Mental Disease*, **155**, 350–355.

Bryan, J. & Luszcz, M.A. (1996). Speed of information processing as a mediator between age and free-recall performance. *Psychology and Aging*, **11**, 3–9.

Burgess, P.W. & Shallice, T. (1996a) Bizarre responses, rule detection and frontal lobe lesions. *Cortex*, **32**, 241–259.

Burgess, P.W. & Shallice, T. (1996b) Response suppression, initiation, and strategy use following frontal lobe lesions. *Neuropsychologia*, **34**, 263–273.

Cermak, L.S. (1972). *Human Memory; Research and Theory*. New York: Ronald Press.

Cicerone, K.D. (1997). Clinical sensitivity of four measures of attention to mild traumatic brain injury. *The Clinical Neuropsychologist*, **11**, 266–272.

Conners, C.K. (1992). *Conners' Continuous Performance Test*. Toronto: Multi-Health Systems.

Conners, C.K. (2000). *Continuous Performance Test II*. Toronto: Multi-Health Systems.

Corwin, J. & Bylsma, F.W. (1993). Translations of excerpts from André Rey's "Psychological examination of traumatic encephalopathy" and P.A. Osterrieth's "The Complex Figure Copy Test". *Clinical Neuropsychologist*, **7**, 4–21.

Craik, F.I.M. & Lockhart, R.S. (1972). Levels of processing: framework for memory research. *Journal of Verbal Learning and Verbal Behavior*, **11**, 671–684.

Crawford, J.R., Sommerville, J. & Robertson, I.H. (1997) Assessing the reliability and abnormality of subtest differences on the Test of Everyday Attention. *British Journal of Clinical Psychology*, **36**, 609–617.

Curran, H.V. (2000). Psychopharmacological approaches to human memory. In M.S. Gazzaniga (ed.), *The New Cognitive Neurosciences*, 2nd edn (pp. 797–804). Cambridge, MA: MIT Press.

Cutting, J. (1990). *The Right Cerebral Hemisphere and Psychiatric Disorders*. Oxford: Oxford University Press.

Damasio, A.R. & Anderson, S.W. (1993). The frontal lobes. In K.M. Heilman & E. Valenstein (eds), *Clinical Neuropsychology*, 3rd edn (pp. 409–460). New York: Oxford University Press.

Damasio, A.R., Damasio, H. & Tranel, D. (1990). Impairments in visual recognition as clues to the processes of memory. In G.M. Edelman et al. (eds), *Signal and Sense. Local and Global Order in Perceptual Maps* (pp. 451–473). New York: Wiley-Liss.

Delis, D.C., Kaplan, E., Kramer, J.H. & Ober, B.A. (2000). *California Verbal Learning Test—Second Edition (CVLT-II) Manual*. San Antonio, TX: The Psychological Corporation/Harcourt Brace Jovanovich.

Delis, D.C., Kramer, J.H., Kaplan, E. & Ober, B.A. (1986). *California Verbal Learning Test*. San Antonio, TX: Psychological Corporation/Harcourt Brace Jovanovich.

Delis, D.C., Kramer, J.H., Kaplan, E. & Ober, B.A. (1983, 1987). *California Verbal Learning Test, Form II (Research edn)*. San Antonio, TX: The Psychological Corporation/Harcourt Brace Jovanovich.

De Luca, J., Barbieri-Berger, S. & Johnson, S.K. (1994). The nature of memory impairments in multiple sclerosis: acquisition vs. retrieval. *Journal of Clinical and Experimental Neuropsychology*, **16**, 183–189.

Diller, L., Ben-Yishay, Y., Gerstman, L.J. et al. (1974). *Studies in Cognition and Rehabilitation in Hemiplegia* (Rehabilitation Monograph No. 50). New York: New York University Medical Center Institute of Rehabilitation Medicine.

Di Stefano, G. & Radanov, B.P. (1996). Quantitative and qualitative aspects of learning in common whiplash patients: a 6-month follow-up study. *Archives of Clinical Neuropsychology*, **11**, 661–676.

Dodrill, C.B. (1978). A neuropsychological battery for epilepsy. *Epilepsia*, **19**, 611–623.

Eslinger, P.J. & Geder, L. (2000). Behavioral and emotional changes after focal frontal lobe damage. In J. Bogousslavsky & J.L. Cummings (eds), *Behavior and Mood Disorders in Focal Brain Lesions* (pp. 217–260). Cambridge: Cambridge University Press.

Fastenau, P.S., Denburg, N.L. & Abeles, N. (1996). Age differences in retrieval: further support for the resource-reduction hypothesis. *Psychology and Aging*, **11**, 140–146.

Fischler, I. (1998). Attention and language. In R. Parasuraman (ed.), *The Attentive Brain* (pp. 381–399). Cambridge, MA: MIT Press.

Freed, D.M., Corkin, S., Growdon, J.H. & Nissen, M.J. (1989). Selective attention in Alzheimer's disease: characterizing cognitive subgroups of patients. *Neuropsychologia*, **27**, 325–339.

Freides, D. & Avery, M.E. (1972). Narrrative and visual spatial recall: assessment incorporating learning and delayed retention. *Clinical Neuropsychologist*, **5**, 338–344.

Fuster, J.M. (1995). *Memory in the Cerebral Cortex*. Cambridge, MA: MIT Press.

Ganor-Stern, D., Seamon, J.G. & Carrasco, M. (1998). The role of attention and study time in explicit and implicit memory for unfamiliar visual stimuli. *Memory & Cognition*, **26**, 1187–1195.

Gasquoine, P.G. (1997). Postconcussion symptoms. *Neuropsychological Review*, **7**, 77–85.

Grant, D.A. & Berg, E.A. (1948). A behavioral analysis of degree of reinforcement and ease of shifting to new responses on a Weigl-type card-sorting problem. *Journal of Experimental Psychology*, **38**, 404–411.

Greenwald, M.L. (2000). The acquired dyslexias. In S.E. Nadeau et al. (eds), *Aphasia and Language. Theory to Practice* (pp. 159–183). New York: Guilford.

Greenwood, P. & Parasuraman, R. (1991). Effects of aging on the speed of attentional cost of cognitive operations. *Developmental Neuropsychology*, **7**, 421–434.

Grigsby, J., Kaye, K. & Busenbark, D. (1994). Alphanumeric sequencing: a report on a brief measure of information processing used among persons with multiple sclerosis. *Perceptual and Motor Skills*, **78**, 883–887.

Gronwall, D.M.A. (1977). Paced auditory serial-addition task: a measure of recovery from concussion. *Perceptual and Motor Skills*, **44**, 367–373.

Gronwall, D.M.A. & Sampson, H. (1974). *The Psychological Effects of Concussion*. Auckland: University Press/Oxford University Press.

Habib, M. (2000). Disorders of motivation. In J. Bogousslavsky & J.L. Cummings (eds), *Behavior and Mood Disorders in Focal Brain Lesions* (pp. 261–284). Cambridge: Cambridge University Press.

Halstead, W.C. (1947). *Brain and Intelligence*. Chicago: University of Chicago Press.

Heaton, R.K., Chelune, G.J., Talley, J.L. et al. (1993). *Wisconsin Card Sorting Test Manual: Revised and Expanded*. Odessa, FL: Psychological Assessment Resources.

Heaton, R.K., Grant, I. & Matthews, C.G. (1991). *Comprehensive Norms for an Expanded Halstead–Reitan Battery: Demographic Corrections, Research Findings, and Clinical Applications*. Odessa, FL: Psychological Assessment Resources.

Hertel, P.T. (1998). Relation between rumination and impaired memory in dysphoric moods. *Journal of Abnormal Psychology*, **107**, 166–172.

Hildebrandt, H., Brand, A. & Sachsenheimer, W. (1998). Profiles of patients with left prefrontal and left temporal lobe lesions after cerebrovascular infarctions on California Verbal Learning Test-like indices. *Journal of Clinical and Experimental Neuropsychology*, **20**, 673–683.

Hinton-Bayre, A.D., Geffen, G. & McFarland, K. (1997). Mild head injury and speed of information processing: a prospective study of professional rugby league players. *Journal of Clinical and Experimental Neuropsychology*, **19**, 275–289.

Hintzman, D.L. (2000). Memory judgments. In E. Tulving & F.I.M. Craik (eds), *The Oxford Handbook of Memory* (pp. 165–177). New York: Oxford University Press.

Howieson, D.B., Kaye, J. & Howieson, J. (1991). Cognitive status in healthy aging. *Journal of Clinical and Experimental Neuropsychology*, **13**, 28.

Huber, S.J. & Shuttleworth, E.C. (1990). Neuropsychological assessment of subcortical dementia. In J.L. Cummings (ed.), *Subcortical Dementia* (pp. 71–86.) New York: Oxford University Press.

Kapur, N. (1988). Pattern of verbal memory deficits in patients with bifrontal pathology and patients with third ventricle lesions. In M.M. Gruneberg, P.E. Morris & R.N. Sykes (eds), *Practical Aspects of Memory: Current Research and Issues*, Vol. 2 (pp. 10–15). New York: Wiley.

Knight, R.T. & Grabowecky, M. (2000). Prefrontal cortex, time, and consciousness. In M.S. Gazzaniga (ed.), *The New Cognitive Neurosciences*, 2nd edn (pp. 1319–1339). Cambridge, MA: MIT Press.

Knoke, D., Taylor, A.E. & Saint-Cyr, J.A. (1998). The differential effects of cueing on recall in Parkinson's disease and normal subjects. *Brain and Cognition*, **38**, 261–274.

Kosslyn, S.M. & Thompson, W.L. (2000). Shared mechanisms in visual imagery and visual perception: Insights from cognitive neuroscience. In M.S. Gazzaniga (ed.), *The New Cognitive Neurosciences*, 2nd edn (pp. 975–985). Cambridge, MA: MIT Press.

Kuehn, S. & Snow, W.G. (1992). Are the Rey and Taylor figures equivalent? *Archives of Clinical Neuropsychology*, **7**, 445–448.

LaBerge, D. (2000). Networks of attention. In M.S. Gazzaniga (ed.), *The New Cognitive Neurosciences*, 2nd edn (pp. 711–724). Cambridge, MA: MIT Press.

LaFleche, G. & Albert, M. (1995). Executive function in mild Alzheimer's disease. *Neuropsychology*, **9**, 313–320.

Laine, M. & Butters, N. (1982). A preliminary study of problem solving strategies of detoxified long-term alcoholics. *Drug & Alcohol Dependence*, **10**, 235–242.

Lezak, M.D. (1979). Recovery of memory and learning functions following traumatic brain injury. *Cortex*, **15**, 63–70.

Lezak, M.D. (1982). The problem of assessing executive functions. *International Journal of Psychology*, **17**, 281–297.

Lezak, M.D. (1994). Domains of behavior from a neuropsychological perspective: the whole story. In W. Spaulding (ed.), *41st Nebraska Symposium on Motivation* (pp. 23–55). Lincoln, NE: University of Nebraska.

Lezak, M.D. (1995). *Neuropsychological Assessment*, 3rd edn. New York: Oxford University Press.

Lines, C.R., Dawson, C., Preston, G.C. et al. (1991). Memory and attention in patients with senile dementia of the Alzheimer's type and in normal elderly subjects. *Journal of Clinical and Experimental Neuropsychology*, **13**, 691–702.

Luria, A.R. (1971). Memory disturbance in local brain lesions. *Neuropsychologia*, **9**, 367–376.

Luria, A.R. (1980). *Higher Cortical Functions in Man*, 2nd edn. New York: Basic Books.

Malec, J.F., Ivnik, R.J. & Hinkeldey, N.S. (1991). Visual spatial learning test. *Psychological Assessment*, **3**, 82–88.

Markowitsch, H.J. (2000). Memory and amnesia. In M.-M. Mesulam (ed.), *Principles of Behavioral and Cognitive Neurology*, 2nd edn (pp. 257–293). New York: Oxford University Press.

Milner, B. (1970). Memory and the medial regions of the brain. In K.H. Pribram & D.E. Broadbent (eds), *Biology of Memory* (pp. 29–50). New York: Academic Press.

Milner, B. (1971). Interhemispheric differences in the localization of psychological processes in man. *British Medical Bulletin*, **27**, 272–277.

Mitrushina, M.N., Boone, K.B. & D'Elia, L.F. (1999). *Handbook of Normative Data for Neuropsychological Assessment*. New York: Oxford University Press.

Morris, J.C., Heyman, A., Mohs, R.C. et al. (1989). The consortium to establish a registry for Alzheimer's disease (CERAD). Part I. Clinical and neuropsychological assessment of Alzheimer's disease. *Neurology*, **39**, 1159–1165.

Morrow, L.A., Robin, N., Hodgson, M.J. & Kamis, H. (1992). Assessment of attention and memory efficiency in persons with solvent neurotoxicity. *Neuropsychologia*, **30**, 911–922.

Moscovitch, M. (1982). Multiple dissociations of function in amnesia. In L.S. Cermak (ed.), *Human Memory and Amnesia* (pp. 337–370). Hillsdale, NJ: Erlbaum.

Nebes, R.D. & Brady, C.B. (1989). Focused and divided attention in Alzheimer's disease. *Cortex*, **25**, 300–315.

Nestor, P.G., Parasuraman, R. & Haxby, J.V. (1991). Speed of information processing and attention in early Alzheimer's dementia. *Developmental Neuropsychology*, **7**, 242–256.

Ogden, J.A. (1996). *Fractured Minds* (pp. 125–153). New York: Oxford University Press.

Parasuraman, R. (1998). Issues and prospects. In R. Parasuraman (ed.), *The Attentive Brain*. (pp. 381–399). Cambridge, MA: MIT Press.

Pachana, N.A., Boone, K.B., Miller, B.L. et al. (1996). Comparison of neuropsychological functioning in Alzheimer's disease and frontotemporal dementia. *Journal of the International Neuropsychological Society*, **2**, 505–510.

Pashler, H.E. (1998*). The Psychology of Attention*. Cambridge, MA: MIT Press.

Peterson, L.R. & Peterson, M.J. (1959). Short-term retention of individual verbal items. *Journal of Experimental Psychology*, **58**, 193–198.

Petrides, M. (1998). Specialized systems for the processing of mnemonic information. In A.C. Roberts, T.W. Robbins et al. (eds), *The Prefrontal Cortex. Executive and Cognitive Functions* (pp. 103–116). London: Oxford University Press.

Pimental, P.A. & Kingbury, N.A. (1989). The injured right hemisphere: Classification of related disorders. In P.A. Pimental & N.A. Kingsbury (eds), *Neuropsychological Aspects of Right Brain Injury* (pp. 19–64). Austin, TX: PRO-ED.

Ponsford J. (1995). *Traumatic Brain Injury*. Hove: Erlbaum.

Ponsford, J. & Kinsella, G. (1992). Attentional deficits following closed-head injury. *Journal of Clinical and Experimental Neuropsychology*, **14**, 822–838.

Posner, M.I. & DiGirolamo, G.J. (2000). In M.S. Gazzaniga (ed.), *The New Cognitive Neurosciences*, 2nd edn (pp. 623–631). Cambridge, MA: MIT Press.

Randolph, J.J., Arnett, P.A. & Higginson, C.I. (2001). Metamemory and tested cognitive functioning in multiple sclerosis. *The Clinical Neuropsychologist*, **15**, 357–368.

Rao, S.M. (1996). White matter disease and dementia. *Brain and Cognition*, **31**, 250–268.

Rao, S.M., Hammeke, T.A., McQuillen, M.P. et al. (1984). Memory disturbance in chronic progressive multiple sclerosis. *Archives of Neurology*, **41**, 625–631.

Raskin, S.A. & Mateer, C.A. (2000). *Neuropsychological Management of Mild Traumatic Brain Injury*. New York: Oxford University Press.

Rey, A. (1964). *L'examen Clinique en Psychologie*. Paris: Presses Universitaries de France.

Robertson, I.H., Ward, T., Ridgeway, V. & Nimmo-Smith, I. (1996) Structure of normal human attention: the Test of Everyday Attention. *Journal of the International Neuropsychological Society*, **2**, 525–534.

Robertson, L.C. & Rafal, R. (2000). Disorders of visual attention. In M.S. Gazzaniga (ed.), *The New Cognitive Neurosciences*, 2nd edn (pp. 633–649). Cambridge, MA: MIT Press.

Rosvold, H.E., Mirsky, A.F., Sarason, I. et al. (1956). A continuous performance test of brain damage. *Journal of Consulting Psychology*, **20**, 343–350.

Rubin, E.H., Storandt, M., Miller, J.P. et al. (1998). A prospective study of cognitive function and onset of dementia in cognitively healthy elders. *Archives of Neurology*, **55**, 395–401.

Ruff, R.M., Light, R.H. & Evans, R.W. (1987). The Ruff Figural Fluency Test: a normative study with adults. *Developmental Neuropsychology*, **3**, 37–52.

Salthouse, T.A. (1996). The processing-speed theory of adult age differences in cognition. *Psychological Review*, **103**, 403–428.

Salthouse, T.A. & Babcock, R.L. (1991). Decomposing adult age differences in working memory. *Developmental Psychology*, **27**, 763–776.

Salthouse, T.A. (1994). Aging associations: influence of speed on adult age differences in associative learning. *Journal of Experimental Psychology: Learning, Memory and Cognition*, **20**, 1486–1503.

Schacter, D.L. & Curran, T. (2000). Memory without remembering and remembering without memory: Implicit and false memories. In M.S. Gazzaniga (ed.), *The New Cognitive Neurosciences*, 2nd edn (pp. 829–840). Cambridge, MA: MIT Press.

Schacter, D.L., Wagner, A.D. & Buckner, R.L. (2000). Memory systems of 1999. In E. Tulving & F.I.M. Craik (eds), *The Oxford Handbook of Memory* (pp. 627–643), New York: Oxford University Press.

Schneider, W. & Shiffrin, R.M. (1977). Controlled and automatic human information processing: I. Detection, search and attention. *Psychological Review*, **84**, 1–66.

Shallice, T. (1982). Specific impairments of planning. In D.E. Broadbent & L.Weiskrantz (eds), *The Neuropsychology of Cognitive Function* (pp. 199–209). London: The Royal Society.

Shimamura, A.P., Janowsky, J.S. & Squire, L.R. (1991). What is the role of frontal lobe damage in memory disorders. In H.M. Levin, H.M. Eisenberg & A.L. Benton (eds), *Frontal Lobe Function and Dysfunction* (pp. 173–195). New York: Oxford University Press.

Shum, D.H.K., Murray, R.A. & Eadie, K. (1997). Effect of speed of presentation of administration of the Logical Memory subtest of the Wechsler Memory Scale—Revised. *Clinical Neuropsychologist*, **11**, 188–191.

Sivan, A.B. (1991). *Benton Visual Retention Test*, 5th edn. San Antonio, TX: Psychological Corporation.

Small, J.A., Kemper, S. & Lyons, K. (2000). Sentence repetition and processing resources in Alzheimer's disease. *Brain and Language*, **75**, 232–258.

Smith, M.L., Leonard, G., Crane, J. & Milner, B. (1995). The effects of frontal- or temporal-lobe lesions on susceptibility to interference in spatial memory. *Neuropsychologia*, **33**, 275–285.

Spreen, O. & Strauss, E. (1998). *A Compendium of Neuropsychological Tests*, 2nd edn. New York: Oxford University Press.

Stebbins, G.T., Gabrieli, J.D., Masciari, F. et al. (1999). Delayed recognition memory in Parkinson's disease: a role for working memory? *Neuropsychologia*, **37**, 503–510.

Storandt, M., Morris, J.C., Rubin, E. (1992). Progression of senile dementia of the Alzheimer's type on a battery of psychometric tests. In L. Baeckman (ed.), *Memory Functioning in Dementia* (pp. 207–226). Amsterdam: Elsevier Science.

Stroop, J.R. (1935). Studies of interference in serial verbal reactions. *Journal of Experimental Psychology*, **18**, 643–662.

Strub, R.L. & Black, F.W. (2000) *Mental Status Examination in Neurology*, 3rd edn. Philadelphia, PA: F.A. Davis.

Stuss, D.T., Alexander, M.P. & Benson, D.F. (1997). Frontal lobe functions. In M.R. Trimble & J.L. Cummings (eds), *Contemporary Behavioral Neurology* (pp. 141–158). Boston, MA: Butterworth-Heinemann.

Stuss, D.T. & Benson, D.F. (1987). The frontal lobes and control of cognition and memory. In E. Perecman (ed.) *The Frontal Lobes Revisited* (pp. 141–158). New York: IRBN Press.

Stuss, D.T., Craik, F.I., Sayer, L. et al. (1996). Comparison of older people and patients with frontal lesions: evidence from word list learning. *Psychology and Aging*, **11**, 387–395.

Stuss, D.T., Stethem, L.L., Hugenholtz, H. et al. (1989). Reaction time after head injury: fatigue, divided and focused attention, and consistency of performance. *Journal of Neurology, Neurosurgery, and Psychiatry*, **52**, 742–748.

Swick, D. & Knight, R.T. (1998). Cortical lesions and attention. In R. Parasuraman (ed.), *The Attentive Brain* (pp. 143–162). Cambridge, MA: MIT Press.

Taylor, R. (1992). Art training and the Rey figure. *Perceptual and Motor Skills*, **74**, 1105–1106.

Tombaugh, T. (1996). *Test of Memory Malingering*. North Tonawanda, NY: Multi-Health Systems.

Trahan, D.E. & Larrabee, G.J. (1988). *Continuous Visual Memory Test*. Odessa, FL: Psychological Assessment Resources.

Vallar, G. & Shallice T. (1990). *Neuropsychological Impairments of Short-Term Memory*. Cambridge: Cambridge University Press.

van Boxtel, M.P., van Beijsterveldt, C.E., Houx, P.J., et al. (2000). Mild hearing impairment can reduce verbal memory performance in a healthy adult population. *Journal of Clinical and Experimental Neuropsychology*, **22**, 147–154.

Vanderploeg, R.D., Schinka, J.A. & Retzlaff, P. (1994). Relationships between measures of auditory verbal learning and executive functioning. *Journal of Clinical and Experimental Neuropsychology*, **16**, 243–252.

Van Gorp, W.G., Miller, E.N., Satz, P. & Visscher, B. (1989). Neuropsychological performance in HIV-1 immunocompromised patients. *Journal of Clinical and Experimental Neuropsychology*, **11**, 763–773.

Verhaeghen, P. & Salthouse, T.A. (1997). Meta-analyses of age-cognition relations in adulthood: estimates of linear and nonlinear age effects and structural models. *Psychological Bulletin*, **122**, 231–249.

Warrington, E.K. (1984). *Recognition Memory Test*. Windsor: National Foundation for Educational Research-Nelson.

Warrington, E.K. & Shallice, T. (1984) Category specific semantic impairments. *Brain*, **107**, 829–854.

Wechsler, D. (1944). *The Measurement of Adult Intelligence*, 3rd edn. Baltimore, MD: Williams & Wilkins.

Wechsler, D. (1945). A standardized memory scale for clinical use. *The Journal of Psychology*, **19**, 87–95.

Wechsler, D. (1955). *WAIS Manual*. New York: Psychological Corporation.

Wechsler, D. (1981). *WAIS-R Manual*. New York: Psychological Corporation.

Wechsler, D. (1987). *Wechsler Memory Scale—Revised: Manual*. San Antonio, TX: Psychological Corporation/Harcourt Brace Jovanovich.

Wechsler, D. (1997). *WAIS-III Administration and Scoring Manual*. San Antonio, TX: Psychological Corporation/Harcourt Brace Jovanovich.

Weintraub, S. (2000). Neuropsychological assessment of mental state. In M.-M. Mesulam (ed.), *Principles of Behavioral and Cognitive Neurology*, 2nd edn (pp. 121–173). New York: Oxford University Press.

Williams, J.M. (1991). *Memory Assessment Scales*. Odessa, FL: Psychological Assessment Resources.

Williams, M.A., LaMarche, J.A., Alexander, R.W. et al. (1996). Serial 7s and alphabet backwards as brief measures of information processing speed. *Archives of Clinical Neuropsychology*, **11**, 651–659.

Wilshire, C.E. & Coslett, H.B. (2000). Disorders of word retrieval in aphasia: theories and potential applications. In S.E. Nadeau, R. Gonzalez, J. Leslie et al. (eds), *Aphasia and Language. Theory to Practice* (pp. 40–81). New York: Guilford.

Wilson, B.A., Alderman, N., Burgess, P.W. et al. (1996). *Behavioural Assessment of the Dysexecutive Syndrome*. Bury St Edmunds: Thames Valley Test Company.

Wrightson, P. & Gronwall, D. (1999). *Mild Head Injury*. Oxford: Oxford University Press.

CHAPTER 10

Management and Remediation of Memory Problems in Brain-injured Adults

Barbara A. Wilson

*MRC Cognition and Brain Sciences Unit, Cambridge, and Oliver Zangwill
Centre for Cognitive Rehabilitation, Ely, UK*

Because I've got a bad memory, it doesn't mean I'm intellectually impaired. People talk down to me, they see the handicap and not the person (Alex, in Wilson, 1999, p. 66).

The statement by the young man quoted above illustrates how people with memory problems can suffer distress caused by the misunderstanding of others. Problems experienced by memory-impaired people in their daily interaction with people who do not have, and perhaps cannot appreciate, the effects of memory loss, can sometimes be regarded as reflecting stupidity or laziness. Too much might be expected from the memory-impaired person—or indeed too little, with the effect, either way, of causing them unhappiness. The situation is compounded by the fact that few people are offered appropriate rehabilitation to help them compensate for their cognitive problems and reduce the social and emotional consequences of brain injury.

There are large numbers of people like Alex in our society. Some 36% of people with severe head injury will have significant and permanent memory impairments. In the UK these figures reflect about 2500 new cases each year, and over four times that number in the USA.

Some 10% of people over the age of 65 years have dementia, with memory impairment an almost inevitable consequence. About 34% of people with multiple sclerosis have moderate or severe memory problems, as do 70% of people with AIDS, 70% of people who survive encephalitis, and 10% of people with temporal lobe epilepsy. In addition, memory impairment is commonly seen after Korsakoff's syndrome and is not uncommon after stroke, cerebral tumour, myocardial infarction, meningitis and carbon monoxide poisoning. Despite these large numbers, and the severity of impairment experienced by people with brain damage, few will receive help in managing problems they will confront each day of

The Essential *Handbook of Memory Disorders for Clinicians.* Edited by A.D. Baddeley, M.D. Kopelman and B.A. Wilson.
© 2004 John Wiley & Sons, Ltd. ISBN 0-470-09141-X.

their lives, few will be given guidance as to how to reduce the effect of their handicap on their everyday functioning.

Among neurologists, and many neuropsychologists working with these patients, the prevailing attitude seems to suggest that little or nothing can be done to alleviate the problems of brain-injured people. In contrast, relatives live in the hope, and sometimes indeed the expectation, that memory functioning can be restored if the right drug or relevant set of exercises can be administered. Neither of these views is correct: although at present it is not possible to *restore* memory functioning in people with organic amnesia once the period of natural recovery is over, it is nevertheless true that these people and their families can be helped to *cope with* everyday difficulties they are likely to experience. The lives of brain-injured people can be made much more tolerable by teaching them, for example, to bypass certain problems, compensate for them, or use their residual skills more efficiently.

THE CONSEQUENCES OF MEMORY PROBLEMS FOR PATIENTS AND THEIR FAMILIES

Not only are memory problems common following brain injury, they are also among the most handicapping of cognitive deficits, often preventing return to work or independent living, and causing considerable stress to brain-injured people and their families. Some brain-injured people feel they are going crazy or believe that other people regard them as insane. They frequently refer to isolation and loneliness. A large proportion of families and caregivers become infuriated, for example, at the constant repetition of a story, joke or question that is proffered by amnesic people who forget they have said the same thing earlier or forget that an answer has been supplied. One mother of a memory-impaired son once said to me, "If he tells me that story once more. I'll kill him". When their loss of memory causes such effects on others who are close to them, it is hardly surprising that some brain-injured people, fearing they might repeat something they have said perhaps on a number of other occasions, end up remaining very quiet. A woman who survived herpes simplex encephalitis said, "In company I'm very quiet. I'm afraid of repeating myself so I don't say anything".

A typical account of the kinds of everyday problems faced by families is provided by the mother of a young man, Jack, whose memory problems followed an attempted suicide by carbon monoxide poisoning. She said:

> He never remembers where the car is parked and gets embarrassed if he has to look in his book. He gets confused about arrangements with his friends. He double-books: e.g. he records one appointment at home and then meets someone in the street and arranges another meeting with that person. He loses everything, pencils, his wallet—everything. It would be worse, except I move things to obvious places. He never remembers what he has spent his money on and he forgets to carry out any plans he has made for himself, like sorting out his video tapes.

Wearing (1992) graphically illustrates the very limited understanding many people, including Health Service staff, have of memory impairments when she writes:

> One mother in Manchester told me that her daughter, amnesic since an aneurysm at age 19, was to attend a day centre at a psychiatric hospital. She spent a couple of hours in discussion with the staff to make sure they understood her daughter's amnesia. After the

first day she went to collect her but arrived to find that she was lost. "Well", explained a staff member, "we told her the way to lunch but she never arrived". Naturally the poor girl had forgotten the directions almost immediately and had no idea where she was supposed to go, or why, or what she was doing there. So she found herself in the alcoholics' clinic and sat there for she knew not how long, in the expectation that somehow her mother would eventually find her [one of very many similar incidents] (Wearing, 1992, pp. 280–281).

Although severe memory impairment is always distressing for family members and carers, their feelings of distress are not always shared by the person with the impairment. Usually, lack of concern on the patient's part is associated with poor insight that can follow from the original injury. Not surprisingly, on the other hand, those with greater awareness of their difficulties are typically distressed and/or depressed. They may feel that their memory disorder looks like stupidity in the eyes of others, or they may believe that other people will regard them as mentally unstable. Some memory-impaired people report that life is like a dream, and one young woman did in fact repeat to me several times each day the words, "This is a dream, I am going to wake up". Some people, aware of the effect they have on others, become very withdrawn and socially isolated because of their reluctance to bore and irritate their families and friends.

Because of the stressful efforts required to cope with daily living and the need to participate in compensatory behaviour in order to get through each day, the effects of amnesia can be exhausting for both relatives and the memory-impaired person. People with amnesia are also frustrated by frequent and sometimes humiliating failures and constant misunderstandings. As one young man said, "Frustration is constantly waiting in the wings". Tate (Chapter 15, this volume) discusses emotional aspects of memory impairment in more detail.

RECOVERY OF MEMORY FUNCTION AFTER BRAIN INJURY

Particularly in the early stages of an insult to the brain, families are keenly if not anxiously interested in the extent of possible recovery and improvement of memory functioning. When asked questions about recovery, however, it is likely that most health service professionals hedge their bets by suggesting that some improvement will take place while avoiding pronouncements on the extent of such improvement.

One problem associated with prognosis in cases of brain injury is that recovery means different things to different people. Some clinicians focus on survival rates, some on biological recovery, such as repair of brain structures, and others are interested in recovery of cognitive functions. The differences do not end there. Some clinicians interpret *recovery* as a complete regaining of identical functions that were lost or impaired as a result of the brain injury (Finger & Stein, 1982). Recovery of memory functioning, in this sense, is rarely achievable for people with brain injury. Others regard good recovery as resumption of normal life, even though there may be minor neurological and psychological deficits (Jennett & Bond, 1975). Such resumption is possible for some memory-impaired people (see for example "Alex" and "Jay", described in Wilson, 1999). Another interpretation of recovery regards it as the reduction of impairments in functioning over time (Marshall, 1985); and this is certainly applicable to the majority of memory-impaired people (see for example Wilson, 1991). Kolb (1995) believes that recovery typically involves partial recovery of function together with considerable *substitution* of function, i.e. learning to do things in a different way. Wilson (1998) defines cognitive recovery operationally as "a complete or partial resolution of cognitive deficits incurred as a result of an insult to the brain" (p. 281).

How does this discussion relate to memory-impaired people referred for help with their memory problems? On the one hand, we have studies that show families reporting a high incidence of memory problems several years after the insult (e.g. Brooks, 1984; Brooks et al., 1987; Oddy, 1984; Stilwell et al., 1999). On the other hand, we have studies showing significant recovery of memory functioning taking place during the first year after brain injury (Lezak, 1979). We know that one densely amnesic patient, H.M., did not show recovery or indeed improvement over a 30 year period (Freed et al. 1998; Scoville & Milner, 1957); and that another patient, T.B., showed a dramatic recovery at least 2 years after insult (Wilson & Baddeley, 1993). Victor et al. (1989) found that 74% of a sample of 104 Korsakoff patients showed some degree of recovery over a 3 year period following admission, and 21% of their sample seemed to show a more or less complete recovery. Kapur & Graham (2002) provide a more comprehensive discussion of recovery of memory functions.

What should we say to those who ask us about improvement or recovery? The answer depends, in part, on the cause of the memory impairment. We would not expect improvement in people with Alzheimer's or Huntington's disease, although it may prove possible to slow down the rate of deterioration, either with drugs or cognitive strategies or a combination of both. Fetal, stem cell or neural transplants, too, may eventually be able to reverse deterioration (for discussion, see Barker & Dunnett, 1999). Caution must be exercised when responding to questions from families, as people with progressive conditions, while failing to improve, may nevertheless be able to learn new skills or information; for example, new learning and maintenance of this learning was observed by Clare et al. (1999, 2000) in patients with Alzheimer's disease (see also Chapter 12, this volume).

In contrast, patients in posttraumatic amnesia (PTA) following head injury may show complete or considerable recovery, depending on the length of PTA (Wilson et al., 1999b). Even when patients are several months postinjury and out of PTA, improvement for some may be considerable. In one study of 43 brain-injured people referred for memory therapy during 1979–1985 and followed up 5–12 years later, just over 30% showed a substantial improvement on memory test scores, 60% remained virtually unchanged and just over 9% had declined. In addition to the 43 seen and reassessed, a further seven had died (including two suicides) three could not be contacted and one refused to take part in the study (Wilson, 1991). Although only one-third had improved since the end of rehabilitation, many had improved *during* rehabilitation. In addition, most subjects were using more aids, strategies and techniques to compensate for difficulties compared to the period before and at the end of rehabilitation. Those people who were using six or more strategies were significantly more likely to be independent (defined as in paid employment or living alone or in full-time education) than those using less than six strategies ($\chi^2 = 10.87$, $p < 0.001$).

Most people in the 1991 study, including those who had improved, were left with residual memory deficits, so they had not achieved their pre-injury levels. Nevertheless, the long-term prognosis was less bleak than had been believed several years earlier. Only nine of the 43 were in long-term care (despite the fact that most of the 43 had very significant cognitive problems), while 15 were in paid employment. Most were coping better than when last seen. These figures should not, however, hide the fact that some individuals in the group were lonely, unhappy and still very handicapped by their brain injury and their memory impairment.

It is probably true to say that people whose memory problems follow encephalitis and anoxia are likely to reach their final level of recovery earlier than those who have sustained a severe head injury, who may continue to show some recovery for a long period. Even with damage that occurred in childhood, little change may be seen. Vargha-Khadem et al. (1997) followed three children with early bilateral hippocampal damage from anoxic episodes for several years. The children showed reasonable levels of language functioning and general knowledge but their memory deficits remained severe. Broman et al. (1997) report on a boy who became severely amnesic following a cardiac arrest when he was 8 years old. He was followed for 19 years and his memory functioning remained severely impaired. He was described as being similar to H.M. (Scoville & Milner, 1957).

An adult patient, C.W., who became densely amnesic following herpes simplex encephalitis in 1985, showed no recovery of memory functioning over a 10 year period (Wilson et al., 1995). Funnell & De Mornay Davies (1996) also report on an encephalitic patient who showed little change over time. On the face of it, then, it looks as if restoration of memory functioning is unlikely following certain types of neurological damage. Kolb (1995) believes that language functions are more likely to show recovery than other cognitive functions, including memory. Yet a paper by Eriksson et al. (1998) suggests that regeneration of hippocampal cells can occur, even in the adult human brain: the authors found post-mortem evidence for neurogenesis in the dentate gyrus of the hippocampus in five patients who died of cancer. The authors were appropriately cautious about the practical implications of their findings and, to date, it is not clear whether such cells can survive in sufficient numbers and integrate in ways to improve everyday functioning.

What is clear, however, is that intervention and rehabilitation can reduce some of the everyday problems faced by people with memory problems. This appears to work through one of the following mechanisms: (a) reducing the load on memory through organizing or structuring the environment; (b) enabling people to learn more efficiently; and/or (c) teaching people to compensate for deficits. Each of these areas will be discussed later.

HELPING MEMORY-IMPAIRED PEOPLE AND THEIR FAMILIES

When first seeing someone who requires memory therapy, a good approach is to begin by formally interviewing the person and one or more relatives. Ask about the precipitating accident or illness and question them about resultant problems as they are manifested in everyday life. Also ask what they hope to achieve as a result of the referral. Questioning along these lines usually opens up an opportunity to explain that, although it may not be possible to restore or retrain memory functioning lost through certain accidents and illnesses, there may well be actions we can take that will help the patient manage his/her everyday life more successfully.

The nature of these actions will depend on a number of factors, including the nature and severity of the deficit (e.g. whether the memory impairment is due to a degenerative condition), the presence or absence of additional cognitive impairments, the current social and vocational situation of the patient, and the environmental demands of the patient's lifestyle.

A neuropsychological assessment will provide a picture of the patient's cognitive strengths and weaknesses (see Howieson & Lezak, Chapter 9, this volume). This should be supplemented by a more direct assessment of everyday problems, using procedures such as interviews, questionnaires, rating scales, checklists, memory diaries and direct observation (see Wilson, Chapter 8, this volume; Wilson, 1999).

Combining information from different assessments will highlight problems that need tackling, thus enabling realistic treatment programmes to be designed in such a way that they are both relevant to the life of the patient and match the neuropsychological demands suggested by cognitive test results. Of course, treatment programmes should be within the capabilities of the patient, therefore we should not expect memory-impaired people to remember arguments made in a previous session about the value of using external memory aids. Neither should we confuse patients having visuospatial difficulties by employing spatial terms when teaching routes. Those who are very ataxic will not be able to write quickly or even at all. People with deep dyslexia will have problems comprehending verbs, prepositions and abstract nouns. The message here is that our own treatment programmes should aim to bypass those areas that might rely on strengths or aptitudes that are themselves damaged in any particular patient.

Having identified particular problem areas and assessed cognitive functioning, a decision has to be made as to which of the problems should be tackled. Apart from the provisos listed immediately above, there is no right or wrong way of doing this. However, treatment planners will be influenced by the wishes of the patient, relatives and other staff members. Some patients are quite specific about the kind of help they want: for example they may say, "I can't remember my partners' names when playing bridge" or "I always forget where I have parked the car". Others are more vague and might say something like, "It's just everything, I can't remember a thing". Yet others will deny they have memory problems: "There's nothing wrong with my memory, it's people like you who are destroying my confidence". Relatives will also vary according to the clarity or vagueness of their descriptions of problems.

Future plans and placement will also influence the choice of problems to be tackled. For people planning to return to education, the choice might involve teaching study techniques to improve verbal recall (see Wilson, 1987a) or teaching the use of one of the electronic personal organizers (see later in this chapter and Kapur et al., Chapter 14, this volume). For someone going into long-term care the focus might be on teaching how to transfer from a wheelchair to an ordinary chair, or teaching the location of the toilet.

Another question concerns the number of problems to be tackled at any one time. This will depend on factors such as the patient's general intellectual level, the level of insight into physical and mental status, degree of motivation, the amount of involvement of others in the programme, and, of course, time available. For a person with a pure amnesia, having good intellectual functioning, good insight and high motivation, and whose family is willing to assist, it might be possible to work on four to six problems at any one time. With someone who is of poor intellectual functioning, with little insight or motivation and without family support, tackling one problem at a time is more appropriate.

When planning a treatment programme to overcome these problems, one can follow a behavioural approach using the steps involved in behaviour modification programmes (for a more detailed discussion, see Wilson, 1992). Working in this way provides a structure for the psychologist or therapist when attempting to get to grips with a difficult area: it enables him/her to measure the problem(s) and to determine whether goals have been achieved. There is a saying that "structure reduces anxiety", and this is true not only for brain-injured patients but also for those treating them.

The behavioural structure is adaptable to a wide range of patients, problems and settings, the goals are small and specific, treatment and assessment are inseparable, and there is continuous monitoring of results. Evidence that this approach is effective has been supplied by Wilson (1987a) and Moffat (1989). The number of steps in a behavioural programme may vary but can include as many as 11:

- Define the problem.
- (An operational definition may be required).
- Set goals (may need both short- and long-term).
- Measure the problem (take baseline).
- Consider reinforcers or motivators.
- Plan treatment.
- Begin treatment.
- Monitor progress.
- Evaluate.
- Change if necessary.
- Plan for generalization.

Examples of successful treatment programmes using this structure can be found in Wilson (1987b, 1992).

Another approach is to follow a holistic programme (Ben-Yishay, 1978; Diller, 1976; Prigatano, 1987, 1999). Followers of this approach believe that rehabilitation should consider cognitive, social and emotional aspects together, so one would not just treat memory problems in isolation but would include accompanying social and emotional consequences. Holistic programmes include group and individual therapies aimed at: (a) increasing awareness of what has happened; (b) achieving acceptance and understanding of one's difficulties; (c) providing cognitive remediation for memory and other deficits; (d) developing compensatory skills; and (e) offering vocational counselling. For further details on how this approach works in practice, see Prigatano (1999) and Wilson et al. (2000). Ben-Yishay (1996) also provides an interesting historical account of the origins of this approach.

MANAGING THE EMOTIONAL CONSEQUENCES OF MEMORY IMPAIRMENT

Clare & Wilson (1997) argue that:

> Memory is a very important part of our sense of who we are ... It is no surprise that memory problems often have major emotional consequences, including feelings of loss and anger and increased levels of anxiety (p. 41).

People with severe memory difficulties may become frightened, isolated, withdrawn or worried about making mistakes. As Jack (already mentioned) wrote in a letter to me:

> I can't perform basic sociable tasks, such as taking orders to buy a round of drinks or noting the names and faces of new acquaintances. In fact, I am sure that on many occasions I have met people who are not aware of my condition, and then upon not recognizing them on a second meeting, will have appeared rude and impolite (Wilson, 1999, p. 42).

Another young man with memory impairment told me that he was exhausted with making an effort to remember, and yet another that trying to be normal wore him out.

Evans & Wilson (1992) found anxiety levels high in people attending a memory group, while Kopelman & Crawford (1996) found depression present in over 40% of 200 consecutive referrals to a memory clinic. Reducing distress, anxiety and depression, together with increasing awareness and understanding, should be part of every memory rehabilitation programme. Giving people the chance to talk, ask questions and express their feelings may ease the distress and frustration and help them to accept the strategies we can offer.

One inexpensive and easily implemented strategy for reducing anxiety is to provide information. Questions such as, "Why does she ask the same question over and over again?" or "Why can he remember things that happened years ago but not what happened this morning?" deserve explanations. Some people are happy with simple explanations, for example "She isn't doing it to annoy you, she has simply forgotten how many times she asked the question" or "old memories are stored differently in the brain from new memories". Others will want access to references providing more detailed information. Simply being reassured that the behaviours seen are normal in people with memory problems may reduce anxiety for both relatives and memory-impaired people. Written information should supplement oral explanations, as even those with good memories find it harder to remember when preoccupied or distressed. Clare & Wilson (1997) wrote a short book for people with memory impairments, their relatives, friends and carers. This book contains general information about memory as well as suggestions as to how to deal with specific problems. A useful reference on self-help and support groups is Wearing (1992).

Relaxation therapy is also useful for people under stress. Even if those with memory problems do not remember that they have taken part in relaxation exercises, the effects may well remain. Individual relaxation therapy is fairly easy to organize and one can make tapes for individuals to take away and practice at home. Group relaxation therapy is sometimes carried out at rehabilitation centres. In addition, memory groups may have an indirect effect on reducing anxiety. Evans & Wilson (1992) felt that reduction in anxiety was one of the main benefits of their memory groups. Reduction in social isolation was another benefit for those attending outpatient groups. Wilson & Moffat (1992) describe the structure of memory groups in more detail.

Depression can also impair memory functioning (see Dalgleish & Cox, 2002). Cognitive-behavioural therapy and psychological support can be offered. Even though memory-impaired people may not remember much of the discussions that take place, they can be given handouts, notes and revision sessions. Group work to increase awareness and reduce emotional stress is common in holistic rehabilitation programmes (Prigatano, 1999).

Reminiscence therapy is a way of encouraging older memory-impaired people to remember experiences and incidents from the past by using reminders, such as old songs, newspaper articles and photographs. Reminiscence groups may also help to reduce anxiety and depression and improve mood. Because remembering old songs, advertisements, newspaper cuttings, etc. are typically easier for older people to recall and to engage in, the enjoyment experienced may improve their mood. Although reminiscence therapy is typically used with older people and in groups, it can be adapted for younger people and/or for individuals.

Finally, psychologists and other therapists engaged in memory therapy can act as a resource for putting families in touch with the right services. Given that emotional problems after a neurological insult may result from loss of income, loss of structure in one's life and loss of enjoyment from leisure or work, there is nothing to stop us telling families how to approach local social services or self-help societies, or how to access the right kind of assessment or treatment packages.

GUIDELINES FOR HELPING PEOPLE WITH MEMORY DIFFICULTIES

In 1991, Berg et al. described a memory group in The Netherlands. The participants were told, "Try to accept that a deficient memory cannot be cured: make a more efficient use of your remaining capacities; use external aids when possible; pay more attention; spend more time; repeat; make associations; organize; link input and retrieval situations" (p. 101). These general guidelines were given to brain-injured people in the form of a textbook and illustrated with examples. In addition, participants tackled real-life problems in their sessions and were given homework to enable them to practise and rehearse the strategies they were taught. For each participant, about three real-life problems were selected and worked on in an 18 session therapy programme. In the short term, participants in the memory rehabilitation group did better than those in the control group, although a follow-up 4 years later showed that the control group had caught up (Milders et al., 1995).

Others have also taught general strategies to memory-impaired people to try to enable them to cope in real-life situation. Lawson & Rice (1989), for example, were working with a 15 year-old boy who had sustained a severe head injury some 4 years earlier. They taught him a strategy to cope with his memory problems. First, he had to recognize that he had memory problems. Then he was taught to say, "I have a plan for helping me to work on a memory problem. It's WSTC". "WSTC" referred to a series of steps to follow: W stood for *What* (what are you asked to do?); this was regarded as the analysis of the problem. S stood for *Select* (select a strategy for the task); this was seen as strategy selection. T stood for *Try* (try out the strategy); this was seen as the strategy initiation stage. Finally, C stood for *Check* (check how the strategy is working); this was seen as the monitoring stage. The young man was able to employ the WSTC strategy in test situations and maintain the ability to do this up to 6 months posttraining. Unfortunately there was no attempt to generalize this training to real-life tasks or to monitor the extent to which he applied the strategy learning to real-life situations. Similar training in strategy application has been used in other areas of cognitive rehabilitation, for example Von Cramon & Matthes-von Cramon (1992) used problem-solving therapy for clients with dysexecutive syndrome, and Levine et al. (2000) used a somewhat similar strategy training programme to help people with memory and attention disorders.

The advantage of general strategy training is that it enables memory-impaired people to deal with whatever difficulties come their way. Ideally, of course, this is what all of us in memory rehabilitation would like. In practice, we may need to set our sights a little lower with those clients who have more widespread cognitive difficulties (say a combination of memory, attention, planning and organizational problems), or who are so severely impaired that it is difficult to teach them to remember to apply a strategy.

There are general guidelines that psychologists, therapists, family members and others can apply to help memory-impaired people *take in*, *store* and *retrieve* information more successfully. While these guidelines will not solve memory problems, they may improve or ease situations for those with impaired memory functioning. The guidelines themselves are the result of theoretical experiments to determine whether the amnesic syndrome is due to a deficit of (a) encoding, or (b) storage, or (c) retrieval). Although accounts to explain amnesia as a failure in only one of these processes are insufficient in themselves, experiments trying to prove or disprove these views have provided us with a number of useful pointers.

People are more likely to encode (i.e. take in) information efficiently if:

- The information is simplified (it is easier to remember short words than long words and jargon should be avoided).
- They are required to remember one thing at a time (do not present three or four names/instructions/words at once).
- The information is understood (ask the memory-impaired person to repeat the information back in his/her own words to check for understanding).
- The information is linked or associated with something already known (for example, when trying to remember the name Molly, you could check if they have an Aunt Molly, or if they know the song "Good Golly Miss Molly" or "Molly Malone".
- The "little and often" or distributed practice rule is followed (have frequent breaks when teaching new information or a new skill).
- The information is processed or manipulated in some way (don't let your memory-impaired clients be passive recipients of the information, instead ask them to think about it, question it, do something with it, to ensure they process the information).

Once the information is encoded, it has to be stored. Rehearsal, practice and testing can all be used to try to ensure the information remains in storage. The method known as "spaced retrieval" (also called "expanding rehearsal") is a good testing procedure to follow. Present the information, test immediately, test again after a very brief delay and so forth. The retention interval is gradually increased. This method will be discussed in more detail later in the chapter.

Another problem, faced at times by all of us, is retrieving the information from memory when it is required. Some memory-impaired people seem to have particular problems with retrieval. If we can provide a hook in the form of a cue or prompt, they may be able to retrieve the information more readily. The first letter of a word or name to be recalled can be a powerful retrieval cue. The problem here, of course, is that someone needs to be available to provide the first letter. Some people, including some memory-impaired people, learn to go through the alphabet systematically to try to find their own first letter cue. Even for these people, however, the system is haphazard and unreliable.

Perhaps the best way to improve retrieval is to avoid context specificity, i.e. if material is learned in one situation, it is recalled better in the same situation (Godden & Baddeley, 1975; Watkins et al.,1976). Most of us will have experienced this phenomenon. You may, for example, know a work colleague very well and be able to greet him/her by name at work without a second thought. However, if you meet that colleague in a different situation, say at a shopping centre, the name may become inaccessible because of the change of context. In rehabilitation it is not uncommon to find clients who use a notebook in occupational therapy but do not use it elsewhere, or who can tell you the name of their physiotherapist in the gym but not elsewhere. The answer here is to avoid such context-specific learning by teaching the use of the notebook not only in occupational therapy but also in a number of other situations. Similarly, the physiotherapist will need to be met and interacted with in other settings.

Another general guideline when working with severely memory-impaired people is to avoid trial-and-error learning. As errorless learning is such a large part of current memory rehabilitation, it deserves a section to itself and will be discussed at some length later.

In the final part of this section on general strategies, a series of steps is provided by Schuri et al. (1996). These are described as the basic steps to follow in memory rehabilitation.

Step 1 Assess the memory functions and associated cognitive deficits. Standardized tests should be used (to understand the client's cognitive strengths and weaknesses) and behavioural measures to see how the problems are manifested in everyday life.

Step 2 Inform the clients and their families and caregivers about the functional deficits and possible consequences in everyday life. Clients should be provided with practical experience relevant to "real-life" situations.

Step 3 Agree on the goals of therapy and on which specific problems should be treated.

Step 4 Select the most appropriate external and/or internal strategies for the specific problems to be treated.

Step 5 Teach the clients to use the strategies themselves, or use the strategies in therapy to achieve a treatment goal (e.g. learn a specific piece of information or change a piece of behaviour).

Step 6 Evaluate treatment effectiveness (in terms of the goals achieved). If necessary, change the procedure.

The next three sections will discuss more specific strategies for improving everyday life situations for people with memory impairment.

ENVIRONMENTAL ADAPTATIONS

One of the simplest ways to help people with memory impairment is to arrange the environment so that they rely less on memory. Examples include labelling doors for a person who cannot remember which room is which, or labelling cupboards in the kitchen or beds in a hospital ward. Other examples include drawing arrows or lines to indicate routes round a building, or positioning objects so they cannot be missed or forgotten (e.g. tying a front door key to a waist belt). Making rooms safer for confused, brain-injured people is also possible by altering the environment.

Sometimes it is possible to avoid irritating or problematic behaviours by identifying and then changing the environmental triggers of the behaviour: people who constantly ask the same question may be responding to something said to them, such as a greeting or request.

There are a few reports of environmental changes in the management of memory problems, for example Harris (1980) describes a geriatric unit where the rate of incontinence was reduced by the simple strategy of painting all lavatory doors a different colour from other doors, thus making them easier to distinguish. Kapur, et al. (Chapter 14, this volume) also discuss environmental adaptations.

Lincoln (1989) reports how one woman was able to keep track of whether she had taken her medication by placing a chart next to the bottle of tablets rather than in another room. Lincoln also provides suggestions for further environmental adaptations. She notes that most hospital staff wear name badges that may be too small for elderly people to read, and contain surnames rather than first names, which are used more frequently on the ward.

The most densely amnesic person seen by the present author is C.W., a musician who developed herpes simplex encephalitis in 1985. The only strategies that seem to help this man are environmental adaptations. He has an unusual form of epilepsy that takes the form of jerking movements and belching. These occur with greater frequency when C.W. is under stress or agitated. A behavioural analysis undertaken by Avi Schmueli (personal communication) showed that the seizures were far more likely to occur when there was a change in activity, for example when changing from one test to another during assessment, or when an additional person entered the room. Although it was not possible or indeed ethical to prevent all such changes in activity or personnel, some changes were introduced to reduce the frequency of this man's seizures.

Because C.W. was unable to remember any of the people involved in his care, he considered them all to be strangers and disliked being treated informally by them as though they were well known to him. Consequently, he was not called by his first name, as was usual with long-stay patients. Demonstrations of affection also caused him fear and distress. For example, one nurse who had known C.W. for 4 years, went on holiday for 2 weeks and on returning she approached C.W. to give him a hug. He saw what was for him a total stranger bear down upon him with open arms and panicked. Again, a more formal approach can reduce the number of occasions resulting in panic.

C.W. also repeats certain phrases scores of times in the course of each day, the most frequent stating that he has just that moment woken up. Every few minutes during a conversation or assessment he says something along the lines of, "This is the first time I've been awake, this is the first taste I've had, the first time I've seen anything or heard anything. It's like being dead. I don't remember you coming into the room but now for the first time, I can see." Sympathizing with these statements or trying to offer explanations seems to increase his agitation and cause an escalation of the number of repetitions. Distracting him by introducing another topic of conversation results in calmer behaviour.

For people with severe intellectual deficits or progressive deterioration or very dense amnesia, environmental adaptations may be the best we can offer to enable them to cope and reduce some of their confusion and frustration. Few studies have discussed ways in which environments can be designed to help people with severe memory impairment, although it would seem to be a fruitful area for psychologists, engineers, architects and designers to join forces.

Modification or restructuring the environment means that problems due to memory impairment can be avoided. The origins of this approach can be found within the field of behaviour modification, especially in the area of severe learning disability (Murphy & Oliver, 1987). Despite being, at times, an effective and rapid way of reducing problems, this approach does not always work. For example, people have to be able to understand the labels and the signposts; some repetitious behaviours are not triggered by external events and the notebook clipped to a belt is no good if it is never used. In addition, one has to be aware of possible ethical considerations of an environment that is too restrictive. Therefore, it might be possible to avoid any demands on memory by placing someone in an environment where every move is supervised by a staff member, leaving the person with memory problems completely unable to exercise any choice. Like other psychiatric and psychological methods of management, environmental control is open to abuse. Nevertheless, there is little doubt that for some people with severe and widespread cognitive impairments, environmental restructuring or modification probably provides the best chance of some degree of independence.

ERRORLESS LEARNING IN REHABILITATION

Errorless learning is a teaching technique whereby people are prevented, as far as possible, from making mistakes while they are learning a new skill or acquiring new information. Instead of teaching by demonstration, which may involve the learner in trial-and-error, the experimenter, therapist or teacher presents the correct information or procedure in ways that minimize the possibility of erroneous responses.

There are two theoretical backgrounds to investigations of errorless learning in people with organic memory impairment. The first is the work on errorless discrimination learning from the field of behavioural psychology, first described by Terrace (1963, 1966). Terrace was working with pigeons and found it was possible to teach pigeons to discriminate a red key from a green key with a teaching technique whereby the pigeons made no (or very few) errors during learning. Furthermore, pigeons learning via errorless learning were reported to show less emotional behaviour than pigeons learning with trial-and-error.

Sidman & Stoddard (1967) soon applied errorless learning principles to children with developmental learning difficulties. They were able to teach these children to discriminate ellipses from circles. Others soon took up the idea (e.g. Cullen, 1976; Jones & Eayrs, 1992; Walsh & Lamberts, 1979).

Cullen (1976) believed that if errors were made during learning it was harder to remember just what had been learned. He also pointed out that more reinforcement occurred during errorless learning as only successes occurred, never failures. To this day errorless learning is a frequently used teaching technique for people with developmental learning difficulties.

The second theoretical impetus came from studies of implicit memory and implicit learning from cognitive psychology and cognitive neuropsychology (e.g. Brooks & Baddeley, 1976; Graf & Schacter, 1985; Tulving & Schacter, 1990; and many others). Although it has been known for decades that memory-impaired people can learn some skills and information normally through their intact (or relatively intact) implicit learning abilities, it has been difficult to apply this knowledge to reduce real-life problems encountered by people with organic memory deficits.

Glisky and colleagues (Glisky & Schacter, 1987; Glisky et al., 1986) tried to capitalize on intact implicit abilities to teach people with amnesia computer terminology, using a technique they called "the method of vanishing cues". Despite some successes, the method of vanishing cues involved considerable time and effort from both experimenters and people with amnesia. Implicit memory or learning, on the other hand, does not involve effort, as it occurs without conscious recollection. This, together with certain other anomalies seen during implicit learning (such as the observation that in a fragmented picture/perceptual priming procedure, if an amnesic patient mislabels a fragment during an early presentation, the error may "stick" and be repeated on successive presentations), led Baddeley & Wilson (1994) to pose the question, "Do amnesic patients learn better if prevented from making mistakes during the learning process?" In a study with 16 young and 16 elderly control participants, and 16 densely amnesic people, employing a stem completion procedure, it was found that every one of the amnesic people learned better if prevented from making mistakes during learning.

Baddeley & Wilson (1994) believed that errorless learning was superior to trial-and-error learning because it depended on implicit memory. As the amnesic people could not use explicit memory effectively, they were forced to rely on implicit memory. This system is not designed to eliminate errors, so it is better to prevent the injection of errors in the first place. In the absence of an efficient episodic memory, the very fact of making an incorrect response may strengthen or reinforce the error.

Errorless learning principles were quickly adopted in the rehabilitation of memory-impaired people. Wilson et al. (1994) described a number of single-case studies in which amnesic people were taught several tasks, such as learning therapists' names, learning to programme an electronic organizer and learning to recognize objects. Each participant was taught two similar tasks in an errorful or an errorless way. In each case errorless was superior to errorful learning. Wilson & Evans (1996) provided further support for these findings. Squires et al. (1996) taught a man with amnesia to use a notebook with an errorless learning procedure. The same group (Squires et al., 1997, 1998) found that errorless learning procedures enabled amnesic people to learn novel associations and to acquire word-processing skills. More recently, these principles have been used successfully for people with Alzheimer's disease (Clare et al., 1999, 2000).

As stated above, Baddeley & Wilson (1994) believed that errorless learning was effective for people with amnesia because it capitalized on their intact implicit memory capacities. Hunkin et al. (1998) believed that errorless learning capitalized on the impoverished, residual, explicit memory capacities. Ongoing and, as yet unpublished, investigations in Cambridge suggest that both these explanations may be correct. For very severely amnesic people with virtually no explicit memory, it would appear that errorless learning is succesful because it capitalizes on their implicit abilities. For those with some, albeit weak, explicit/episodic memory, then errorless learning is beneficial for both memory systems.

OTHER WAYS OF IMPROVING LEARNING

There are a number of strategies that can help memory-impaired people learn more efficiently. These include spaced retrieval (otherwise known as expanding rehearsal) and mnemonics.

Spaced retrieval involves the presentation of material to be remembered (e.g. a new telephone number) followed by immediate testing. People with a normal digit span will, for example, be able to repeat back a seven figure number. The tester then waits for a second or two and requests the number again. The test interval is very gradually increased until the number is learned. New names, short addresses, items of general knowledge can also be taught in this way. Spaced retrieval is a form of distributed practice, i.e. distributing the learning trials over a period of time rather than massing them together in one block. Massed practice is a less efficient learning strategy than distributed practice (Baddeley, 1999), a phenomenon that has been known since the 1930s (Baddeley & Longman, 1978; Lorge, 1930). Landauer & Bjork (1978) showed that name learning proceeds faster with expanding rehearsal/spaced retrieval and from that time the procedure has been used in memory rehabilitation (Camp, 1989; McKitrick & Camp, 1993; Moffat, 1989; Schacter et al., 1985). Although most published studies describe using spaced retrieval with people with dementia, the technique has been used with people with other conditions, such as traumatic brain injury (see Wilson, 1989).

Mnemonic systems are those that enable people to organize, store and retrieve information more efficiently. Sometimes the term "mnemonics" is used to refer to anything that helps people to remember, including external memory aids. Usually, however, the term is used for methods involving mental manipulation of material; for example, in order to remember how many days there are in each month, most people use a mnemonic. In the USA and the UK this is typically the rhyme, "Thirty days hath September, April, June and November..." and so forth. In other parts of the world people use their knuckles and the dips in between to remember the long and the short months, or else they have different suffixes and prefixes to distinguish them. Every country using our calendar system appears to have a mnemonic for remembering the long and the short months. Mnemonics are also employed to learn notes of music, colours of the rainbow, cranial nerves, and other ordered material.

Mnemonics can be employed to help people with memory impairments learn new information (see Wilson, 1987a, for a series of studies using a variety of mnemonics). It is usually best for the psychologist, therapist or carer to work out the mnemonic (perhaps together with the memory-impaired person) and work through this together. People with organic memory deficits often find it difficult to devise their own mnemonics, or they may forget to employ them, or forget to use them spontaneously in novel situations. This is not always the case, as some people can be taught to use them in new situations (Kime et al., 1996). The real value of mnemonics, however, is that they are useful for teaching new information to people with memory difficulties, and they almost always lead to faster learning than rote rehearsal (Clare et al., 1999; Moffat, 1989; West, 1995; Wilson, 1987a). Clare et al. (1999) employed a combination of strategies, including a visual mnemonic, spaced retrieval and errorless learning to reteach the names of people at a social club to a man with Alzheimer's disease.

EXTERNAL MEMORY AIDS

Helping people to compensate for their memory deficits through the use of external memory aids is one of the most effective methods of rehabilitation. External memory aids enable us to remember by using systems to record or access information. Diaries, notebooks, lists, alarm clocks, wall charts, calendars, tape recorders and personal organizers are all examples of external memory aids. Almost every one of us makes use of these at one time or another. Such aids are likely to be the most helpful method of compensating for difficulties encountered by memory-impaired people (Wilson, 1991), but, unfortunately, it is often difficult for memory-impaired people to learn to use these aids, because they forget to record or access information. They may use the aids in a disorganized way or they may be embarrassed to use aids in the presence of others. The trouble with external memory aids is that their use involves memory. Thus, the very people who need external memory aids the most have the greatest difficulty in learning to use them.

Despite these problems, there is evidence that some memory-impaired people use external aids effectively, for example people with a pure amnesic syndrome tend to be able to use them reasonably well (Wilson & Watson, 1996). A good example is J.C. (see Wilson et al., 1997a), who had a haemorrhage caused by a ruptured posterior cerebral artery aneurysm when he was 20 years old. As a result he became severely amnesic and remains so to this day, 15 years later. Despite this, he is able to live alone, earn his own living, complete his own tax forms and remain completely independent. He developed (and continues to develop) a sophisticated system of compensatory strategies. Soon after his haemorrhage he started writing notes on scraps of paper. Over the years he has progressed to using a number of different aids. The most often used include a databank watch, a personal organizer and a small tape recorder. These are supported by a number of additional strategies, used less often. J.C. records most information he needs to remember in at least two systems, so that if he fails to access it one way, he has a back-up.

The first 10 years of the development of his system is described in Wilson et al. (1997a). It was possible to describe this natural history of a compensatory system, as J.C. kept a journal over this period; his aunt kept details of how she helped J.C., and I kept records of my assessments. By combining information from these three sources, we were able to trace the increasing sophistication of J.C.'s use of strategies.

Another study describing how a densely amnesic young woman was taught to use a memory notebook is that of Kime et al. (1996). The young woman became amnesic following status epilepticus. After 20 months she was admitted to a rehabilitation programme. A complex memory book was provided for her and over a period of weeks she was taught to use the book, containing details of her programme, local transport, important people, locations in the neighbourhood, a things-to-do list and so forth. Initially, the woman was never allowed to fail (so inadvertently an errorless learning approach was employed). She was always prompted and guided to go to the right section and do the right thing. Gradually, the prompts were faded out until she was using the book reliably and systematically. Furthermore, she demonstrated generalization of this behaviour by employing the aids in new environments and for new problems. Following discharge from rehabilitation she was able to obtain paid employment and use the memory book effectively.

One recently developed and successful memory aid that has been helping people with widespread cognitive deficits is NeuroPage® (Hersh & Treadgold, 1994). NeuroPage® is a simple and portable paging system with a screen that can be attached to a belt. Larry Treadgold, the engineer father of a head-injured son, and Neil Hersh, a neuropsychologist, combined their skills to produce a programmable messaging system that utilizes an arrangement of microcomputers linked to a conventional computer memory and, by telephone, to a paging company.

The scheduling of reminders or cues for each individual is entered into the computer and from then on no further human interfacing is necessary. On the appropriate date and time, NeuroPage® accesses the user's data files, determines the reminder to be delivered, transmits the information by modem to the terminal, where the reminder is converted, and transmits, as a wireless radio signal, to only that receiver corresponding to the particular user. The user is alerted to an incoming reminder by a flashing, light-emitting diode and an audible "chirp". The reminder is graphically displayed on the screen of the receiver. Once the message appears, users are requested to telephone a person or an answer service to confirm the message. Without this confirmation, the message is repeated.

Users of NeuroPage® can control everything with one rather large button, easy to press even for those having motor difficulties. It avoids most of the problems of existing aids. It is highly portable, unlike many computers. It has an audible alarm that can be adapted to vibrate if required, together with an accompanying explanatory message, unlike many watch alarms. It is not embarrassing for the majority of users and indeed may convey prestige. Perhaps the biggest advantage of the NeuroPage® is that once it has been programmed it is easy to use. Most other systems require considerable time for memory-impaired people to learn how to handle them.

We began evaluating NeuroPage® in the UK in 1994. Using an ABA single case experimental design, we started with 15 neurologically impaired people, all of whom had

significant everyday memory problems because of organic memory impairment or because
of problems with planning and organization resulting from frontal lobe damage. We found a
statistically significant improvement between the baseline and treatment phases for each of
the 15 clients. In this study, clients selected their own target behaviours (e.g. "take medication; feed the dog; pack your spectacles for work"). The mean success rate for the group as
a whole was just over 37% of targets achieved during a 4–6 week baseline. This rose to over
85% during the 12 week treatment phase, i.e. when subjects were provided with a pager
and reminded to carry out the target behaviours. During the second (posttreatment) baseline
phase, the overall percentage of targets achieved was 74%. In fact, some clients learned their
routines during the baseline while others did not. This suggests that for some clients, the
pager may only be needed for a short while in order to establish certain behaviours. Others,
particularly those with executive deficits, may need the reminding service on a longer-term
basis.

We have also published two single case studies using NeuroPage®. The first (Evans
et al., 1998) is a treatment study with a stroke patient who had considerable problems with
planning and organization. The second (Wilson et al., 1999a) is an account of a very amnesic
young man who was enabled to live independently with the help of NeuroPage®. Health
and Social Services saved considerable amounts of money on these clients following the
implementation of the pager (Wilson & Evans, 2002).

Following the success of the pilot study (Wilson et al., 1997b), we carried out a further
investigation with NeuroPage® (Wilson et al., 2001) involving 143 clients, even more
impaired (as a group) than those in the pilot study. Some were referred by other therapists
who were feeling some desperation because all else had failed. We employed a randomized
control trial in the larger study whereby, following a 2 week baseline, clients were allocated
to either the treatment group (pager) or to a waiting list control group. After a further 7
weeks, those on the waiting list were given a pager and those who had been using the pager
were taken off the paging service. After a further 5 weeks, target behaviours were monitored
for a final 2 weeks. The results can be seen in Figure 10.1.

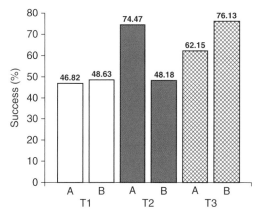

Figure 10.1   Percentage success rate for participants in Group A (pager first) and Group B
(pager later) at Time 1 (baseline); Time 2 (weeks 8 and 9) and Time 3 (weeks 15 and 16).
Reproduced from Wilson et al. (2001). © 2001, BMJ publishing group

There were no significant differences between groups A and B during baseline. Group A then went on to receive the pager while group B members were on the waiting list. At time 2 (weeks 6 and 7), following the end of baseline, there was a significant difference in favour of group A. Group B participants were then given a pager with group A returning their pagers. At time 3 (weeks 6 and 7 following the changeover), there was a significant difference in the number of target behaviours achieved in favour of group B. The main findings then were broadly similar to those in the pilot study.

One big advantage of a system like NeuroPage® is that it is adaptable and suitable for a wide range of people and problems, from different diagnostic groups and at different times postinsult. The main disadvantage is that people cannot programme the system themselves and have to telephone or otherwise contact a centre so that the messages can be entered on to a computer and, on the right date and time, be transmitted to the individual pager.

There are, of course, systems to bypass these problems, for example "Reminder system" (Davis, D., personal communication, 16 July 1999) enables people to programme their own messages via the World Wide Web. A study comparing two different keyboards of microcomputers found some people preferred one system while others preferred the other. Both, however, allowed clients to programme their own reminders (Wright et al., 2000, 2001).

The use of pagers, computers and other technological aids in memory rehabilitation is likely to expand in the future, given the current growth in information technology. One of the first studies to use an electronic aid with a brain-injured person was that of Gouvier (1982). A small portable timer was used to remind a memory-impaired man to check his memory book. More sophisticated technology in the form of computers came later in the 1980s. Although computers have been used in cognitive rehabilitation since the 1970s, these were used, on the whole, to provide exercises, in the belief that exercising an impaired function such as memory would lead to an improvement in that function (Gianutsos, 1980; see also Wilson, 1997, for a critique of this approach). Computers as a compensatory aid arrived a little later (see for example Bergman, 1991; Kim et al., 1999; Kirsch et al., 1987, 1992). Another series of studies using computers is that of Glisky and colleagues (Glisky, 1995; Glisky & Schacter, 1986, 1987, 1989). The very latest in technology is the use of virtual reality systems in rehabilitation (see Brooks et al., 1999; Rizzo et al., 1997; Rose, et al., 1996). Kapur et al., (Chapter 14, this volume) discusses the use of computers and other external memory aids in detail.

In conclusion to this section, compensating for memory problems is probably one of the best strategies for improving quality of life for people with significant memory impairment. The principle here is to try to find an alternative means to achieve a goal. This idea can be traced back to Zangwill (1947), when he discussed his principle of compensation, and is also similar to Luria's (1963) principle of functional adaptation, i.e. if you cannot achieve something one way, try to find an alternative way to achieve the goal. Frequently, however, psychologists and therapists need to spend time finding the best aids for a particular client and then teaching the use of those aids. One paper describing in some detail how to teach use of a memory aid is that of Sohlberg & Mateer (1989), in which they describe a three-stage procedure for teaching the use of compensatory memory books. The three stages are acquisition, application and adaptation. The authors state correctly that often compensatory notebooks are provided with minimal instruction or without formal training in their use. Furthermore, memory books are frequently rejected by clients or only used for a short time. Sohlberg & Mateer believe that the notebook must be tailored for the individual client, so the content or sections of the book will differ; for example, some clients will require an orientation section containing personal, autobiographical information and details about the brain injury, whereas others will not need this.

In the acquisition stage clients learn the different sections and the purpose of each section. A question-and-answer format is used to teach this and 100% success is required before moving to the second stage—application. In this stage clients learn appropriate methods of recording in their notebooks. Role-play situations are used to teach the skill and success is defined as 100% accuracy in three role-play situations without cueing on two consecutive days. The final stage is adaptation. Here clients have to demonstrate appropriate notebook use in naturalistic settings. Training is in the community (e.g. a shop or cafeteria) and a certain score from the clinician accompanying the client is required on two consecutive days before the client is considered to be efficient at this stage.

The Sohlberg & Mateer (1989) description is clinically useful, flexible and suitable for a wide range of clients. They provide ideas on how to adapt the training to inpatients in the acute stage and for clients who are unable to write. This paper is important in stressing that many, if not most, memory-impaired people will need to undergo training if they are to use their compensatory strategies or external aids efficiently.

In a study comparing four different memory improvement strategies, namely written rehearsal, verbal rehearsal, acronym formation and memory notebook logging, Zencius et al. (1991) found that only memory notebook logging was effective in increasing recall of classroom material. A more recent account of training in the use of memory journals, using a five-step approach, can be found in Donaghy & Williams (1998). Ownsworth & McFarland (1999) also found diary training with self-instructional training led to better diary use than diary training alone.

So, do memory-impaired people use aids in their everyday lives and, if so, what aids are used? In the long-term follow-up study mentioned earlier (Wilson, 1991), it was found that most subjects were using more aids, strategies and techniques to compensate for their difficulties, compared with the numbers they were using before and immediately at the end of rehabilitation. Of the 44 people for whom information was available, 38 of them were using compensations. The remaining six, who were not using anything, were all in long-term care. A further three people in long-term care were using memory compensations. Those using six or more aids, strategies or techniques were significantly more likely to be independent (i.e. in paid employment, or living alone or in full-time education) than those using five or less.

A more recent study interviewed 94 people with memory problems (Evans et al., 2003) and once again found that 92 of the participants were using at least some form of memory aid or strategy, and use of these correlated with independence, i.e. people who used six or more aids were significantly more likely to be independent. This confirmed the results of the earlier study by Wilson & Watson (1996). The number and type of aids used by people in the Evans et al. (2003) study can be found in Table 10.1.

In the first edition of *The Handbook of Memory Disorders*, Kapur (1995) said:

> The contribution of aids to memory rehabilitation holds considerable promise but many questions remain unanswered. We need to know which memory aids benefit which memory problems in which memory-disordered clients. Memory aids may often best be used in combination and we need to know the optimal combinations for particular clinical needs. We also need to know if the magnitude of any benefit to clients is significant and makes a meaningful difference to their everyday adjustment, if the change is permanent and if it is cost-effective in terms of money and in therapists' time (p. 550).

Table 10.1 Number of participants using particular memory aids/strategies

Remembering strategy	Number of sample using the strategy ($n = 94$)
Wall calendar/wall chart	68
Notebook	60
List	59
A diary	51
Asking others to remind	46
Mental retracing	45
Alarm clock (wake up)	38
Objects in unusual places	33
Notes in special places	32
Repetitive practice	28
Writing on hand	23
Making associations	20
Watch with date/timer	17
Daily routine	17
Personal organizer	16
Journal	15
Daily timetable	14
Alarm clock/timer	9
Visual imagery	9
Weekly routine	9
Alphabetic searching	7
Electronic organizer	7
TV guide (annotated)	7
First-letter mnemonics	5
Pager	5
Recipe cards or books	5
Pleasantness rating	3
Key chain	3
Pocket phone book	3
Mobile phone	3
Dictaphone/tape recorder	2
Rhymes	2
Knot in handkerchief	2
Orientation of medication	2
Dictionary	2
Chunking	1
Phone numbers/address on key ring	1
Home filing system	1
Home accounts	1
Information for work on wall	1
Organizer handbag	1
Buying small quantities	1
Clock–calendar combination	1

While endorsing Kapur's views, examples such as J.C. and the Kime et al. (1996) client, described above, would appear to be cost-effective in that both these young people were in paid employment. Nevertheless, we need to address Kapur's point in future studies of external aids in rehabilitation (see Chapter 14, this volume).

GENERALIZATION ISSUES

Generalization of principles, techniques and strategies practised or learned in rehabilitation to situations outside rehabilitation is of crucial importance. There are several kinds of generalization, such as across subjects, across behaviours or across settings. Our concern here is with generalization as it refers to transfer of training, i.e. generalization across settings and generalization across behaviours.

Generalization across settings refers to a situation where a strategy taught in one setting is applied to other settings. An example would be where a patient is taught to use an electronic aid or particular mnemonic in one setting (say in the clinical psychology department) and then uses the aid or the mnemonic at home or at school.

Generalization across behaviours refers to situations in which a strategy taught to help with one problem is used to assist with another problem. An example would be teaching a person to use a technique for remembering current events in the newspapers, and finding that the person used the method for school work. Once again, there is little evidence that this occurs spontaneously in adults with acquired brain damage. If generalization is considered desirable (as it usually is in treatment), then it should be built into the treatment programme in the same way as it is built into programmes with people with developmental learning difficulties (Zarkowska, 1987).

To promote generalization across settings we can use a variety of places as part of the treatment. For example, when teaching the use of a personal organizer, we might begin in the clinical psychology department and, once the patient is proficient at recording and referring to the organizer in this setting, the psychologist could see the patient in the occupational therapy department and, if necessary, reteach the use of the organizer there. The next step might be to repeat the procedure in physiotherapy, then speech therapy, on the ward, at home and so forth. The wider the range of settings, the more likelihood there is of the strategy generalizing to other settings (Zarkowska, 1987).

Similarly, to encourage generalization across behaviours, a patient could be taught how to use a strategy for remembering some of the content in newspaper articles, then encouraged or taught to use that same strategy for remembering magazine stories, then chapters in books, and even studying for examinations.

Persuading patients to put into practice strategies they have been taught may be more difficult. Again several options are open. It is possible to put some patients on a behaviour programme to reinforce the use of memory aids and mnemonics. Practical goals could be formulated in ways similar to the following examples: "Teaching Mrs X to refer to her notebook after each meal" or "Increasing the number of times Mr Z uses a particular study technique spontaneously when he is revising for examinations". The use of timers, together with prompting and fading, would perhaps be one way of achieving success, for example a timer could be set to ring at the end of each meal. Initially, when the timer sounds the therapist or psychologist may need to prompt (or remind) Mrs X to check her notebook. Gradually the verbal reminders could be abbreviated and eventually stopped. Later still, the timer could be omitted as the meal-time setting itself becomes the reminder to check the notebook. Alternatively, a chaining method could be used whereby a particular task is broken down into a series of smaller units and taught one at a time, thus if a patient is required to learn a new route, it should be possible to break the route down into sections. One section of the route could be taught, then section two added to section one, then section three added to sections one and two, and so forth.

In other cases it might be necessary to allow more time before expecting strategies to be used spontaneously. Some patients who are slow to start can sometimes begin to put into practice the skills they have been taught previously when they are given sufficient time. One amnesic man frequently argued with his wife over whether or not he had taken a bath. Because of his amnesia he could not remember and therefore insisted he had bathed recently. His wife knew better but could not convince him. It was suggested that he kept a "bath diary" in which he recorded dates and times of baths. However, he kept forgetting to record times. With the help of his wife, frequent reminding and keeping the diary above the sink in the bathroom, he began to note his bath times and now he continues to bathe regularly.

It may be necessary to abandon a particular strategy in favour of another if a patient shows signs of distress when participating in therapy; one man hated visual imagery and his comment every time he worked with imagery was, "Where's the logic in that?". Although he learned the names of staff by using imagery, he became angry whenever the method was presented. He was much happier using first-letter cueing, as he could see "the logic in it". In his case, visual imagery was not recommended to his relatives when the time came for his discharge from the centre. At what point a therapist abandons a strategy in favour of another will usually be guided by observation, clinical experience and intuition, but there is little doubt that a method that causes a patient some discomfort and even distress will be unlikely to produce a favourable outcome.

In ending this section on generalization, it should be emphasized again that generalization must not be expected to occur automatically. When it does occur spontaneously it is a bonus, but to increase the chances of it happening more regularly we must ensure that planning for generalization is always part of any treatment programme. If it is not possible to teach generalization, then relatives and staff can be taught to implement the procedure if necessary. In the use of visual imagery for names, it can be explained to the relatives that if the memory-impaired person needs to learn, for example, the names of neighbours, they can teach these names by converting each name into a picture, drawing the picture, and teaching one name at a time. The principles of errorless learning and expanding rehearsal can be explained too, so these can be incorporated. Finally, all explanations should be written down for the relatives as they, too, are likely to forget what has been said to them.

SUMMARY AND FUTURE DIRECTIONS

Although people with memory impairment and their families should not be led to believe that significant improvement in memory can occur once the period of natural recovery is over, they can nevertheless be helped to understand, manage, cope with or bypass problems arising from the impairment. Such help will normally be given to individual patients and their families by therapists and psychologists. They can also be put in touch with local and national self-help groups.

Indirect or emotional consequences of brain injury and cognitive deficit should be addressed by counsellors, psychologists and psychotherapists, so that anxiety management and cognitive therapy programmes can be introduced. When planning for a memory therapy programme, results from a neuropsychological assessment should be combined with more direct assessment of everyday problems, obtained by observation, interviewing, rating scales and questionnaires. Neuropsychological assessment will identify cognitive strengths and weaknesses, while direct assessment will highlight everyday problems requiring treatment.

In addition to treatment of specific problems revealed by neuropsychological assessment, more general guidelines are recommended to improve encoding, storage and retrieval. In view of the findings of recent research studies, which indicate that people learn better when prevented from making errors, it is probably best to avoid trial-and-error learning for people with organic memory deficits.

Specific problems can be dealt with in a number of ways, including environmental adaptations, teaching the use of external aids as compensatory strategies and using mnemonics as a faster route to learning new information. Planning and imagination should be brought into play when teaching the use of external aids. Although mnemonics may not be used spontaneously by memory-impaired people, their teachers, therapists and psychologists can use them to enhance learning by the memory impaired.

Memory groups have certain advantages. They are useful in reducing anxiety and depression, in increasing social contacts, and in introducing and practising the use of external aids. Memory-impaired group members may be more willing to imitate their peers than the non-impaired professionals running a group.

People with severe memory problems will probably need help in generalizing from one setting to another, and from one problem to another. It is therefore recommended that the teaching of generalization is an integral part of any rehabilitation programme.

At present, drugs are of rather limited value in enhancing memory functioning. However, this disappointing situation may change in the future. If it does, a combination of pharmacological and psychological treatments is likely to enhance performance in everyday life. It is also possible that neural transplants in people with Huntington's disease may lead to better memory performance, although here again the recipients may need to be taught to use their memories to the best advantage by employing memory rehabilitation strategies.

In the immediate future advances are likely to be made in better design and implementation of external aids and better structuring of the environment, hence reducing the load on memory. Meanwhile, further development of the errorless learning technique described above, and perhaps other ways of improving learning, can be implemented to teach people to use their prosthetic memory more efficiently.

REFERENCES

Baddeley, A.D. (1999). *Essentials of Human Memory*. Hove: Psychology Press.

Baddeley, A.D. & Longman, D.J.A. (1978). The influence of length and frequency of training sessions on the rate of learning to type. *Ergonomics*, **21**, 627–635.

Baddeley, A.D. & Wilson, B.A. (1994). When implicit learning fails: amnesia and the problem of error elimination. *Neuropsychologia*, **32**, 53–68.

Barker, R.A. & Dunnett, S.B. (1999). *Neural Repair, Transplantation and Rehabilitation*. Hove: Psychology Press.

Ben-Yishay, Y. (ed.) (1978). *Working Approaches to Remediation of Cognitive Deficits in Brain-damaged Persons* (Rehabilitation Monograph). New York: New York University Medical Center.

Ben-Yishay, Y. (1996). Reflections on the evolution of the therapeutic milieu concept. *Neuropsychological Rehabilitation*, **6**, 327–343.

Berg, I.J., Koning-Haanstra, M. & Deelman, B.G. (1991). Long-term effects of memory rehabilitation: a controlled study. *Neuropsychological Rehabilitation*, **1**, 97–111.

Bergman, M.M. (1991). Computer-enhanced self sufficiency: Part 1. Creation and implementation of a text writer for an individual with traumatic brain injury. *Neuropsychology*, **5**, 17–24.

Broman, M., Rose, A.L., Hotson, G. & Casey, C.M. (1997). Severe anterograde amnesia with onset in childhood as a result of anoxic encephalopathy. *Brain*, **120**, 417–433.

Brooks, D.N. (1984). *Closed Head Injury: Psychological, Social and Family Consequences*. Oxford: Oxford University Press.

Brooks, B.M., McNeil, J.E., Rose, D.F. et al. (1999). Route learning in a case of amnesia: a preliminary investigation into the efficacy of training in a virtual environment. *Neuropsychological Rehabilitation*, **9**, 63–76.

Brooks, D.N. & Baddeley, A.D. (1976). What can amnesic patients learn? *Neuropsychologia*, **14**, 111–122.

Brooks, D.N., Campsie, L. & Symington, C. (1987). The effects of severe head injury upon patient and relative within seven years of injury. *Journal of Head Injury Trauma Rehabilitation*, **2**, 1–13.

Camp, C.J. (1989). Facilitation of new learning in Alzheimer's disease. In G. Gilmore, P. Whitehouse & M. Wykle (eds), *Memory and Aging: Theory, Research and Practice* (pp. 212–225). New York: Springer.

Clare, L. & Wilson, B.A. (1997). *Coping with Memory Problems: A Practical Guide for People with Memory Impairments, Relatives, Friends and Carers*. Bury St Edmunds: Thames Valley Test Company.

Clare, L., Wilson, B.A., Breen, E.K. & Hodges, J.R. (1999). Errorless learning of face-name associations in early Alzheimer's disease. *Neurocase*, **5**, 37–46.

Clare, L., Wilson, B.A., Carter, G. et al. (2000). Intervening with everyday memory problems in dementia of Alzheimer type: an errorless learning approach. *Journal of Clinical and Experimental Neuropsychology*, **22**, 132–146.

Cullen, C.N. (1976). Errorless learning with the retarded. *Nursing Times*, 25 March.

Dalgleish, T. & Cox, S.G. (2002). Memory and emotional disorder. In A.D. Baddeley, M.D. Kopelman & B.A. Wilson (eds), *Handbook of Memory Disorders*, 2nd edn (pp. 437–450). Chichester: Wiley.

Diller, L.L. (1976). A model for cognitive retraining in rehabilitation. *Clinical Psychologist*, **29**, 13–15.

Donaghy, S. & Williams, W. (1998). A new protocol for training severely impaired patients in the usage of memory journals. *Brain Injury*, **12**, 1061–1076.

Eriksson, P.S., Perfilieva, E., Bjork-Eriksson, T. et al. (1998). Neurogenesis in the adult human hippocampus. *Nature Medicine*, **4**, 1313–1317.

Evans, J.J., Emslie, H. & Wilson, B.A. (1998). External cueing systems in the rehabilitation of executive impairments of action. *Journal of the International Neuropsychological Society*, **4**, 399–408.

Evans, J.J. & Wilson, B.A. (1992). A memory group for individuals with brain injury. *Clinical Rehabilitation*, **6**, 75–81.

Evans, J.J., Wilson, B.A., Needham, P. & Brentnall, S. (2003). Who makes good use of memory-aids: results of a survey of 100 people with acquired brain injury. *Journal of the International Neuropsychological Society*, **9**, 925–935.

Finger, S. & Stein, D.G. (1982). *Brain Damage and Recovery: Research and Clinical Perspectives*. New York: Academic Press.

Freed, D.M., Corkin, S. & Cohen, N.J. (1998). Forgetting in H.M.: a second look. *Neuropsychologia*, **25**, 461–471.

Funnell, E. & De Mornay Davies, P. (1996). JBR: a reassessment of concept familiarity and a category-specific disorder for living things. *Neurocase*, **2**, 461–474.

Gianutsos, R. (1980). What is cognitive rehabilitation? *Journal of Rehabilitation*, **1**, 37–40.

Glisky, E.L. (1995). Computers in memory rehabilitation. In A.D. Baddeley, B.A. Wilson & F.N. Watts (eds), *Handbook of Memory Disorders*, 1st edn (pp. 557–575). Chichester: Wiley.

Glisky, E.L. & Schacter, D.L. (1986). Long-term retention of computer learning by patients with memory disorders. *Neuropsychologia*, **26**, 173–178.

Glisky, E.L. & Schacter, D.L. (1987). Acquisition of domain-specific knowledge in organic amnesia: training for computer-related work. *Neuropsychologia*, **25**, 893–906.

Glisky, E.L. & Schacter, D.L. (1989). Extending the limits of complex learning in organic amnesia: computer training in a vocational domain. *Neuropsychologia*, **27**, 107–120.

Glisky, E.L., Schacter, D.L. & Tulving, E. (1986). Computer learning by memory impaired patients: acquisition and retention of complex knowledge. *Neuropsychologia*, **24**, 313–328.

Godden, D. & Baddeley, A.D. (1975). Context-dependent memory in two natural environments: on land and under water. *British Journal of Psychology*, **66**, 325–331.

Gouvier, W.D. (1982). Using the digital alarm chronograph in memory retraining. *Behavioral Engineering*, **7**, 134.

Graf, P. & Schacter, D.L. (1985). Implicit and explicit memory for new associations in normal and amnesic subjects. *Journal of Experimental Psychology: Learning, Memory, and Cognition*, **11**, 501–518.

Harris, J.E. (1980). We have ways of helping you remember. *Concord: The Journal of the British Association of Service to the Elderly*, **17**, 21–27.

Hersh, N. & Treadgold, L. (1994). NeuroPage: the rehabilitation of memory dysfunction by prosthetic memory and cueing. *NeuroRehabilitation*, **4**, 187–197.

Hunkin, M.M., Squires, E.J., Parkin, A.J. & Tidy, J.A. (1998). Are the benefits of errorless learning dependent on implicit memory? *Neuropsychologia*, **36**, 25–36.

Jennett, B. & Bond, M. (1975). Assessment of outcome after severe brain injury. *Lancet*, **1**, 480–484.

Jones, R.S.P. & Eayrs, C.B. (1992). The use of errorless learning procedures in teaching people with a learning disability. *Mental Handicap Research*, **5**, 304–312.

Kapur, N. (1995). Memory aids in the rehabilitation of memory disordered patients. In A.D. Baddeley, B.A. Wilson & F.N. Watts (eds), *Handbook of Memory Disorders*, 1st edn (pp. 533–556). Chichester: Wiley.

Kapur, N. & Graham, K.S. (2002). Recovery of memory function in neurological disease. In A.D. Baddeley, M.D. Kopelman & B.A. Wilson (eds), *Handbook of Memory Disorders*, 2nd edn (pp. 233–248). Chichester: Wiley.

Kim, H.J., Burke, D.T., Dowds, M.M. & George, J. (1999). Utility of a microcomputer as an external memory aid for a memory-impaired head injury patient during inpatient rehabilitation. *Brain Injury*, **13**, 147–150.

Kime, S.K., Lamb, D.G. & Wilson, B.A. (1996). Use of a comprehensive program of external cuing to enhance procedural memory in a patient with dense amnesia. *Brain Injury*, **10**, 17–25.

Kirsch, N.L., Levine, S.P., Fallon-Krueger, M. & Jaros, L.A. (1987). The microcomputer as an "orthotic" device for patients with cognitive deficits. *Journal of Head Trauma Rehabilitation*, **2**, 77–86.

Kirsch, N.L., Levine, S.P., Lajiness O'Neill, L. & Schnyder, M. (1992). Computer assisted interactive task guidance: facilitating the performance of a simulated vocational task. *Journal of Head Trauma Rehabilitation*, **7**, 13–25.

Kolb, B. (1995). *Brain Plasticity and Behavior*. Mahwah, NJ: Erlbaum.

Kopelman, M. & Crawford, S. (1996). Not all memory clinics are dementia clinics. *Neuropsychological Rehabilitation*, **6**, 187–202.

Landauer, T.K. & Bjork, R.A. (1978). Optimum rehearsal patterns and name learning. In M.M. Gruneberg, P.E. Morris & R.N. Sykes (eds), *Practical Aspects of Memory* (pp. 625–632). London: Academic Press.

Lawson, M.J. & Rice, D.N. (1989). Effects of training in use of executive strategies on a verbal memory problem resulting from closed head injury. *Journal of Clinical and Experimental Neuropsychology*, **11**, 842–854.

Levine, B., Robertson, I.H., Clare, L. et al. (2000). Rehabilitation of executive functioning: an experimental–clinical validation of Goal Management Training. *Journal of the International Neuropsychological Society*, **6**, 299–312.

Lezak, M.D. (1979). Recovery of memory and learning functions following traumatic brain injury. *Cortex*, **15**, 63–72.

Lincoln, N.B. (1989). Management of memory problems in a hospital setting. In L.W. Poon, D.C. Rubin & B.A. Wilson (eds), *Everyday Cognition in Adulthood and Late Life* (pp. 639–658). Cambridge: Cambridge University Press.

Lorge, I. (1930). *Influence of Regularly Interpolated Time Intervals upon Subsequent Learning*. Quoted in H.H. Johnson & R.L. Solso (1971) *An Introduction to Experimental Design in Psychology: A Case Approach*. New York: Harper & Row.

Luria, A.R. (1963). *Restoration of Function after Brain Injury*. New York: Pergamon.

Marshall, J.F. (1985). Neural plasticity and recovery of function after brain injury. *International Review of Neurobiology*, **26**, 201–247.

McKitrick, L.A. & Camp, C.J. (1993). Relearning the names of things: the spaced-retrieval intervention implemented by a caregiver. *Clinical Gerontologist*, **14**, 60–62.

Milders, M.V., Berg, I.J. & Deelman, B.G. (1995). Four-year follow-up of a controlled memory training study in closed head injured patients. *Neuropsychological Rehabilitation*, **5**, 223–238.

Moffat, N. (1989). Home-based cognitive rehabilitation with the elderly. In L.W. Poon, D.C. Rubin & B.A. Wilson (eds), *Everyday Cognition in Adulthood and Late Life* (pp. 659–680). Cambridge: Cambridge University Press.

Murphy, G. & Oliver, C. (1987). Decreasing undesirable behaviour. In W. Yule & J. Carr (eds), *Behaviour Modification for People with Mental Handicaps* (pp. 102–142). London: Croom Helm.

Oddy, M. (1984). Head injury and social adjustment. In D.N. Brooks (ed.), *Closed Head Injury: Psychological, Social and Family Consequences*. Oxford: Oxford University Press.

Ownsworth, T.L. & McFarland, K. (1999). Memory remediation in long-term acquired brain injury: two approaches in diary training. *Brain Injury*, **13**, 605–626.

Prigatano, G. (1999). *Principles of Neuropsychological Rehabilitation*. New York: Oxford University Press.

Prigatano, G.P. (1987). Recovery and cognitive retraining after craniocerebral trauma. *Journal of Learning Disabilities*, **20**, 603–613.

Rizzo, A.A., Buckwalter, J.G. & Neumann, U. (1997). Virtual reality and cognitive rehabilitation: a brief review of the future. *Journal of Head Trauma Rehabilitation*, **12**, 1–15.

Rose, F.D., Attree, E.A. & Johnson, D.A. (1996). Virtual reality: an assistive technology in neurological rehabilitation. *Current Opinion in Neurology*, **9**, 461–467.

Schacter, D.L., Rich, S.A. & Stampp, M.S. (1985). Remediation of memory disorders: experimental evaluation of the spaced-retrieval technique. *Journal of Clinical and Experimental Neuropsychology*, **7**, 79–96.

Schuri, U., Wilson, B.A. & Hodges, J. (1996). Memory disorders. In T. Brandt, L.R. Caplan, J. Dichgans et al. (eds), *Neurological Disorders: Course and Treatment* (pp. 223–230). San Diego, CA: Academic Press.

Scoville, W.B. & Milner, B. (1957). Loss of recent memory after bilateral hippocampal lesions. *Journal of Neurology, Neurosurgery, and Psychiatry*, **20**, 11–21.

Sidman, M. & Stoddard, L.T. (1967). The effectiveness of fading in programming simultaneous form discrimination for retarded children. *Journal of Experimental Analysis of Behavior*, **10**, 3–15.

Sohlberg, M.M. & Mateer, C. (1989). Training use of compensatory memory books: a three-stage behavioural approach. *Journal of Clinical and Experimental Neuropsychology*, **11**, 871–891.

Squires, E.J., Aldrich, F.K., Parkin, A.J. & Hunkin, N.M. (1998). Errorless learning and the acquisition of word processing skills. *Neuropsychological Rehabilitation*, **8**, 433–449.

Squires, E.J., Hunkin, N.M. & Parkin, A.J. (1996). Memory notebook training in a case of severe amnesia: generalising from paired associate learning to real life. *Neuropsychological Rehabilitation*, **6**, 55–65.

Squires, E.J., Hunkin, N.M. & Parkin, A.J. (1997). Errorless learning of novel associations in amnesia. *Neuropsychologia*, **35**, 1103–1111.

Stilwell, P., Stilwell, J., Hawley, C. & Davies, C. (1999). The National Traumatic Brain Injury Study: assessing outcomes across settings. *Neuropsychological Rehabilitation*, **9**, 277–293.

Terrace, H.S. (1963). Discrimination learning with and without "errors". *Journal of Experimental Analysis of Behavior*, **6**, 1–27.

Terrace, H.S. (1966). Stimulus control. In W.K. Honig (ed.), *Operant Behavior: Areas of Research and Application* (pp. 271–344). New York: Appleton-Century-Crofts.

Tulving, E. & Schacter, D.L. (1990). Priming and human memory systems. *Science*, **247**, 301–306.

Vargha-Khadem, F., Gadian, D.G., Watkins, K.E. et al. (1997). Differential effects of early hippocampal pathology on episodic and semantic memory. *Science*, **277**, 376–380.

Victor, M., Adams, R.D. & Collins, G.H. (1989). *The Wernicke–Korsakoff Syndrome and Related Neurological Disorders Due to Alcoholism and Malnutrition*, 2nd edn. Philadelphia, PA: F.A. Davis.

von Cramon, D.Y. & Matthes-von Cramon, G. (1992). Reflections on the treatment of brain injured patients suffering from problem-solving disorders. *Neuropsychological Rehabilitation*, **2**, 207–230.

Walsh, B.F. & Lamberts, F. (1979). Errorless discrimination and fading as techniques for teaching sight words to TMR students. *American Journal of Mental Deficiency*, **83**, 473–479.

Watkins, M.J., Ho, E. & Tulving, E. (1976). Context effects in recognition memory for faces. *Journal of Verbal Learning and Verbal Behavior*, **15**, 505–517.

Wearing, D. (1992). Self-help groups. In B.A. Wilson & N. Moffat (eds), *Clinical Management of Memory Problems*, 2nd edn (pp. 271–301). London: Chapman & Hall.

West, R.L. (1995). Compensatory strategies for age-associated memory impairment. In A.D. Baddeley, B.A. Wilson & F.N. Watts (eds), *Handbook of Memory Disorders*, 1st edn (pp. 481–500). Chichester: Wiley.

Wilson, B.A. (1987a). *Rehabilitation of Memory*. New York: Guilford.

Wilson, B.A. (1987b). Single-case experimental designs in neuropsychological rehabilitation. *Journal of Clinical and Experimental Neuropsychology*, **9**, 527–544.

Wilson, B.A. (1989). Models of cognitive rehabilitation. In R.L. Wood & P. Eames (eds), *Models of Brain Injury Rehabilitation* (pp. 117–141). London: Chapman & Hall.

Wilson, B.A. (1991). Long-term prognosis of patients with severe memory disorders. *Neuropsychological Rehabilitation*, **1**, 117–134.

Wilson, B.A. (1992). Memory therapy in practice. In B.A. Wilson & N. Moffat (eds), *Clinical Management of Memory Problems*, 2nd edn (pp. 120–153). London: Chapman & Hall.

Wilson, B.A. (1997). Cognitive rehabilitation: how it is and how it might be. *Journal of the International Neuropsychological Society*, **3**, 487–496.

Wilson, B.A. (1998). Recovery of cognitive functions following non-progressive brain injury. *Current Opinion in Neurobiology*, **8**, 281–287.

Wilson, B.A. (1999). *Case Studies in Neuropsychological Rehabilitation*. New York: Oxford University Press.

Wilson, B.A. & Baddeley, A.D. (1993). Spontaneous recovery of digit span: does comprehension recover? *Cortex*, **29**, 153–159.

Wilson, B.A., Baddeley, A.D., Evans, J.J. & Shiel, A. (1994). Errorless learning in the rehabilitation of memory impaired people. *Neuropsychological Rehabilitation*, **4**, 307–326.

Wilson, B.A., Baddeley, A.D. & Kapur, N. (1995). Dense amnesia in a professional musician following Herpes Simplex Virus encephalitis. *Journal of Clinical and Experimental Psychology*, **17**, 668–681.

Wilson, B.A., J.C. & Hughes, E. (1997a). Coping with amnesia: the natural history of a compensatory memory system. *Neuropsychological Rehabilitation*, **7**, 43–56.

Wilson, B.A., Emslie, H., Quirk, K. & Evans, J. (1999a). George: learning to live independently with NeuroPage®. *Rehabilitation Psychology*, **44**, 284–296.

Wilson, B.A. Emslie, H.C., Quirk, K. & Evans, J.J. (2001). Reducing everyday memory and planning problems by means of a paging system: a randomised control crossover study. *Journal of Neurology, Neurosurgery, and Psychiatry*, **70**, 477–482.

Wilson, B.A. & Evans, J. (2002). Does cognitive rehabilitation work? Clinical and economic considerations and outcomes. In G. Prigatano (ed.), *Clinical Neuropsychology and Cost–Outcome Research: An Introduction*. Hove: Psychology Press.

Wilson, B.A. & Evans, J.J. (1996). Error-free learning in the rehabilitation of individuals with memory impairments. *Journal of Head Trauma Rehabilitation*, **11**, 54–64.

Wilson, B.A. Evans, J., Brentnall, S. et al. (2000). The Oliver Zangwill Centre for Neuropsychological Rehabilitation: a partnership between health care and rehabilitation research. In A.-L. Christensen & B.P. Uzzell (eds), *International Handbook of Neuropsychological Rehabilitation* (pp. 231–246). New York: Kluwer Academic/Plenum.

Wilson, B.A., Evans, J.J., Emslie, H. et al. (1999b). Measuring recovery from post traumatic amnesia. *Brain Injury*, **13**, 505–520.

Wilson, B.A., Evans, J.J., Emslie, H. & Malinek, V. (1997b). Evaluation of NeuroPage: a new memory aid. *Journal of Neurology, Neurosurgery, and Psychiatry*, **63**, 113–115.

Wilson, B.A. & Moffat, N. (1992). The development of group memory therapy. In B.A. Wilson & N. Moffat (eds), *Clinical Management of Memory Problems*, 2nd edn (pp. 243–273). London: Chapman & Hall.

Wilson, B.A. & Watson, P.C. (1996). A practical framework for understanding compensatory behaviour in people with organic memory impairment. *Memory*, **4**, 465–486.

Wilson, B.A., Watson, P.C., Baddeley, A.D. et al. (2000). Improvement or simply practice? The effects of twenty repeated assessments on people with and without brain injury. *Journal of the International Neuropsychological Society*, **6**, 469–479.

Wright, P., Bartram, C., Rogers, N. et al. (2000). Text entry on handheld computers by older users. *Ergonomics*, **43**, 702–716.

Wright, P., Rogers, N., Bartram, C. et al. (2001). Comparison of pocket-computer aids for people with brain injury. *Brain Injury*.

Zangwill, O.L. (1947). Psychological aspects of rehabilitation in cases of brain injury. *British Journal of Psychology*, **37**, 60–69.

Zarkowska, E. (1987). Discrimination and generalisation. In W. Yule & J. Carr (eds), *Behaviour Modification for People with Mental Handicaps* (pp. 79–94). London: Croom Helm.

Zencius, A., Wesolowski, M.D., Krankowski, T. & Burke, W.H. (1991). Memory notebook training with traumatically brain-injured clients. *Brain Injury*, **5**, 321–325.

CHAPTER 11

Assessment and Management of Memory Problems in Children

Judith A. Middleton
Radcliffe Infirmary, Oxford, UK

The assessment of memory and learning in children has changed considerably in the last 15 years or so since more reliable and valid tests of children's memory, which have been well standardized on large numbers of children, have become available. Previous to that, scaled-down versions of adult assessments were often the only available measures, or tests specifically constructed for research purposes, both of which were often unsuitable for use with a clinical population of children. With the advent of new assessment batteries, it is now possible to look at children's memory development and disorders more appropriately. Whether the aim of assessment is to: (a) research into the nature of brain–behaviour links; (b) describe the nature of the impairment; (c) contribute to diagnosis and decisions about treatment; (d) monitor change over time; or (e) plan rehabilitation, it is vital that tests should fulfil the strict standard criteria in order to make them appropriate and meaningful.

ISSUES OF NEUROPSYCHOLOGICAL ASSESSMENT OF MEMORY IN CHILDREN

The basis of a good clinical neuropsychological assessment of memory should be based on six lines of enquiry:

1. Where known, the underlying neuropathology.
2. The child's age, developmental level and cultural background.
3. General level of cognitive functioning and co-morbid difficulties.
4. Functional information gleaned from careful clinical interviewing.
5. Observations of how children complete (or fail) memory and learning tasks, and perform generally.
6. The results of psychometric tests.

The Essential *Handbook of Memory Disorders for Clinicians.* Edited by A.D. Baddeley, M.D. Kopelman and B.A. Wilson.
© 2004 John Wiley & Sons, Ltd. ISBN 0-470-09141-X.

Major errors can occur when inferences and conclusions are drawn from only the first and last sources of information in isolation. In other words, wrong assumptions can be made about direct brain–behaviour links when the child's age and development, cultural context, clinical history and careful observations of how they go about performing tasks are omitted in forming hypotheses.

A second important point to remember is that young children rarely complain of memory problems themselves if the problem is acquired in infancy, unlike older children (and adults) who have an acquired memory problem, or adults who may know that their memory is not what it used to be. While normal children will be able to discuss memory from a young age (for further discussion, see Joyner & Kurtz-Costes, 1997) their metamemory or understanding that they have memory, that they are able to forget and that they are able to know that they have forgotten what they have known at one time, does not develop until later childhood. Indeed, even older children whose memory may have been poor for a number of years may not know that they have a problem, never having been consciously aware that they did not have a fully functioning memory.

Generally it is parents or teachers who first raise concerns about problems of memory in children. Here again, it may be that it is not a child's poor memory that is described, but that they are failing to learn and make progress that is the presenting problem. This is again a major difference with adults, who will have had the experience of a normal memory for many years. Even if they have lost insight into their problem, their family and associates will notice a loss or difference in them which gives rise to concern. With young children there may be little against which to compare their present memory capacity or processing, so there may not be a sense of loss of memory function, but rather a failure to make progress as expected over time. In older children the loss of memory may be a presenting problem, depending on the aetiology.

CAUSES OF MEMORY PROBLEMS

Neuropathology

Damage to the temporal lobes, hippocampus, amygdala, mammillary bodies, thalamus and frontal lobes, those parts of the brain mostly commonly associated with memory problems, may broadly arise from necrosis, injury, inflammation (meningitis and encephalitis), atrophy (following febrile convulsions in childhood), oedema, cerebral haemorrhage, tumours (whether malignant or benign), calcification (e.g after radiotherapy for central nervous system [CNS] involvement in leukaemia), other treatment (surgery or medication), disease (epilepsy) or displacement (i.e. following tumours, bleeds or infection elsewhere in the brain causing midline shift) (for further discussion of this see Tranel & Damasio, 2002). In addition, there may be developmental disorders where the brain is malformed and consequently memory and learning are compromised. However, a number of case histories highlight that children may present with specific memory problems in the absence of any definite neuropathology (Casalini et al., 1999; Temple, 1997).

Psychological

There are also some instances where there may be no documented neuropathology, but children still have reported problems in learning and memory in general, but with less specificity than in the above cases. As part of a good clinical assessment, it is important to consider whether there may be psychological causes. Children who are anxious and depressed may be preoccupied with their own concerns and present with complaints about their distractedness, failure to learn and frequent forgetting, both at home and in school. Careful clinical interviews of the child and family are needed to exclude such issues. Lack of motivation and cooperation in the assessment may also be the cause of test failure. There is also evidence that children with post-traumatic stress disorder (PTSD) may also present with memory problems (Canterbury & Yule, 1997), and it is therefore crucial, when a child has had a head injury, that both psychological and neuropathological causes are considered.

AGE, DEVELOPMENTAL LEVEL AND AGE AT LOSS

Irrespective of whether we are assessing memory and learning in children for clinical or research purposes, it is important that there is an appreciation that the model most commonly assumed for adults may be inappropriate when applying it to children, or at least to very young children. As the chapter on the development of memory will have illustrated (Chapter 5, this volume), infants are not born with a fully developed memory system or memory capacity, and will not have the same complexity for encoding, storing and retrieving information at birth that is present in adults. In addition, the means that we have to assess memory in preverbal children and in children with developing but immature language systems is consequently compromised and different paradigms need to be employed. Importantly, children are maturing very rapidly, so assessments at any one age have to be specific to the child's developmental level. Comparisons between assessments at different ages may give unexpected results if their memory capacity, speed of processing and age-appropriate strategies are not understood.

In addition, the age of acquisition of memory loss is crucial in understanding children's memory problems. Younger children are more vulnerable than older children, however the injury is acquired (e.g. head injuries, Levin et al., 1995; or central nervous system radiation, Said et al., 1989).

Fletcher & Taylor (1984) propose a developmental model of assessment whereby the starting point is exploration of the presenting or manifest behaviour, rather than the neuropathology. They argue that brain–behaviour links based on adult models can be misleading, as children are rapidly developing and may use different strategies to adults to carry out tasks. They support a model in which assessment of the specific processing difficulties is based on the manifest problems within a wider assessment of ability. This precedes making a possible link to the known or suspected neuropathology.

CO-MORBID PROBLEMS

It is particularly important in children to ensure that an apparent memory problem is not the result of other physical and/or cognitive problems about which the child may not be able to articulate. Visual and hearing problems are obvious areas to exclude. Delayed language development will mean that test instructions and test content may not be understood, even in nonverbal memory tests. Failure to focus attention on test materials, distractibility and short attention span may also result in deviant memory test scores. As Lezak (1995) points out (p. 429), problems that appear to be related to poor memory may be more to do with difficulties in attention or mental tracking. Perceptual organization problems may be the root difficulty for children with a poor visuospatial memory. If children are only able to process information slowly, then failure on some memory tests where information is presented rapidly, or where there is a set time for them to respond, may be related to this rather than to a memory problem *per se*, although functionally the problem emerges as a difficulty with learning.

Children's general level of cognitive functioning will also impact on their performance in memory tasks. This is especially so in younger children, where memory is more closely correlated to intelligence than in older children (Cohen, 1997). It is not unknown clinically for children with memory problems to be referred for assessment, who, when tested comprehensively, are found to be functioning at the bottom of the normal range on standard assessments of cognitive development and academic achievement, although teachers have reported that the child is functioning reasonably in school. Consequently, any assessment of memory problems needs to start with a formal assessment of general cognitive functioning.

ETHNIC AND CULTURAL CONTEXT

Mistry (1998) has discussed the issue that the development of remembering will be influenced by children's cultural environment. For a start, many assessments have been standardized on USA populations, matching the census data for ethnicity. However, it is worthwhile remembering that when used in the UK there are different minority ethnic groups compared to the USA populations, which may make the assessment batteries less relevant for these children, with the content and process being less familiar to some groups than others. More importantly, Mistry (1998) points out that different cultural backgrounds will place different emphasis on the practice of remembering (p. 364). Children who have been to schools where memory and organizational strategies have been integrated into normal classroom instruction may be at an advantage in assessments compared to those who have not (see Bjorklund & Douglas, 1998). Finally, in some cultures, rote learning of special texts (e.g. the Koran in Muslim cultures) may mean that children from these backgrounds have a specific strength in those tasks where rote learning is crucial. Of course, poor rote learning in these children may have profound cultural implications.

CLINICAL INTERVIEW

A great deal can be learnt from the clinical interview in forming initial hypotheses about the cause and nature of memory problems. A clinical finding has been that some referrals may speak of children losing skills, in other words failing to retain information that they had learnt and been able to retrieve before. If there is known neuropathology (such as localized damage from a cerebral haemorrhage, focal head injury or tumour) this can occur, but in some conditions (such as generalized seizures or diffuse closed head injury) it is often that parents and schools are concerned that the gap between their child and his/her peers is widening, either from a slower or uneven acquisition of knowledge or of a failure to learn at all. Of course, virtually every child will develop to some degree, and those with memory problems still learn to carry out many activities of everyday life and form relationships with their families, all based on implicit procedural learning, frequent repetition and multisensory input. Sometimes their difficulties seem to be related to, or at least may first emerge as, problems relating to explicit memory and learning. In other words they may have difficulties in acquiring skills and knowledge that need to be specifically taught, such as reading, writing and mathematics. Studies by Vargha-Khadem et al. (1997) and Broman et al. (1997) have also described cases of children with specific and profound episodic memory problems arising from bilateral hippocampal pathology, where children attended mainstream school and attained low to low-average levels of functioning in speech and language, literacy and factual knowledge, suggesting that episodic and semantic memory are partly dissociable.

It is critical in all neuropsychological assessments of children to carry out a full clinical and developmental interview with parents, even when there is documented evidence of neuropathology, which could directly explain problems in learning and memory. In acquired problems, premorbid cognitive functioning and behaviour may indicate cognitive style and earlier difficulties which could interact with, and directly affect how to manage, the presenting memory and learning problems. In addition, information about the family history may show that there are specific or general learning difficulties implicating slow learning in other family members, which can give a fuller picture of the child's problem. More specifically, clinical assessment of the problem should include the child's perspective to the extent that he/she can explain what he/she feels is wrong, as well as the perspective of both parents if at all possible. However, younger children tend to overestimate their memory skills and may not see that there is a problem. Older children with frontal damage may lack insight and accurate monitoring of their difficulties. There may be occasions when parents have very differing views as to the aetiology of any difficulties, or when one parent does not acknowledge that there is a problem. While this may not directly affect the assessment procedure and the analysis of the problem, parental disagreement can have major implications for management and rehabilitation.

Areas to consider include: (a) capacity (how much can be remembered); (b) content (verbal/visual: concrete/abstract): (c) type (declarative/procedural, episodic/semantic); (d) speed of acquisition; (e) rate of loss of information after a delay; and (f) process (storage, encoding or retrieval). Useful clinical questions should consider whether children can:

- Remember requests to carry out activities in the future.
- Remember and execute a number of instructions at any one time.
- Be sent shopping, with or without a shopping list (at an appropriate age).
- Remember if they have homework and, if so, what it consists of.
- Remember to take their homework back to school once completed.
- Find their clothes and possessions around the house
- Keep track of their equipment, coat, etc. at school.
- Know the way to school.
- Know their way round the block to neighbours.
- Remember rules in games.

- Remember which team they are on when they play team games.
- Remember arrangements to meet friends after school.
- Remember to pass on information between home and school in connection with meetings, school outings, etc.
- Remember secrets and that secrets are secret.
- Get into trouble at school or home for telling fanciful stories, where fiction is embroidered onto a semblance of the truth.
- Relate what has been happening at school, or to talk with peers or teachers about specific home activities after the weekend or holidays.
- Improve their memory if information is given more slowly, in a simplified form, or if it is repeated.
- Remember something they have been told for an hour, a day, a week.

These questions are not exclusive but serve to illustrate the scope of what needs to be covered in relation to general everyday activities (for further examples, see Ylvisaker & Gioia, 1998, pp. 165–167).

Beyond this, information gathering should become more specific about school performance on different subjects and about a range of functional school activities. Consequently, it is important to include the opinion of teachers within the assessment. Questions that can be illuminating relate to the subjects or areas where there are particular problems, whether there have been any previous attempts to help a child through organizing work, prompting, or cuing a child who has been slow to learn or cannot remember from one day to the next what has been taught. Parents and teachers may complain that, for instance, specific spellings can be repeatedly taught and retained for a week but will be forgotten by the end of the following week, when new material has been learnt. In addition, it is possible that some teaching styles may include organizational strategies or a study skill component which may have been helpful to children (Bjorklund & Douglas, 1998), so classroom observations can be illuminating.

ASSESSMENT VARIABLES

The assessment of memory in children crucially needs to take into account three major sets of variables:

1. *Test variables*, including test selection, standardization, suitability of the test for the population and suitability of the test to answer a specific question for the child.
2. *Testing variables*, i.e. rate of presentation, mode of presentation, mode of response, response elicitation (i.e. cued, prompted or free recall or recognition). These include stimulus properties and characteristics, meaningfulness and familiarity to the child (see Figure 11.1).
3. *Situational and presentation variables*, such as distractions, quietnes and the structure of the assessment session.

Before going on to consider assessment of young children and adults, it is important to consider the assessment of infant memory.

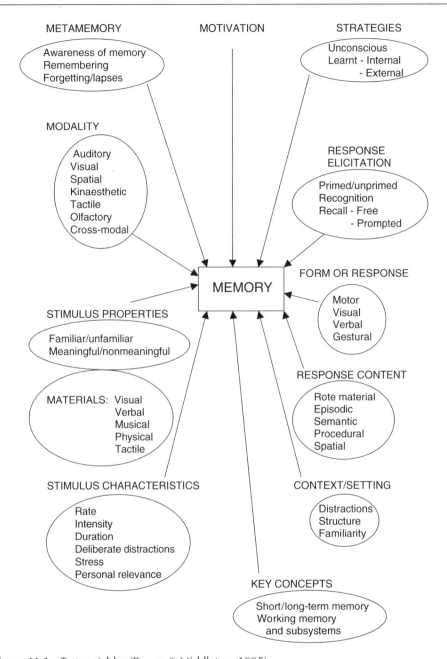

Figure 11.1   Test variables (Berger & Middleton, 1995)

ASSESSMENT OF INFANT MEMORY AND LEARNING

Memory and learning are innate capacities of the human brain. From the moment of birth, and before, infants are learning from and about the external world. It is, therefore possible to observe and assess memory and learning from the very earliest periods of an infant's life. Early in life, recognition is context-dependent because of infants' lack of speech. It is necessary to create a similar setting to allow an infant to recognize what he/she has experienced before. As infants grow older, the importance of language as a primary mediator in memory and learning will grow, and with this the development of a verbal memory system which begins to correspond to that of adults and which allows them to begin to hold semantic and abstract information in memory (Rovee-Collier & Gerhardstein, 1997; Temple, 1997).

Infant memory can be assessed through a number of different paradigms, such as paired-comparison, habituation, and classical and operant conditioning (for detailed discussion, see Rovee-Collier & Gerhardstein, 1997). For instance, Walton, Bower & Bower (1992) indicate that infants may show a visual preference for their mother within 12 hours of birth and certainly within a day (Bushnell, et al., 1983, in Blass, 1999). This implies very early recognition and learning. By 20 days they can learn to blink at an auditory signal to prevent a puff of air on their cornea (Little et al., 1984, in Rovee-Collier & Gerhardstein, 1997, p. 17). Within the first few weeks of life, infants will recognize the smell of their mother's breast milk and the sound of novel sounds. Using an operant kicking paradigm, they can be taught to operate a mobile at 3 months (Rovee-Collier et al., 1980). The development of casting and searching play indicates that children are beginning to obtain object permanency; and failure to achieve this and apparently miss their primary caregivers when they are absent at age-appropriate levels may be explored to see whether there is a failure to learn and retain information.

Clinical assessment using formal developmental measures can be used judiciously. For example, one or two items in the Bayley Scales of Infant Development (Bayley, 1993), such as comparing checkerboard patterns or hiding a small toy under one of two cups with the infant having to search for the toy after a set time limit can begin to be used to look at memory and learning formally. However, interpreting failure in these tasks as being indicative of problems with memory and learning needs to be done with caution.

ASSESSMENT OF OLDER CHILDREN AND ADOLESCENTS

Qualitative Assessment

Although observations cannot be standardized and should, therefore, be treated with some caution, watching how children go about completing memory and learning tasks and assessment in general, provides extremely important information about the kinds of problems they may have, and how weaknesses can be managed. In addition, it is combining this information with test results and the picture gathered from the clinical interview, that will make most sense of the data and inform how problems may be best managed.

As at all times, it is important to remember the child's age and developmental level when observing them complete tasks. Work by Hulme & Mackenzie (1992) has shown that the speed of processing of verbal material in tasks like word recall is linearly related to age, with more words being recalled with increased speech rate in 7-year-olds compared to 4-year-olds and 10-year-olds compared to 7-year-olds. Thus, children whose speed of processing is slow, both from observations during assessment and on speed of information processing tasks in the Wechsler Intelligence Scale for Children, 3rd edn (WISC-III; Wechsler, 1991) or British Ability Scales, 2nd edn (BAS-II; Elliott et al., 1983), are likely to do badly in memory tasks where information is presented quickly (see below for a discussion of the various specific demands on a range of tasks purportedly assessing similar abilities). Frequent requests for questions or instructions to be repeated (e.g. in Arithmetic in the WISC-III), or the need for children to check with the model every few seconds (e.g. in Coding, WISC-III) may, but not necessarily, mean that they cannot hold the image or words in their short-term memory for long.

Close clinical observations of children as they complete assessments, and asking them about how they have gone about tackling items, may also indicate whether they are automatically using strategies, whether the strategies are developmentally appropriate and how helpful they are to the child. Bjorklund et al. (1997) have discussed the utilization deficiencies in memory-training studies in normal children. The effectiveness of strategy use is not an all-or-nothing affair and strategy use is dependent on age, other (e.g. frontal) problems, level of general cognitive functioning, motivation, insight and self-monitoring the efficacy of the strategy. Not only is the complexity of the material a factor in what and how much children of different ages can recall, but also the strategies that they could use to help them remember emerge at different stages in their development (Bjorklund et al., 1997). This is important for management of memory problems and will be discussed below in more detail.

Test Selection

Issues of reliability and validity generally will not be discussed in detail here, but it is crucial to consider the psychometric properties of each test carefully. It is important that the assessments are sensitive to strengths and weaknesses in memory, as well as being sufficiently stable over time to pick up subtle changes. As with testing in general, but particularly with memory, repeated assessments will give rise to specific problems relating to practice effects. None of the major batteries (except the Rivermead Behavioural Memory Test) have more than one version, although there are shortened forms for younger children and some have different stories at different ages. With children in particular, it is crucial to bear in mind that they are rapidly developing in a way that adults are not. There should be improvement with time, so failure to develop better memory skills is an extremely important marker that there may be serious problems.

Assessments of General Cognitive Functioning

Hypotheses about a memory problem can be formed not only during clinical interview, but when completing a full assessment of general cognitive functioning. Using Kaufman's (1994) information-processing model in analysing the Wechsler Intelligence Scale for Children, 3rd edn (WISC-III), comparatively lower scores in Arithmetic and Digit Span may suggest short-term verbal memory problems, while lower Information and Vocabulary subtests may be indicative of poor semantic or long term verbal memory. Picture Completion in the performance Scale could be indicative of problems with long-term visual memory. Qualitative observations of both Coding and Symbol Search may indicate short-term visual memory difficulties if children are seen to refer to the test material repeatedly and do not seem to remember the codes/symbols easily. These can only be tentative hypotheses, as weaknesses in these subtests and in the strategies that children use may be due to factors other than memory problems. The corollary is that if children do well in these subtests, it does not mean they do not have real memory problems. Similar analyses can be made of specific subtests in the Wechsler Pre-school and Primary Scales of Intelligence, Revised (WPPSI-R; Wechsler, 1993) or the British Ability Scales, 2nd edn (BAS-2), where there are three short term visual memory tasks, which will be discussed later. The McCarthy Scales (McCarthy, 1972) have a memory index, which can be a useful starter in making hypotheses.

Specific Memory Batteries

There are a number of major test batteries for assessing memory, each with its own relative strengths and weaknesses. The selection of which assessment battery to use may be academic in many departments where there has been the purchase of a single memory battery only. It is, however, essential to look carefully at whatever assessments are used to ensure that they assess what they purport to assess; for example, so-called visual learning subtests in the Wide Range Assessment of Memory and Learning (WRAML; Sheslow & Adams, 1990) and in the Test of Memory and Learning (TOMAL; Reynolds & Bigler, 1994) are, in fact, spatial learning tasks. Children do not have to remember whether or not a pattern is present, but rather where it is placed on a matrix. Some tests are more explicit in describing the response modality, for example the BAS-2 has verbal and spatial recall of pictures of objects on a matrix.

What follows is, first, a description of some of the most frequently used assessment batteries in terms of their breadth and standardization, and a discussion of what their advantages or disadvantages may be. Second, there is an analysis of some of the major components of these batteries, showing that there may be very real differences in factors influencing performance by a child in tests that apparently assess the same function.

Children's Memory Scale (CMS) (Cohen, 1997)

This is becoming one of the most popular assessments to evaluate memory and learning in children aged 5–16 years in the UK. It was standardized on a stratified sample of 1000 children in the USA divided into 10 age bands. Of these 1000 children, 300 were also administered the WISC-III or WPPSI-R. Correlation's between the various CMS and WISC-III indices indicated that: (a) generally, memory and the WISC-III were strongly correlated; and (b) that intelligence has a "small-to-moderate impact" (p.117). on children's memory. The correlations between the WPPSI-R and CMS differed from these. Although the sample size was smaller and the stratification was different, the results did suggest that in younger children memory may be more closely linked to verbal abilities than in older children.

The CMS was also correlated with other ability scales, such as the Differential Ability Scales (DAS; Elliott, 1990); and with various achievement tests, including the Wechsler

Individual Achievement Test (WIAT; Wechsler, 1995). In addition correlations with a number of executive functioning tests were made, such as the Wisconsin Card Sorting Task (WCST; Heaton et al., 1993) and the Children's Category Test (CCT; Boll, 1993); with language assessments, for example the Clinical Evaluation of Language Fundamentals, 3rd edn (CELF-3; Semmel et al., 1995); and with other memory assessments, such as the WRAML, Wechsler Memory Scale, 3rd edn (WMS-III; Wechsler, 1997) and the California Verbal Learning Test—Children's Version (CVLT-C; Dean et al., 1994).

The general memory index of the CMS includes measures of verbal and visual memory (immediate and delayed). In addition, there are measures of attention and concentration, learning, and delayed verbal recognition. A disappointment is the use of word pairs as part of the core memory index rather than the word list, also included but as a supplementary subtest. However, generally this test is colourful and child-friendly, with good conversion tables so that actual memory scores can be compared with those predicted from the WISC-III and WPPSI-R.

Test of Memory and Learning (TOMAL)

The TOMAL was designed and standardized on a stratified sample of 1342 children and adolescents, and had extensive piloting based on the 1990/1992 US census demographic characteristics. There are a number of studies quoted in the manual, where it has been correlated with tests such as the Kaufman Assessment Battery for Children (K-ABC; Kaufman & Kaufman, 1984); the Wide Range Achievement Test—Revised (WRAT-R; Jastak & Wilkinson, 1993); the Californian Achievement Test (CAT) and the Wechsler Intelligence Scale for Children—Revised (WISC-R; Wechsler, 1974). It essentially consists of two scales each (verbal and nonverbal memory), with five subtests leading to a composite memory scale. Both a selective reminding word list and word pairs are included in the verbal scale. There is also a composite delayed memory index (made up of four subtests). Supplementary subtests include letters forward and backwards, digits backwards, and manual imitation. As well as the core indices, supplementary indices include sequential recall, free recall, associative recall, learning and attention/concentration. Although of relatively weak validity, they are useful in leading to more specific hypotheses.

This test battery is in the range 5–19.11 years, giving it the advantage over all other memory batteries of having the longest age span. However, because of its US standardization, some of the stories contain words that are less common to UK populations, and need small adaptations. This, of course, interferes to a mild extent with the standardization. Generally it is not a particularly child-friendly battery, with all visual material only being in black and white, which means that younger children in particular are less engaged by it.

Wide-Range Assessment of Memory and Learning (WRAML) (Sheslow & Adams, 1990)

The WRAML was one of the earlier batteries to be developed to look comprehensively at children's memory and learning. It was standardized on a stratified sample of 2363 children and young people in the USA and covers an age range of 5–16 years. Reliability in terms of internal consistency and stability appears good. It has been correlated against other measures of memory. These are the memory index from the McCarthy Scales of Children's Ability (MCSCA); the Wechsler Memory Scale—Revised (WMS-R; Wechsler, 1987) and the memory scale of the Stanford–Binet test 4th edn. In addition correlations with the WISC-R and the WRAT-R are also included, and, as predicted, the correlations are moderate.

The battery comprises three indices (verbal, visual and learning). Issues for the UK relate to the American English in two of the three stories, with Story C requiring quite extensive adaptations for English children. Strengths include the sound/symbol learning test, which clinical experience suggests is useful in looking at phoneme–grapheme problems in children with poor reading skills. Another is the "visual" learning subtest already discussed, which is a test of spatial rather than visual learning. However, its simple, bright designs and general format are extremely child-friendly and it is almost always enjoyed by children—a strength in any test. Sentence repetition and a visual span (finger location) are also included.

The WRAML's main failure, however, is its lack of a good measure of delayed memory, and it is best thought of as a battery of immediate memory and learning. The delayed scores are merely calculated by taking a delayed score from the immediate or the last of the learning trial scores. Scores are then compared to broad bands rather than more specific standardized scores. The major problem is that, for example, an immediate score of 10 in stories with a delayed score of 8 (resulting in a score of 2) would be seen as indicating a poorer delayed memory score compared to someone with an immediate and delayed memory score of 3 (score of 0). It is perhaps an indication of forgetting, but still a poor measure.

Rivermead Behavioural Memory Test for Children (5–10 Years) (RBMT-C) (Wilson et al., 1991)

The RBMT-C was developed out of the Rivermead Behavioural Memory Test (RBMT) (Wilson et al., 1985), which in itself can be used with children above the age of 11 years (Wilson et al., 1990). The standardization for the RBMT-C was undertaken in the UK, using a total of 335 children within the normal range of intelligence, and roughly split equally between boys and girls, from three urban, three suburban and three rural schools in the south of England. Scores are converted to standard profile scores, and fall within the normal, borderline or impaired ranges. The battery was correlated with subtests from the BAS and WISC-R. Intelligence and the RBMT-C only correlated in younger but not in older children.

The RBMT-C is made up of a number tasks, including story recall, recognition of faces and pictures, remembering someone's name, a route around a room, instructions to do something on hearing a cue and some orientation questions. Children who fail the RBMT-C will have substantial difficulties in memory in everyday life situations, but falling within the normal range does not exclude memory and learning problems in academic work.

A specific advantage of the RBMT-C (and RBMT) is that there are four parallel versions, which makes it the only one of the tests of children's memory to have this feature. Thus there is an opportunity to use this test serially to monitor early memory recovery in hospital after a head injury etc., or to assess a child at close and regular intervals. This is also one of the rare memory tests that has been standardized in the UK.

NEPSY: A Developmental Neuropsychological Assessment (NEPSY) (Korkman et al., 1998)

The NEPSY is a comprehensive neuropsychological assessment for children aged 3–12 years, and consists of core and expanded assessments, which includes a memory and learning domain. The battery was standardized in the USA using a stratified sample of 1000 cases in 10 age groups. As with the CMS, TOMAL and WRAML, the sample was matched to the US population census, taking into account sex, race/ethnicity, geographical region and parent education.

The test was correlated with the WPPSI-R, WISC-III and WIAT. In addition, correlations were carried out with the Benton Neuropsychological Tests (BNT), the Multilingual Aphasia Examination (MAE; Benton & Hamsher, 1989) and the CMS, with moderate to high correlations with the last of these.

The benefit of this memory and learning index is that it can be compared to the other domains or indices of the NEPSY, namely attention and executive functioning, language, sensorimotor functions and visuospatial processing. This is a distinct advantage compared to the other batteries, as such comparisons cannot be made on a similar sample. For children aged 3–4 years, only two core subtests are used in the memory domain, narrative recall and sentence repetition, with supplementary tests comparing free and cued recall. For the older group (5–12 years), subtests include memory for faces, and for names, narrative memory and sentence repetition. There are supplementary subtests for delayed scores for memory for faces and names, as well as list learning.

The pictures in facial memory subtests are printed in black and white, and pen and ink drawings are used for the memory of names, which can be less attractive to children. However, a major disadvantage in the NEPSY is that there is no delayed recall of the story.

Other Tests of Memory and Learning

Recall of Designs

- *Rey–Osterreith Complex Figure* (Osterreith, 1944; Rey, 1941). This can be used with children and the Meyers & Meyers (1995) version has good norms for children from the age of 4–16 years. With immediate recall, delayed recall and delayed recognition, it is an extremely useful test to look at children's ability to recall complex abstract visual material. Observations of the way children copy the figure can give clues as to why they may find recall difficult. Those that draw it piecemeal or first draw the outline, thus distorting the general figure, tend to have greater difficulty in recall than those who draw the main component parts. This may suggest that poor performance is due to weak organizational and planning skills as much as recall *per se*.
- *Benton Visual Retention Test* (Benton & Sivan, 1995). There are norms for children in this immediate recall test, which is simpler than the Rey and gives both error and accuracy scores.
- *BAS-2*. There are three explicit memory tests in the BAS-2. These are Visual Recognition, Recall of Designs and Recall of Pictures, and, unlike the above two tests, they have obviously been standardized on a stratified sample of British children. The Visual

Recognition test has black and white drawings of real objects in a single category (e.g. vehicles, chairs/stools or shells, etc.) which are exposed for 5 s. Children then have to identify them from a larger array. The advantage of this subtest is that the age range is wide (2.6–17.11 years) and it is relatively nonthreatening to younger or nervous children, as they merely have to respond by pointing. Recall of Designs is, in many ways, similar to the Benton. The extended age range is 5–17.11 years. Recall of pictures comprises a sheet with 20 coloured pictures of objects (e.g. hat, bird, clock, etc.), which is exposed for 40 s. Children then have 60 s to name as many pictures as they can recall. After this the sheet is exposed on two further occasions, but this time for only 20 s, and they have only 40 s in which to recall the pictures. The immediate score is the total number of pictures recalled on all three trials. After these three trials, children are given a grid and asked to place 20 cards with the pictures (in a specific order) on the grid in the same layout as the stimulus. There is a delay of 10–30 min when they are again asked to recall the pictures and then place the cards on the grid, as before. The advantage with these tests is that they are part of a general ability assessment against which to compare problems, but the failure to include story recall in the battery is a real weakness in terms of assessing memory. In addition, despite the learning trials in Picture Recall, there has been no standardization of the learning curve, which is a disappointment.

Test Variables—The Difficulty of Comparisons

A comprehensive assessment of memory in children should always include, at least, story recall and recall of designs, but most core batteries include facial recognition, spatial memory and word lists in some form or another. Where it is possible to make a choice, it is worthwhile considering the different specific test variables that could influence results. This is especially so when different tests have been used over time with a particular child, as what appears to be a change in memory functioning may in fact relate to specific test variables with regard to the stimulus, the timing, and to the way in which a response is elicited. Such differences are, of course, over and above differences in the standardization of the various assessment batteries. What follows is a breakdown of the five assessment batteries described, looking at these four components to highlight differences.

Story Recall

Each of the five assessment batteries includes story or narrative recall. The Oxford stories (Bearsdworth and Bishop, 1994) are also included as one of the early tests to be standardized on English children, and, like the RBMT-C, they have multiple versions. However, as a quick view of Table 11.1 will show, there is some variation between what is demanded of children in each of the six story tests. The amount children are required to recall varies from one to three stories. In the NEPSY there is no delayed recall, but in the CMS, WRAML and TOMAL there is a 30 min interval before delay. RBMT-C has an interval of 15–20 min and the Oxford stories 45 min.

It is often the qualitative way by which children recall stories that gives important clues as to how their memory deficit may affect them functionally, and which may, in some cases, hint at the underlying neuropathology. For instance, stories may be recalled generally, with

Table 11.1 Story recall

Test	Stories to recall (n)	Versions (Nos)	Versions (years)	Age range (years)	Delay to recall (min)	Prompts	Delayed version	Detail/ theme	Recognition
TOMAL	3	1–3	(5–8)	5–19	30	Name Story	Yes	D	No
		2–4	(9–11)						
		3–5	(12–19)						
CMS	2	1–2	(5–8)	5–16	30	Name Story	Yes	D/T	Yes
		3–4	(9–12)						
		5–6	(12–16)						
WRAML	2	1 & 2	(6–8)	6–16	30	Name Story	Yes	D	Yes
		2 & 3	(9–16)						
RBMT-C	1	4		4–10	15–20	Picture	Yes	D	Yes
NEPSY	1	1		3–12	N/A	Cues IM	No	D	Yes (IM)
Oxford	2	3		8–12	45	Name Story	No	D	Yes

TOMAL, Test of Memory and Learning; CMS, Children's Memory Scale; WRAML, Wide Range Assessment of Memory and Learning; RBMT-C, Rivermead Behavioural Memory Test—Children; NEPSY, A Developmental Neuropsychological Assessment; Oxford, Beardsworth and Bishop (1994).

children remembering the theme quite well but being unable to recollect exact details. Other children will recall the beginning and/or the end word-for-word, but will have failed to understand the story because they have been unable recall the middle section at all. This may lead to poor delayed recall. Furthermore, others will repeat small sections, or just say a few of the key words but in no specific order, in a way that does not hang together semantically. Only the CMS has a standardized measure of both the detailed and thematic recall. Depending on the age of the child, it can be reasonable to hypothesize that, if the impairment in recall is disorganized, it is affected by inefficient storage or retrieval strategies and thus may be affected by frontal pathology.

Aldrich & Wilson (1991) found that prompts with younger children (i.e. 5–7 year-old) affected recall considerably. Beardsworth & Bishop (1994) also reported that, although children may have difficulties in recalling stories, cues (the name of the story) enhanced recall, suggesting that this is often a retrieval rather than a storage problem. Beardsworth & Bishop (1994) go on to argue that cued recall is a better measure of delayed memory than free recall, and point out that failure to recall after a prompt may indicate a serious problem with memory.

The TOMAL does not have a recognition trial at all, but in the CMS and WRAML stories there is a recognition trial which is scored separately from delayed recall. The RBMT-C uniquely provides a picture while the story is being read, and this is used as a prompt in recall, while the others only name the story. In addition, there are differences in how delayed recall and recognition trials are scored. In the NEPSY, the immediate recall and recognition scores are combined in the core battery (although separated as supplementary scores) and in the RBMT-C the immediate and delayed recall combines free recall with the prompted scores. The way in which recognition questions are posed also differs, for example: in the CMS children are asked whether or not a statement about the story is true, in the WRAML they are given a forced choice, and in the NEPSY and RBMT-C Stories they are asked more open questions (e.g. "What was the name of the dog ?"). Beardsworth & Bishop (1994) raised the issue of how different types of retrieval cues might affect recall, and the question still seems to be unanswered. Temple (1997, p. 98) suggests that the position of questions in a question series may affect performance, which could be because there is either a better initial organization of the story structure or because there is more rapid decay of information.

Word Lists, Paired Words and Verbal Selective Reminding

List learning, etc., is the other major verbal component of most memory batteries. The advantage of word lists and selective reminding tasks compared to word pairs is that it is possible to see whether children begin to impose their own structure or strategy in recalling words. In the case of the Californian Verbal Learning Test—Children's Version (CVLT-C; Dean et al., 1994), it is also possible to see whether they make spontaneous use of given categories once these have been suggested to them in a learning trial. Failure to structure and use a strategy to help recall, and instead randomly recall words in any order over trials, may suggest a frontal component contributing to a memory problem. The CVLT-C allows for comparison both serial-order and semantic strategies, but this can be considered in any list-learning task.

It is interesting to see how each of the five measures listed in Table 11.2 shows that no two have exactly the same parameters. The RBMT-C does not have a list-learning component. The WRAML has word lists with a recognition trial, the CMS and CVLT-C have interference tasks in the form of a List B but the WRAML and TOMAL do not. Word pairs in the CMS and TOMAL have three or four trials respectively, but in the former lists are longer for both the younger and older children, and the latter does not have a recognition trial. On the other hand, TOMAL and CMS use a verbal selective reminding subtest with a recognition trial, but there is no formal way of comparing long-term retrieval, long term store and consistent long-term retrieval, as in the original Buschke & Fuld (1974) selective reminding task. One of the disappointments of the CMS are that word-pairs are included in the core battery making up the general memory index, but list learning is only a supplementary test. The number of learning trials for list-learning differs in each of the four batteries, ranging from three to six.

Facial Recognition

Four of the assessment batteries, but not the WRAML, include a facial recognition task, but it is in this task above all others where there are major differences in both presentation and response variables. Table 11.3 illustrates this very clearly.

The number of faces for recognition ranges from five to 16. The CMS has large coloured faces of people (12 for younger children and 16 for the older group), presented one at a time at a fast rate of one every 2 s. In the other three batteries, there are black and white photographs of faces, either small (NEPSY and TOMAL), or large (RBMT-C). In the NEPSY and the RBMT-C they are presented one at a time. In the TOMAL there is an increase from 1 to 12 over subsequent trials, but a response is elicited after each trial, rather than at the end of the total exposure. Exposure in the NEPSY is 5 s for each picture, in the RBMT-C for 5 s, during which time the child is asked to identify the sex and whether it is an old or young face, and in the TOMAL 5–20 s, depending on the number of faces exposed at any one time.

It will be seen that the speed of presentation and number of faces to be remembered differs quite considerably across batteries. Consequently, memory capacity and speed of

Table 11.2 Word lists/paired words/selective reminding

Test	Type	Words/pairs n (years)	Learning trials	Interference list	Time to delay (min)	Delayed recall			Recognition trial
						Free	Verbal cue	Visual cue	
CMS	Word pairs	10 (5–8) 14 (9+)	3	No	30	yes	No	No	Yes
	Word lists	10 (5–8) 14 (9+)	4	Yes	30	yes	No	No	Yes
NEPSY	Word lists	15 (9+)	5	Yes	30	yes	No	No	No
TOMAL	Word pairs	6 (5–8) 8 (9+)	4	No	N/A	No	No	No	No
	Selective reminding	8 (5–8) 12 (9+)	8	yes	30	Yes	Yes	Yes	Yes
WRAML	Word lists	(6–8) (9+)	3	No	30	Yes	No	No	No
RBMT-C	Not available								
CVLT-C	Word lists	15 (5–16)	5	Yes	Short and 20	Yes	Category	No	Yes

CMS, Children's Memory Scale; NEPSY, A Developmental Neuropsychological Assessment; TOMAL, Test of Memory and Learning; WRAML, Wide Range Assessment of Memory and Learning; RBMT-C, Rivermead Behavioural Memory Test—Children; CVLT-C, Californian Verbal Learning Test—Child Version.

Table 11.3 Facial recognition

Test	Presentation						Response		
	B/W or colour	Size	Type	Exposure(s)	Single/multiple	Learning trials	Y/N Ind.	Mult. Choice	Delayed
CMS	Colour	Large	Photo	2	One at a time	No	Yes		After 30 mins
NEPSY	B/W	Small	Drawing	5	One of three	3	No	One of three	After 30 mins
TOMAL	B/W	Small	Photo	Varies	1–12 rising	No	No	One 3–30	After 30 mins
RBMT-C	B/W	Large	Photo	5 s while child identifies sex/age	One at a time	No	Yes		Not available
WRAML	Not available								

CMS, Children's Memory Scale; NEPSY, A Developmental Neuropsychological Assessment; TOMAL, Test of Memory and Learning; RBMT-C; Rivermead Behavioural Memory Test—Children; WRAML, Wide Range Assessment of Memory and Learning.

information processing are crucial variables, with some children failing the CMS subtest if they take in the information slowly or if they become distracted once presentation begins. In the TOMAL children may use the strategy of trying to remember just a few faces each time when a larger number are exposed simultaneously, rather than scan them all quickly. Thus, they control the amount of time they may take on looking at individual faces, a strategy that cannot be used in other tests.

Second, the recognition trials are all quite different. Both the CMS and RBMT-C require children to make a decision as to whether they have seen a single face before (or whether they were asked to remember it [CMS]), but in the NEPSY they are asked to decide which of three faces they have seen before. In all three they wait until all the faces have been exposed before being asked to recall any. The TOMAL, however, requires children to recall which of a number of faces they have seen immediately after exposure, but in the last immediate recall trial, this amounts to 12 faces to find in an array of 30. All but the RBMT-C (which has a short delay between presentation and test) have delayed trials (30 min later).

Spatial Recall

Finally in this analysis of different forms of purportedly similar tests, it is worth looking at spatial recall. As has already been mentioned in this chapter, both the TOMAL and the WRAML have subtests called "visual recall" that are really spatial memory tests. Again, each assessment battery varies in terms of how spatial memory is measured. The NEPSY has no spatial memory task. In the RBMT-C, children are asked to watch as the examiner walks round the room describing the route, and they then have to follow the route as well as remember to pick up a message and leave it in a specific place. There is a delayed trial after about 15–20 min. This task is unique in terms of its face validity, but in fact there are usually not many different options where a child may make an error, and clinically it would seem that errors tend to be in relation to the sequence of the route.

Table 11.4 shows that in CMS, TOMAL and WRAML tasks differ in a number of subtle ways. "Dot location" makes up part of the core battery in the CMS, with children having to place dots (6–8) on a grid after an exposure of 5 s. There are three learning trials and a delayed trial after 30 min. Clinical experience suggests that it is an easy test to administer and, coming at the beginning of the battery, apparently not very challenging to children, who often seem unaware how poorly they do if they find this difficult. There is a supplementary test (Picture Location) without learning trials, where children look at coloured pictures placed on a page for 2 s and they have to point to where they were on a grid. Location memory is also included in a Family Pictures test where, after exposure, children have to locate members of a family in a quadrant of a picture as well as identify who they were and what they were doing.

TOMAL has a selective nonverbal reminding task (to parallel the verbal selective reminding task), where children watch the examiner point to one of five dots in each of 6–8 grids, which they then have to repeat. Errors are corrected and there are seven more learning trials as well as a delayed trial after 30 min. Of all the spatial memory tasks, this subtest would clinically seem to be the one most likely to lead to examiner error, particularly if children respond very quickly. Children can also become dispirited if they find it difficult, and may give up quickly. A separate Memory for Location test is also part of the nonverbal

Table 11.4 Spatial recall

Test	Task	Versions	No. of stimuli n (years)	Exposure time (s)	No. of Trials	B/W or colour	Time to delay (min)
CMS	Dot location (all dots on grid)	1	6 (5–8) 8 (9+)	5	3	Blue	30 min
	Picture location (grid)	1	1–5 (5–8) 1–8 (9+)	2	1	Col	N/A
TOMAL	"Visual" selective reminding (1 of 5 dots in small grid)	1	6 (5–8) 8 (9+)	6 8	8	B/W	30 min
	Memory for location	1	1–9 (5–8)	5	1	B/W	N/A
WRAML	"Visual" learning (covered) grid with each pattern exposed separately	1	12 (5–8) 14 (9+)	2 each	3	Col.	30 min
RBMT-C	Route round room (child observes examiner walk round room)	4	5	20–30	1	N/A	15–20 s
NEPSY	Not available						

CMS, Children's Memory Scale; TOMAL, Test of Memory and Learning; WRAML, Wide Range Assessment of Memory and Learning; RBMT-C, Rivermead Behavioural Memory Test—Children; NEPSY, A Developmental Neuropsychological Assessment.

memory index, with children having to point to a grid after a short exposure of up to nine dots on a 4 × 4 grid.

In the WRAML "visual" selective learning task, 12–14 brightly coloured abstract patterns on a 4 × 4 grid are exposed one at a time before being covered. Children then have to recall the position of an individual pattern. After their response, the target pattern is shown. There are three learning and one delayed trial. Even when children are doing poorly on this task, they seem to enjoy it and can be motivated to continue, even if they make multiple errors. As with the other delayed trials in the WRAML, the delayed scoring strategy is weak.

Summary

It will be obvious from the above discussions that comparisons of a child's performance on different occasions, using the same or another test or test battery, can cause major problems in interpretation in terms of both stability and sensitivity to change over time. If the same test is used, where there is no alternative version, it is likely that there will be practice effects, which will enhance performance and hide continuing weaknesses or failure to develop as expected. Using another battery gives rise to three problems. First, there is the issue of the *different standardization procedures* and the *different populations* upon which the standardization was carried out. Second, despite superficially appearing similar, the *composition of the core index* in different batteries may differ enormously. Third, the above analysis of four core subtests of the major memory batteries for children (narrative recall, word lists, facial recognition and spatial recall) has indicated that making comparisons between test performance on different batteries is, if not virtually impossible, extremely difficult, due to the *multiple differences in subtest variables*. Where there is no alternative, interpretation should be qualified and the problems in interpretation should be made explicit.

These issues also underline the importance of including a wide range of nontest data in understanding an individual child's assessment, for example poor performance on facial memory is not always consistent with parents' or teacher's evidence. This may be because of differences in the ability to recognize familiar and unfamiliar faces. Nor do some children seem to be aware they have a problem, although they may have learnt ways to compensate for problems with facial recognition of which they are unaware. It may also be that facial memory is not a problem but there are difficulties with a lower level of processing. Thus, failure in, for example, the CMS, where faces are only exposed for 2 s, may be related to slow speed of processing rather than in a problem with facial memory *per se*. Consequently, the final question to ask in all assessments of memory is related to the ecological validity of the assessment and results in the light of what is else is known about the child.

ISSUES IN THE MANAGEMENT OF MEMORY AND LEARNING PROBLEMS IN CHILDREN

In devising interventions for memory problems in children, the need for generalization of skills beyond the specific training task, and the continuation of improvements after the intervention stops, are crucial outcomes. Ylvisaker & Gioia (1998) have argued that in managing memory and other problems following traumatic brain injury, assessment and management needs to be theory-based, ongoing, contextualized, collaborative and on a hypothesis-testing basis. This approach is not exclusive to head injury and should apply to all children with neurological damage. Consequently, following on from comprehensive interviews, observations and psychometric assessment, a crucial question to ask is how the findings functionally relate to the child's problem. Some of this information will have already been gleaned from clinical interviews and reports, but further hypotheses based on formal assessments can be tested out when reporting back to parents and schools.

In the space allowed here, it is not possible to do more than briefly describe in outline of the kind of interventions that are possible. A number of programmes included in the rehabilitation and management of adults are likely to be appropriate in working with children, particularly older children and adolescents, provided that interventions are suitably adapted to the child's age and level of development.

One major difference compared to adults is the long-term impact of memory problems on children's education and their failure to gain knowledge that will enable them to live independently. There is evidence, however, that children with bilateral hippocampal but no other cortical damage have intact semantic memory and can attain reasonable knowledge in school (Vargha-Khadem et al., 1997), although they still have major problems with episodic memory. Wider CNS involvement leading to both semantic and episodic memory problems can have a profound effect. Adults with an acquired memory loss *may* be able to access the basic information and skills needed for everyday life, which they had acquired and used premorbidly. For children with acquired loss of both episodic and semantic memory, particularly younger children, the effect of problems with memory, and particularly learning and integrating new information into what they know already, may be very debilitating in attempts to add to their knowledge base. This may mean that the effects of memory problems only emerge slowly as children "grow into a deficit" (Mateer et al., 1997). Because they may be able to access premorbid skills and knowledge, initially they may appear to perform well enough for the problem to be thought negligible in school. However, their failure to learn becomes apparent as they slowly slip increasingly behind. These difficulties will be in addition to the daily effects of any episodic memory problems.

Ylvisaker et al. (1998) propose eight intervention premises as the foundation for rehabilitation of memory in children and adolescents following head injury (pp. 182–183):

- Problems with organization and memory are common after traumatic brain injury and have long-term effects.
- Different types of injury can effect organization and memory differentially.
- Organization and memory are intimately related.
- Normal development of organization and memory give insight into how intervention strategies may be effective.
- There are many approaches, all of which are appropriate at some time for some individuals in relation to specific goals.
- Everyday functional activities are the preferred context for intervention.
- Cognitive rehabilitation is collaborative.
- Problems with organization and memory are often misdiagnosed, resulting in inappropriate interventions.

This approach is relevant however memory problems are acquired.

Interventions

Children with memory and learning problems may be helped through a variety of interventions, ranging from specific individual strategies to more general management approaches. These are: (a) informing parents, teachers and, where appropriate, the child of what the problem is; (b) arranging that clinical reports go forward to the Local Educational Authority to get extra help in school and special conditions in examinations; (c) external memory aids and environmental adaptations; (d) direct instruction; and (e) internal memory strategies.

1. *Information and explanation.* A major component in the assessment of memory and learning in children is in informing and advising parents and teachers of the functional implications of having specific memory and learning difficulties, how they affect a child now, and how they can best be managed in the future. Although it might be expected that most parents and children do not understand brain–behaviour links, teachers would also appear to have little in their training that prepares them for working with children with such difficulties, and this may mean that basic information about the neuroanatomical underpinnings of memory and memory problems needs to be explained. Consequently, initial interventions with schools and families, may be in explaining the neuropsychological basis of a child's specific problem, and dispelling any possible misconceptions, for example:

   > *Case*: A teacher complained that, 2 years after he had undergone a left temporal lobectomy for intractable epilepsy, J was still forgetting what he was told, despite the resolution of his epilepsy and being off all medication. It was necessary to explain that the surgery, which had very successfully resolved the epilepsy, had removed that part of J's brain involved in verbal memory, and that her difficulties and awkward behaviour arising from this were directly related to the neuropathology.

   Although such simple information may appear a low-level intervention, helping to explain the aetiology and reframing a problem may in itself make a considerable difference to teaching approaches and attitudes, and thus to children with these difficulties. If they are old enough to be part of the explanation, this knowledge may also enhance children's self-esteem, as they may realise that they are not "stupid" as they may have felt, but have a specific difficulty for which they can receive some help. This information may lead them to become more involved and adhere to rehabilitation interventions, particularly when they are older. More particularly, teachers and schools can begin to appreciate that if a child can remember some things but not others, this may not be due to laziness, lack of motivation or oppositional behaviour, and consequently the need for external adaptations and adapted teaching methods, etc., can be accepted and subsequently planned and implemented. Parents, too, benefit from careful explanation, understanding that their child is not necessarily being naughty or careless when he/she loses clothes and equipment at school, or repeatedly forgets what he/she has been told to do.

2. *Contribution to Statements of Special Educational Need and special concessions in examinations.* A second way in which a child can benefit from a careful neuropsychological assessment is if the report becomes part of the contribution to a child's Statement of Special Educational Needs. Not only can the above explanations of the aetiology and functional implications be used in drawing up a child's Individual

Educational Plan in school, but children may be able to get extra help in the form of one-to-one support in the classroom to help cope with specific problems. Second, this kind of information may be used to request extra time in examinations, so that children can reread the questions more than once if they begin to forget what they have read, as well as track back through their own written answers a number of times if they have forgotten what they have put down already.

3. *External Adaptations and Memory Aids.* As the rate of information technology develops, there are an increasing number of everyday devices that older children and adolescents can be trained to use to help them compensate for poor memory. Diaries, schedules and notebooks in which to write down anything that has to be remembered are simple compensatory methods, but some older children feel it is unacceptable to use them, and there is always the need for a bag in which to carry them, which may also be felt to be inappropriate.

Electronic organizers, however, have more kudos with older children and adolescents, and they are now easily available in the high street stores. They can act as a diary and note pad, and be programmed to act as an alerting system with a bleep. Bleeper watches with message dials are also available, which can be programmed via a link-up with personal computers. In addition, there are small electronic memo recorders, which can store up to 60–100 messages. These are probably more appropriate for older children and adolescents to record brief messages about something they have to do in the future, or information to pass on later.

If problems relate to episodic rather than procedural memory, then children can learn how to programme these devices themselves, but training is needed in using external memory aids whatever these may be (Sohlberg and Mateer, 1989). However, instruction may need to be over extensive periods. With electronic devices, the programming is more likely to be carried out by parents or teachers for younger compared with older children and adolescents, so instruction in this should include everyone who is involved. If children are to use any of these devices effectively, then teachers and parents need to be committed to, and consistent in, supporting the children and ensure that they have the device, whether it is a bleeper watch or memory book, with them at all times. This is why it is so important to assess parents' and teachers' understanding of the problem, and to inform and advise them of rehabilitation strategies, for without their support any intervention is likely to fail. Physical attachment of the device to a child, either by a chain or string to clothing, or carried in a shoulder bag, or pouch, or attached round the waist, may prevent the external device being mislaid, which is not an uncommon problem.

In severe cases of memory problems, less complex support may be extremely helpful. Children may need to have drawers or cupboards labelled, daily schedules and notices to remind them of the order of carrying out basic tasks, such as the morning routine, etc. More frequently, however, they may need adaptations, such as written homework instructions, questions and worksheets and a home–school diary, maps around the school and clear timetables. Families and teachers may need to ensure that routines are set up to help in relearning old and learning new tasks, although this can be particularly difficult in school, where there are many demands on teaching staff in large classes.

4. *Direct Instruction and Compensatory Strategies.* Errorless learning, first developed by Terrace (1963, 1966) and then used by Sidman & Stoddard (1967) for children with developmental learning disabilities, as well as fading behavioural cues, have both

been strategies used effectively in teaching children with learning difficulties for many years. Glisky et al. (1986) used a similar method called "the Method of Vanishing Cues". These methods have been more recently adapted for rehabilitation, for example by Wilson et al. (1994; see Chapter 10, this volume). This method ensures that children do not guess at solutions, as if wrong they can find it very difficult to unlearn the error. Using behavioural methods, skills can be taught by example, guiding, verbal instruction and, finally prompts. In addition, teaching and giving instructions and feedback in a simple, positive and unambiguous manner can be helpful, as well as emphasizing what is important. Asking children to repeat what has been said will enhance learning. Mateer et al. (1997) list task analysis, modelling, shaping and positive reinforcement of success consistently over long periods as adjuncts to the rehabilitation process. For further detailed suggestions for a full range of compensatory strategies, see Ylvisaker et al. (1998).

5. *Training Internal Memory Strategies.*   There is little evidence that drilling or practice can restore memory, but some strategy training has been tried. Bjorklund et al. (1997) have carried out an extensive review on how and why children fail to benefit from training in strategies devised to improve their memory, or at best only experience minimal benefit, termed as utilization deficiencies. Although the children in these studies did not have memory problems *per se*, the review is pertinent in considering how children's ability to access different strategies successfully develops with age and suggests why training children in using strategies may fail. Thus, the importance of careful observations of how a child goes about completing memory tests, in order to see whether or not they are using a strategy spontaneously, is critical. As these authors point out, many children carry out a task but achieve it via a different route to the one in which they were trained.

Mateer et al. (1997) point out that there is considerable evidence to suggest that learning internal strategies to enhance memory has limited success, whatever the strategy used. Harris (1996) has looked at "thinking aloud" or verbal rehearsal to help list-learning in children with head injuries. Her results suggested that strategies differ between those children with closed head injury and those without. The severely injured (but not the mildly injured or the control group) showed not only impaired verbal recall but also inefficient rehearsal strategies, poor self-monitoring and a weaker judgement in deciding which strategy might be more effective (metamemory). Bjorklund et al. (1997) propose that memory strategy training in normal children was more effective if children were given a single rather than multiple strategies with task variables, including sorting, clustering and rehearsal, and training variables covering verbal instruction, demonstration and rationale. Their review indicated that a number of child variables also needed to be considered when considering training strategies, such as level of intelligence, age, insight, temperament, motivation and underlying pathology. In addition, children may have difficulties in integrating strategies, shifting from one strategy to another, or inhibiting the use of a previously ineffective strategy, which relate to a lack of insight and consequently poor adherence to strategy use. Such difficulties may be related to frontal lobe pathology, which is frequently present following head injury and which is closely linked to memory problems. In general, however, the lack of support for training internal strategies is likely to be due to many factors, including the fact that the stratetgies are often taught in abstract or at a very specific level and not within context, so that generalization does not take place and any benefit quickly fades after training ends. It should be remembered that internal strategies lead to faster learning for specific pieces of information. Most people with memory problems do not use them spontaneously and maybe we should expect this. For certain things, however, and with help from parents/teachers/therapists, internal strategies can be helpful in teaching some useful everyday information.

SUMMARY AND CONCLUSIONS

Management and rehabilitation of memory can be effective if appropriate and individualized programmes are set up which take into account the many variables discussed above. As in all rehabilitation, specific goals need to be set, put into operation and monitored, with clear steps from the introduction of a programme to its final achievement. As Ylvisaker et al. (1998) recommend, devising programmes and managing their implementations should be within everyday contexts, and be a collaborative venture if they are to be effective. Consequently, careful assessment, not just of the memory problems but of the child generally, as well as his/her environment, is crucial. In addition, the resources and the restrictions of those who are most likely to carry out the management of programmes, in other words families and teachers, should be assessed and understood to achieve the best possible outcome.

REFERENCES

Aldrich, F. & Wilson, B.A. (1991). Rivermead Behavioural Memory Test for Children: a preliminary evaluation. *British Journal of Clinical Psychology*, **30**, 161–168.

Bayley, N. (1993). *Bayley Scales of Infant Development*, 2nd edn. San Antonio, TX: Psychological Corporation/Harcourt Brace & Co.

Beardsworth, E. & Bishop, D. (1994). Assessment of long-term verbal memory in children. *Memory*, **2**, 129–148.

Benton, A.L. & Hamsher, K. de S. (1989). *Multilingual Aphasia Examination*. Iowa City, IO: AJA Associates.

Benton, A.L. & Sivan, A. (1995). *Benton Visual Retention Test*, 5th edn. San Antonio, TX: Psychological Corporation/Harcourt Brace & Co.

Berger, M. & Middleton, J.A. (1995). Figure presented at talk on Assessment of Memory, Charney Manor, Oxford, November.

Bjorklund, D.G. & Douglas, R.N. (1997). The development of memory strategies. In N. Cowan (ed.), *The Development of Memory in Childhood* (pp. 201–246). Hove: Psychology Press.

Bjorklund, D.F., Miller, P.H., Coyle, T.R. & Slawinski, J.L. (1997). Instructing children to use memory strategies: Evidence of utilization deficiencies in memory training studies. *Developmental Review*, **17**, 411–441.

Blass, E.M. (1999). The ontogeny of human infant face recognition: orugustatory, visual and social influences. In P. Rochat (ed.), *Early Social Cognition. Understanding Others in the First Months of Life* (pp. 35–66). London: Erlbaum.

Boll, T. (1993). *Children's Category Test*. San Antonio, TX: Psychological Corporation/Harcourt Brace & Co.

Broman, M., Rose, A.L., Hotson, G. & Casey, C.M. (1997). Severe anterograde amnesia with onset in childhood as a result of anoxic encephalopathy. *Brain*, **120**, 417–433.

Buschke, H. & Fuld, P.A. (1974). Evaluating storage, retention and retrieval in disordered memory and learning. *Neurology*, **11**, 1019–1025.

Canterbury, R. & Yule, W. (1997). The effects on children of road accidents. In M. Mitchell (ed.), *The Aftermath of Road Accidents* (pp. 59–69). London: Routledge.

Casalini, C., Brizzolara, D., Cavallaro, M.C. & Cipriani, P. (1999). Developmental dysmnesia: a case report. *Cortex*, **35**, 713–727.

CCTB Macmillan/McGraw Hill (1988). *Californian Achievement Test*. Monterey, C.A: Macmillan/McGraw Hill.

Cohen, M. (1997). *Children's Memory Scale*. San Antonio, TX: Psychological Corporation/Harcourt Brace & Co.

Cowan, N. (ed.) (1997). *The Development of Memory in Childhood*. Hove: Psychology Press.

Dean, C.D., Kramer, J.H., Kaplan, E. & Ober, B.A. (1994). *California Verbal Learning Test—Children's Version*. San Antonio, TX: Psychological Corporation Harcourt Brace & Co.

Elliot, C. (1990). *Differential Ability Scales*. San Antonio, TX: The Psychological Corporation/Harcourt Brace & Co.

Elliot, C.D., Murray, D.J. & Pearson, L.S. (1993). *British Ability Scales*. Windsor: NFER Nelson.

Fletcher, J.M. & Taylor, H.G. (1984). Neuropsychological approaches to children: Towards a developmental neuropsychology. *Journal of Clinical Neuropsychology*, **6**, 39–56.

Glisky, E.L., Schacter, D.L. & Tulving, E. (1986). Computer learning by memory impaired patients: Acquisition and retention of complex knowledge. *Neuropsychologia*, **24**, 313–328.

Harris, J.R. (1996). Verbal rehearsal and memory in children with closed head injury: a quantitative and qualitative analysis. *Journal of Communication Disorders*, **29**, 79–93.

Heaton, R.K., Chelune, G.J., Talley, J.L. et al. (1993). *Wisconsin Card Sorting Test*. Odessa, FL: Psychological Assessment Resources.

Hulme, C. & MacKenzie, S. (1992). *Working Memory and Severe Learning Difficulties*. Hove: Erlbaum.

Jastak, J.F. & Wilkinson, G.S. (1993). *Wide Range Achievement Test*, 3rd edn. Wilmington: Jastak Associates.

Joyner, M.H. & Kurtz-Costes, B. (1997). Metamemory development. In N. Cowan (ed.), *The Development of Memory in Childhood* (pp. 275–301). Hove: Psychology Press.

Kaufman, A.S. (1994). *Intelligent Testing with the WISC-III*. New York: Wiley.

Kaufman, A.S. & Kaufman, R.W. (1984). *Kaufman Assessment Battery for Children*. Circle Pines, MN: American Guidance Service.

Korkman, M., Kirk, U. & Kemp, S. (1998). *NEPSY : A Developmental Neuropsychological Assessment*. San Antonio, TX: Psychological Corporation/Harcourt Brace & Co.

Levin, H.S., Ewing-Cobbs, L. & Eisenberg, H.M. (1995). Neurobehavioral outcome of pediatric closed head injury. In S.H. Broman & M.E. Michel (eds), *Traumatic Brain Injury in Children* (pp. 70–94). Oxford: Oxford University Press.

Lezak, M.D. (1995). Neuropsychological Assessment, 3rd edn. New York: Oxford University Press.

Little, A.H., Lipsitt, L.P. & Rovee-Collier, C.K. (1984). Classical conditioning and rentention of the infant's Evelid response: effects of age and interstimulus interval. *Journal of Experimental Child Psychology*, **37**(3), 512–524.

Mateer, C.A., Kerns, K.A. & Eso, K.L. (1997). Management of attention and memory disorders following traumatic brain injury. In E.D. Bigler, E. Clarke & J.E. Farmer (eds), *Childhood Traumatic Brain Injury: Diagnosis, Assessment and Intervention*. Austin, TX: Pro-Ed.

McCarthy, D. (1972). *McCarthy Scales of Children's Abilities*. San Antonio, TX: Psychological Corporation/Harcourt Brace & Co.

Meyers, J.E. & Meyers, K.R. (1995). *Rey Complex Figure Test and Recognition Trial: Professional Manual*. Odessa, FL: Psychological Assessment Resources Inc.

Mistry, J. (1998). The development of remembering in cultural context. In N. Cowan (ed.), *The Development of Memory in Childhood*. Hove: Psychology Press.

Osterreith, P.A. (1944). Le test de copie d'une figure complexe. *Archives de Psychologie*, **30**, 206–356.

Rey, A. (1941). L'examen psychologique dans le cas d'encephalopathie traumatique. *Archives de Psychologie*, **28**, 286–340.

Reynolds, C.R. & Bigler, E.D. (1994). *Test of Memory and Learning*. Austin, TX: Pro-Ed.

Rovee-Collier, C. & Gerhardstein, P. (1997). The development of infant memory. In N. Cowan (ed.), *The Development of Memory in Childhood* (pp. 5–40). Hove: Psychology Press.

Rovee-Collier, C., Sullivan, M.W., Enright, M.K. et al. (1980). Reactivation of infant memory. *Science*, **208**, 1159–1161.

Said, J.A., Waters, B.G.H., Cousens, P. & Stevens, M.M. (1989). Neuropsychological sequelae of central nervous system prophylaxis in survivors of childhood acute lymphoblastic leukaemia. *Journal of Consulting and Clinical Psychology*, **57**, 251–256.

Semmel, E., Wiig, E. & Secord, W. (1995). *Clinical Evaluation of Language Fundamentals*, 3rd edn. San Antonio, TX: Psychological Corporation/Harcourt Brace & Co.

Sheslow, D. & Adams, W. (1990). *Wide Range Assessment of Memory and Learning*. Delaware: Jastak Associates, Inc.

Sidman, M. & Stoddard, L.T. (1967). The effectiveness of fading in programming simultaneous form discrimination for retarded children. *Journal of Experimental Analysis of Behavior*, **10**, 3–15.

Sohlberg, M.M. & Mateer, C.A. (1989). Training use of compensatory memory books: a three stage behavioral approach. *Journal of Clinical and Experimental Neuropsychology*, **11**, 871–891.

Temple, C. (1997). *Developmental Cognitive Neuropsychology*. Hove: Psychology Press.

Terrace, H.S. (1963). Discrimination learning with and without "errors". *Journal of Experimental Analysis of Behavior*, **6**, 1–27.

Terrace, H.S. (1966). Stimulus Control. In W.K. Honig (ed.), *Operant Behavior; Areas of Reserach and Application*. New York: Appleton-Century-Crofts.

Tranel, D. & Damasio, A.R. (2002). Neurobiological foundations of human memory. In A.D. Baddeley, M.D. Kopelman & B.A. Wilson (eds), *The HandBook of Memory Disorders*, 2nd edn (pp. 17–56). Chichester: Wiley.

Vargha-Khadem, F., Gadian, D.G., Watkins, K.E. et al. (1997). Differential effects of early hippocampal pathology on episodic and semantic memory. *Science*, **277**, 376–380.

Walton, G.E., Bower, N.J.A. & Bower, T.G.R. (1992). Recognition of familiar faces by newborns. *Infant Behavior and Development*, **15**, 265–269.

Wechsler, D. (1974). *Wechsler Intelligence Scale for Children—Revised*. San Antonio, TX: Psychological Corporation/Harcourt Brace & Co.

Wechsler, D. (1987). *Wechsler Memory Scale—Revised*. San Antonio, TX: Psychological Corporation/ Harcourt Brace & Co.

Wechsler, D. (1991). *Wechsler Intelligence Scale for Children*, 3rd edn. San Antonio, TX: Psychological Corporation/Harcourt Brace & Co.

Wechsler, D. (1993). *Wechsler Pre-School and Primary Scale of Intelligence—Revised*. San Antonio, TX: Psychological Corporation/Harcourt Brace & Co.

Wechsler, D. (1995). *Wechsler Individual Achievement Test*. San Antonio, TX: Psychological Corporation Harcourt Brace & Co.

Wechsler, D. (1997). *Wechsler Memory Scale*, 3rd edn. San Antonio, TX: Psychological Corporation/ Harcourt Brace & Co.

Wilson, B.A., Baddeley, A., Evans, J. & Shiel, A. (1994). Errorless learning in the rehabilitation of memory impaired people. *Neuropsychological Rehabilitation*, **4**, 307–326.

Wilson, B.A. Cockburn, J. & Baddeley, A.D. (1985). *The Rivermead Behavioural Memory Test*. Bury St. Edmunds: Thames Valley Test Company.

Wilson, B.A., Forester, S., Bryant, T. & Cockburn, J. (1990). Performance of 11–14 year-olds on the Rivermead Behavioural Memory Test. *Clinical Psychology Forum* (30), 8–10.

Wilson, B.A., Ivani-Chalian, R. & Aldrich, B. (1991). *Rivermead Behaviour Memory Test for Children*. Bury St. Edmunds: Thames Valley Test Company.

Ylvisaker, M. & Gioia, G.A. (1998). Cognitive assessment. In M. Ylvisaker (ed.), *Traumatic Brain Injury Rehabilitation*, 2nd edn. Boston, MA: Butterworth-Heinemann.

Ylvisaker, M., Szekeres, S.F. & Haarbauer-Krupa (1998). Cognitive rehabilitation: organisation, memory and language. In M. Ylvisaker (ed.), *Traumatic Brain Injury Rehabilitation*, 2nd edn. Boston, MA: Butterworth-Heinemann.

CHAPTER 12

Assessment and Intervention in Dementia of Alzheimer Type

Linda Clare

Sub-department of Clinical Health Psychology, University College London, UK

Dementia is a major cause of disability and accounts for a considerable proportion of health care expenditure in developed countries (Whitehouse et al., 1993). Prevalence estimates vary, but dementia is thought to affect about 5% of all people over 65 and to increase in prevalence with advancing years, so that over 20% of people over 80 are affected (Woods, 1996a). Dementia with onset before the age of 65 is also a matter of concern (Cox & Keady, 1999; Harvey, 1998). Although "dementia" is a Western diagnostic category, the phenomenon it describes is thought to be universal (Pollitt, 1996). Within the broad disease spectrum of dementia, dementia of the Alzheimer type (DAT) is the most frequently diagnosed subcategory and is said to account for 75% of all dementia diagnoses confirmed at post mortem examination (J.C. Morris, 1996), although estimates of prevalence and incidence vary considerably (Brayne, 1994; Kay, 1991). Behind these figures, striking in themselves, lie the profound personal costs arising from what has been described as "one of the cruellest diseases to assail the human spirit" (Heston & White, 1991).

DEMENTIA OF ALZHEIMER TYPE: A BRIEF OVERVIEW

Consensus diagnostic criteria for DAT are provided by DSM-IV (American Psychiatric Association, 1995), ICD-10 (World Health Organization, 1992) and NINCDS–ADRDA (McKhann et al., 1984). The NINCDS–ADRDA criteria for probable DAT occurring in persons aged 40–90 specify that dementia should be established by clinical examination, documented by Mini-Mental State Examination (MMSE; Folstein et al., 1975) or equivalent screening measure, and confirmed by neuropsychological tests. There should be deficits in at least two areas of cognitive functioning, with progressive deterioration. There should be no disturbance of consciousness, and the possibility of the problems being due to any other disorder should be ruled out. Where there is a second systemic or brain disorder sufficient

The Essential *Handbook of Memory Disorders for Clinicians.* Edited by A.D. Baddeley, M.D. Kopelman and B.A. Wilson.
© 2004 John Wiley & Sons, Ltd. ISBN 0-470-09141-X.

to produce dementia but not considered to be the cause of dementia, or where there are variations in onset, presentation, or course, a diagnosis of possible AD is made. A diagnosis of definite AD can only be made where the clinical criteria for probable AD are met and there is additional histopathological evidence obtained from biopsy or autopsy.

Use of criteria such as these is said to have improved the reliability of diagnosis when tested against post mortem findings, and estimates of accuracy range from 80% to 95% (J.C. Morris, 1996; Burns & Förstl, 1994; Hodges, 1994; Reifler & Larson, 1990). Burns & Förstl (1994) comment, however, that the improvement in accuracy gained by adhering to these criteria is relatively slight, and Henderson & Sartorius (1994) point out that even with a clearly agreed set of criteria there is still variability in the way in which the criteria are applied by different assessors. It should also be noted that the interpretation of histological changes in the brain observed at post mortem, held up as the "gold standard" by which accuracy of clinical diagnosis is assessed, is "by no means uncontroversial", since the process is not entirely free of subjective judgment (Burns & Förstl, 1994).

A defining element in all diagnostic criteria for DAT is the observation of progressive changes in memory and cognitive function. Memory is usually the first cognitive function to be affected by the onset of DAT, although impairments are initially evident only in certain memory systems, particularly episodic memory (Fox et al., 1998; Greene et al., 1996). Attention (Perry & Hodges, 1999), executive function (Greene et al., 1995; Miller, 1996; R.G. Morris, 1996) and word finding (Hamilton, 1994; Miller, 1996; R.G. Morris, 1996) may also be compromised. As the disorder progresses, deficits in these areas become more extensive, psychomotor function is affected and a decline in global cognitive functioning becomes evident (Morris & McKiernan, 1994; Miller, 1996). Visuospatial perception is usually affected only in the later stages, although in atypical cases it may be observed as one of the earliest symptoms (Morris & McKiernan, 1994). Considerable heterogeneity of presentation has been observed in DAT (Wild & Kaye, 1998; Storandt et al., 1992; Neary et al., 1986).

Heterogeneity is evident, not only in initial presentation, but also in the course and progression of DAT. Consequently, models that emphasize clear stages in the progression of DAT have been criticized for implying a degree of temporal order that is belied by the heterogeneity of individual experience (Gubrium, 1987). However, three broad stages are commonly distinguished (Schneck et al., 1982; J.C. Morris, 1996). These are an early or mild stage, a middle or moderate stage, and an advanced end stage. In research studies, stage or degree of severity is commonly defined either in terms of scores on cognitive screening tests, such as the Mini-Mental State Examination (MMSE; Folstein et al., 1975), although this approach has important limitations (Clarke et al., 1999; Little & Doherty, 1996), or with reference to scores on a global rating of functional level, such as the Clinical Dementia Rating (CDR; Hughes et al., 1982).

Conceptualizing DAT

Situating the concept of dementia within an historical and anthropological context serves as a reminder that both dementia in general and dementia of Alzheimer type (DAT) should be viewed as constructed phenomena (Pollitt, 1996; Berrios, 1994a). The concept of dementia in the sense currently accepted in Western societies was constructed during the nineteenth century (Berrios, 1994a, 1994b), while the so-called "Alzheimerization" of dementia was developed and encouraged during the 1970s (Kitwood, 1997). At present, a disease model of dementia predominates in Western thought and practice, that views DAT as a discrete disease category (Roth, 1994). There is, however, a continuing debate about whether the pathological changes in DAT are qualitatively different to those seen in normal ageing, or form a continuum with normal ageing (Huppert, 1994).

While the disease model has produced valuable advances in understanding and treatment, it has been criticized for a number of reasons (Kitwood, 1997). The key forms of neuropathology in DAT appear in the brains of some healthy older people, while some people may show all the symptoms of DAT but lack any observable pathology at post mortem (see for example Sevush & Leve, 1993). Kitwood (1997) argues that this calls into question the notion of DAT as a "disease", since it is not clear that there is any consistent association between symptoms and biological markers. Furthermore, there are considerable difficulties associated with diagnosis and classification (see for example Christensen et al., 1997; Small et al., 1997; Kitwood, 1997; Cohen, 1996; J.C. Morris, 1996; O'Connor, 1994; Burns & Förstl, 1994) and DAT has been described as a "diagnostic category of uncertain boundaries" (Pollitt, 1996). DAT is essentially a diagnosis of exclusion, and there may be frequent failures to distinguish different subtypes of dementia (Woods, 1996a). Differential diagnosis of dementia and depression is also problematic (Small et al., 1997) and recent research on white matter lesions in depression calls into question the traditional distinction between organic and functional disorder (O'Brien et al., 1996, 1998). Most importantly, the disease model fails to account for "excess disability", whereby functioning is worse than the degree of impairment would predict (Reifler & Larson, 1990) for periods of "rementing", where functioning improves or stabilizes (Kitwood, 1996; Sixsmith et al., 1993), or for the rapid deterioration that often follows adverse events, such as temporary hospitalization (Kitwood, 1996). Psychosocial factors are likely to be relevant in these situations, and it is therefore necessary to address issues of coping and adjustment and to consider DAT from the perspective of the person with dementia (R.G. Morris, 1996; Cottrell & Schulz, 1993).

For these reasons, it is suggested that a broader model, which incorporates the role of psychological and social variables, is required (Kitwood, 1997). An "alternative paradigm" has been most clearly articulated by Kitwood (1996, 1997), although related ideas have been presented in social constructionist accounts (Sabat, 1994, 1995; Sabat & Harré, 1992; Sabat et al., 1984). Kitwood (1996, 1997) proposes a dialectical model of dementia. The term "dialectical" reflects the emphasis on interactions between variables operating at the biological and psychosocial levels. The aim of this "alternative paradigm" is to present an account of the process of dementia that bridges these two levels (Kitwood, 1996, 1997). It is suggested that the manifestation and progression of DAT in any one individual is influenced by the interplay of neurological impairment, physical health and sensory acuity, personality, biographical experience and social psychology, in terms of environment, communication and interaction. Where the social psychology is "malignant", the result is an involutional spiral of deterioration. Social interactions and care processes that are undermining and discouraging, and fail to take account of personality and life history, lead to a reduction in self-efficacy which in turn attracts further damaging interactions (Sabat, 1994). It is suggested that a pervasive malignant social psychology might contribute to structural changes in the brain, while a benign social psychology coupled with an enriched environment might facilitate some regeneration (Arendt & Jones, 1992), and some evidence is available to support this view (Bråne et al., 1989; Karlsson et al., 1988).

The dialectical model has clear implications for assessment, intervention and care. It indicates that the primary aim should be to maximize well-being and optimize functioning for the person with dementia and to support and foster positive elements in the surrounding social system. To be effective, care should be person-centred, based on an individualized formulation that takes into account all the relevant biological, psychological and social factors, and delivered in a way that promotes a benign rather than malignant social psychology.

ASSESSMENT IN DAT

In keeping with this broad perspective, assessment of memory and other aspects of cognitive functioning aimed at detecting the presence of DAT should form part of a comprehensive, multidisciplinary assessment alongside information on physical health status and current medication, results of medical tests and neuroimaging data. Other information required to complete the picture includes a full history, an assessment of mood and well-being, an evaluation of functional ability, and a consideration of the social and environmental context, including the needs of close family members. Information should be obtained not only from the individual but also, wherever possible, from someone who knows the person well, such as a partner or relative, and from any other professionals involved in the person's care.

While neuropsychological tests form an essential component of the assessment, the results should be interpreted with caution, bearing in mind the range of factors that may affect performance. These may be related to the individual, e.g. sensory loss, pain, restricted mobility or anxiety about the testing situation; to the testing environment, e.g. distracting noise or uncomfortable seating; or to the tests themselves, e.g. requirements for unrealistic levels of mobility or dexterity, or lack of sensitivity to cultural difference. Neuropsychological assessment can often be an aversive experience for the older person, and care should be taken to create a situation that provides a positive and worthwhile experience. The amount of testing should be limited to the minimum necessary to answer the relevant questions satisfactorily, and practical, constructive feedback should be offered to the individual and family.

Assessment Measures

It is necessary to distinguish screening tests (sometimes described as "cognitive" tests) from neuropsychological tests. Screening tests are often used to provide an indication of whether there is cognitive impairment, and can be valuable provided their limitations are clearly understood. They are not, however, a substitute for full neuropsychological assessment.

Screening Measures

The most widely-used cognitive screening measure is the MMSE, which is brief and simple to administer, but which does not properly sample the cognitive functions known to be affected in early-stage DAT. Administration procedures can vary considerably, although a standardized version is available (Molloy et al., 1991). Varying cut-offs are used for presence and degree of impairment and the constraints of test–retest reliability, which indicate that a change of least four points in a given direction is required before one can state confidently that there has been an improvement or a decline, are frequently ignored. Additionally, where the MMSE is administered repeatedly at fairly short intervals, practice effects result in artificial inflation of scores, and it has been suggested that the MMSE should only be administered at intervals of 3 years or more (Clarke et al., 1999). MMSE scores are heavily influenced by education, so that highly educated people may score highly despite severe problems in episodic memory; similarly, results are influenced by ethnicity. Therefore, although a low score (24/30 or below) strongly suggests the presence of impairment, results should always be treated with caution. Furthermore, the MMSE can be seen as rather patronizing and perhaps demeaning in its approach to the older person, so that professionals may feel embarrassed to use it (van Hout et al., 2000) and patients may feel affronted.

Some of the limitations of the MMSE are addressed by the CAMCOG, which is a component of the CAMDEX system for diagnosis of dementia in older people (Roth et al., 1999). The CAMCOG incorporates the MMSE items into a more extensive cognitive screening assessment that does attempt to sample all the relevant cognitive functions. However, none of the relevant functions is assessed in depth. Other widely-used screening measures include the Middlesex Elderly Assessment of Mental State (MEAMS; Golding, 1989) and the Kendrick Scales (Kendrick & Watts, 1999).

Neuropsychological Tests

Where neuropsychological assessment is indicated, the following domains of cognitive functioning should be considered:

- *General cognitive functioning*—both current and estimated prior IQ.
- *Long-term memory*—episodic, semantic, autobiographical and prospective. It is useful to consider memory functions (learning, forgetting), modalities (visual, verbal, sensory), time periods (recent, remote), relation to onset of problems (anterograde, retrograde) and testing methods (recall vs. recognition, immediate vs. delayed recall).
- *Working memory, attention and executive function.*
- *Perception*—object perception, spatial perception.
- *Language*—expressive and receptive.

Table 12.1 provides examples of tests that may be used, in whole or in part, to assess various cognitive functions in older people presenting with possible DAT. As well as tests suitable for use in general neuropsychological assessment, the list includes some tests that can be used to explore further and more specific hypotheses within a cognitive neuropsychological framework. For reviews of specific neuropsychological tests and information on the availability of additional age-specific norms, see Spreen & Strauss (1998) and Lezak (1995). The assessment of memory functioning is discussed in detail by Wilson (Chapter 8, this volume).

Non-cognitive Measures

It is useful to consider including some non-cognitive measures in the assessment; for example mood might be assessed using the Geriatric Depression Scale (Yesavage et al., 1983) or Hospital Anxiety and Depression Scale (Snaith & Zigmond, 1994). Measures of functional ability are reviewed by Carswell & Spiegel (1999) and Little & Doherty (1996). When

Table 12.1 Neuropsychological assessment in DAT

Previous IQ	National Adult Reading Test or Cambridge Contextual Reading Test
Reading ability	Schonell Graded Word Reading Test
Current IQ	WAIS short form Verbal or Full-scale IQ Ravens Coloured or Standard Progressive Matrices
Attention	Test of Everyday Attention Behavioural Inattention Test
Working memory	Digit Span from WAIS or Wechsler Memory Scale WMS Visual Span
Executive function	Trail-making Test Controlled Oral Word Association Test—letter fluency (FAS) Category fluency Modified Wisconsin Card Sorting Test Stroop Test Weigl sorting task Behavioural Assessment of the Dysexecutive Syndrome
Visuospatial perception	Visual Object and Space Perception Battery Benton Judgment of Line Orientation Benton Unfamiliar Face Matching Birmingham Object Recognition Battery
Semantic memory	Pyramids and Palm Trees Graded Naming Test Birmingham Object Recognition Battery Famous faces and names
Long-term memory *Recall, immediate and delayed*	WMS Logical Memory and Visual Reproduction
Recognition	Camden Memory Tests; Recognition Memory Test; Doors and People Test
Everyday memory	Rivermead Behavioural Memory Test; Rivermead Behavioural Memory Test—Extended Version
Autobiographical	Autobiographical Memory Interview
Learning and forgetting	WMS Paired Associate Learning; California Verbal Learning Test; Rey Auditory–Verbal Learning Test; Doors and People Test
Language comprehension	Naming from description Token Test Test for the Reception of Grammar PALPA
Language expression	Graded Naming Test COWA and category fluency Boston Diagnostic Aphasia Examination PALPA
Calculation	WAIS Arithmetic
Praxis	WAIS Block Design
Functioning in moderate or severe dementia	Rivermead Behavioural Memory Test Severe Impairment Battery

gathering information from an informant who is in the role of caregiver, it is useful to assess whether the informant is experiencing high levels of caregiver burden (Gilliard & Rabins, 1999); a number of appropriate measures are reviewed by Vitaliano et al. (1991).

Detecting Dementia

Making the diagnosis of dementia is reasonably straightforward in the moderate and severe stages, but it can be problematic to distinguish the early stages of DAT from "normal" ageing or depression, although recent work has helped to clarify which neuropsychological tests discriminate most effectively (Welsh et al., 1991, 1992; Christensen et al., 1997). Most people who present with concerns about memory problems do not in fact have dementia, and it is also important to note that in specialist clinical practice professionals see an atypical group of patients. O'Connor (1994) found that only 3% of people identified in a community survey as having mild dementia had been referred to specialist services, along with 18% of those with moderate dementia and 33% of those with severe dementia.

Early Detection

Interest in the early detection of DAT has increased with the recent licensing of anti-cholinesterase inhibiting medication as a treatment for the cognitive impairment of early-stage DAT (Rogers et al., 1998a, 1998b; Rogers & Friedhoff, 1998; Corey-Bloom et al., 1998). The detection of early-stage DAT is increasingly undertaken in the context of multidisciplinary memory clinics (Wilcock et al., 1999; Thompson et al., 1997; Wright & Lindesay, 1995; van der Cammen et al., 1987), where neuropsychological assessment plays a critical role in establishing a diagnosis. Early detection of DAT offers the possibility of introducing psychosocial and pharmacological interventions at an early stage. It has been demonstrated that memory clinics can provide an effective focus for early intervention and for the development of integrated psychosocial approaches (Moniz-Cook & Woods, 1997; Moniz-Cook et al., 1998). Early detection of DAT remains a challenge, however, and there are a number of barriers to early detection. People with dementia, and their families, may interpret memory difficulties as part of normal ageing (O'Connor, 1994) or deny that there have been any changes (Cohen & Eisdorfer, 1986), and rates of detection by general medical practitioners are low (O'Connor, 1994; Iliffe, 1997; Rait et al., 1999; van Hout et al., 2000).

Distinguishing Dementia from "Normal" Ageing

The boundaries between dementia and normal forgetfulness appear somewhat fluid, and it remains unclear how the difference between dementia and normal ageing should be conceptualized. Although many older people and their families expect to observe a decline in memory functioning, there is a great deal of variation in the general population as regards the kinds of memory changes seen as part of "normal" ageing, and the issue is compounded by cohort effects. A broad overview suggests that, although memory functioning becomes less efficient from about 67 years onwards, there is no general decline in memory ability and no uniform decline across the range of different memory tasks. Memory functioning is relatively more affected in the very old, so that diagnostic criteria do not allow for a dementia diagnosis made after the age of 90. The following general observations can be made with regard to memory changes in healthy older people (Cohen, 1996):

- Working memory may be affected.
- Episodic memory is affected to a much greater degree than semantic or procedural memory.
- Immediate recall is affected more than delayed recall, while recognition memory is unaffected.
- Retrieval is slower and less efficient, with more rapid and extensive forgetting.
- Prospective memory remains as good as that of younger people if external aids and reminders can be used, but is poorer if no such aids are available.
- Autobiographical memory does *not* show the stereotypical discrepancy between vivid memories of the distant past and hazy memories of more recent events; instead, memories across the lifespan show loss of detail and become more vague.
- Alterations in memory functioning can be offset by intelligence, expertise and use of compensatory strategies, enabling the person to cope well despite any changes.

The Boundaries between Dementia and "Normal" Ageing

As a general rule, the lower the score on cognitive tests, the more likely it is that the person has dementia. However, Storandt & Hill (1989) found that scores of patients with very mild Alzheimer's overlapped considerably with those of both normal older people and people with mild Alzheimer's. Furthermore, even where people do show some degree of memory impairment, progression to dementia is not inevitable (Bowen et al., 1997; Reisberg et al., 1982).

The area of uncertainty between "normal" ageing and dementia has attracted a number of attempts to define diagnostic categories. Among the diagnostic labels suggested are age-associated memory impairment (AAMI), mild cognitive impairment, benign senescent forgetfulness, and minimal or questionable dementia. These concepts remain controversial, and practice varies regarding their use. The category of AAMI, for example, would include large numbers of older people, and it is questionable whether changes that are essentially normative should be labelled in this way (Woods, 1996a).

Which Tests Are Useful in Discriminating between Dementia and Normal Ageing?

The CERAD studies (Welsh et al., 1991, 1992) suggest that the best discriminator is performance on delayed recall tasks. A 10-word list presented in three learning trials and tested after a 5–8 min delay correctly classified 94% of controls and 86% of patients with mild dementia, using a cutting score of 2 SDs below the control group mean. Performance on naming tests was found to be useful as an adjunctive measure. If patients have impairment in delayed recall and problems in naming or verbal fluency, this is a very strong indicator for dementia. Other studies have also emphasized the value of delayed recall. Tierney et al. (1996) found that problems in delayed recall and attention were the best predictors of whether people with mild memory problems would go on to develop Alzheimer's disease.

Distinguishing between Dementia and Depression

Depression in older people often presents somewhat differently to depression in younger adults. Somatic and sleep-related symptoms are less helpful as indicators of depression in older people, since such changes are more widespread in this age group. Factors such as retirement, bereavement, health problems, pain, poor housing, financial hardship and limited social support all contribute to depression, and these form part of the lives of many older people; however, rates of depression are not thought to increase significantly with age. Depression is still an important problem nevertheless, as a substantial number of older people do not recover, and many others relapse. Unfortunately, while depression may affect cognitive functioning, treatments for depression may also have adverse effects in this respect.

The effects of depression on cognitive functioning appear very variable. Some older people with depression show no cognitive impairment, while others perform poorly on cognitive tests. In general, the effects of depression on cognitive test performance are relatively small (e.g. Feehan et al., 1993); the term "depressive pseudodementia" can therefore be misleading, as this represents the extreme case of severe depression. Effects of depression on test performance appear to result more from a conservative response bias and a reluctance to guess for fear of being wrong than from inability to respond. Thus, response to the process of assessment may be a key factor in alerting the clinician to the likelihood of depression. A further important difference is that people with depression are more likely to report subjective concerns about cognitive dysfunction, especially problems with memory and concentration, whereas in the case of people with dementia, it is much more likely to be family members who are worried and who initiate the referral.

The Overlap between Dementia and Depression

The distinction between dementia and depression is not clear-cut. People with depression appear to have a slightly increased risk of getting dementia. Older people with depression, while not having dementia, may show cognitive impairments that prove not to be fully reversible once the depression is treated; these may be accompanied by some structural changes in the brain. People who have dementia frequently display at least some depressive symptoms, and depression is a significant source of excess disability in dementia (Ross et al., 1998); it is also possible that depressive symptoms could represent a prodrome of dementia.

Which Tests Can Help to Discriminate between Depression and Dementia?

Christensen et al. (1997) present a meta-analysis of studies assessing differences in performance between older people with depression and older people with dementia. These can be summarized as follows:

- Depression gave rise to moderate deficits on almost every type of test (with scores on average 0.64 of a SD below control performance) but the extent of the deficits varied according to type of task. People with dementia showed much larger deficits than people with depression, especially on memory tasks.

- Depression led to greater deficits on timed and speeded tasks than on untimed or non-speeded tasks. People with dementia did much worse on nonspeeded tasks than people with depression.
- For people with depression, performance tests were affected more than verbal tests, and there were difficulties in problem-solving.
- People with dementia were more likely to make false-positive errors on recognition memory tasks.
- People with depression did better on memory tasks with depressive content (where the information to be remembered was mood-congruent) than on memory tasks with neutral or pleasant content, whereas people with dementia did not show this differential effect.
- As regards specific tests, the best discriminators were paired associate learning, naming, block design and anomalous sentence repetititon.

Distinguishing Different Types of Dementia

Where it is evident that dementia is present, it is important to determine the specific type of dementia, as this has implications for intervention and care.

Alzheimer's, Vascular Dementia and Dementia with Lewy Bodies

DAT is not easily distinguished from vascular dementia or dementia with Lewy bodies on the basis of neuropsychology, and attempts to differentiate are made with reference to the history, presentation and results of medical investigations. People with vascular dementia have a history of stepwise progression, which contrasts with the gradual onset of DAT, and risk factors for vascular illness are usually present; it is important to note, though, that vascular dementia and DAT may coexist. People who have dementia with Lewy bodies show fluctuating levels of cognitive functioning and typically report characteristic types of visual hallucination which are not seen in DAT.

Alzheimer's and Frontotemporal Dementia

Neuropsychological assessment is helpful, however, in distinguishing between DAT and the frontal and temporal variants of frontotemporal dementia. The key neuropsychological and behavioural features that are observed in the early stages of each of these three forms of dementia are summarized by Hodges et al. (1999). Whereas people with early-stage DAT show severe impairments in episodic memory, mild impairments in semantic memory, verbal letter fluency, attention, executive function and working memory, and may also have subtle impairments in visuospatial perception, the profile of impairments differs markedly in the early stages of frontotemporal dementia. In the frontal variant, impairments are observed in some aspects of executive function, with mild impairments in episodic memory and verbal letter fluency, and there are progressive changes in behaviour and personality, but semantic memory and visuospatial perception are intact. In the temporal variant (often termed "semantic dementia"), there are severe impairments in semantic memory, accompanied by anomia, surface dyslexia and progressive loss of vocabulary, and these may interfere with performance on tests of other cognitive functions, but episodic memory, working memory, visuospatial perception and nonverbal problem-solving are intact, along with behaviour and personality.

Blacker et al. (1994) note, however, that the distinction is made more complex by the observation of "atypical" cases of DAT, where the first symptoms may be in word-finding, perception or praxis, with memory being much less affected than one would normally expect. Early prominent behavioural changes, however, strongly suggest that the problem is *not* DAT, but is much more likely to be frontal dementia. Where the first symptoms observed are language difficulties, the question arises as to whether this is atypical DAT or frontotemporal dementia. Blacker et al. (1994) suggest that these people should be given a diagnosis of Alzheimer's disease if the presentation is otherwise typical, but not if there are behavioural changes or other atypical features.

Components of an Assessment Battery

A good neuropsychological assessment battery aimed at distinguishing between normal ageing, depression and dementia and between different types of dementia might therefore encompass the following components, with an emphasis on nonspeeded tasks:

- Delayed recall—preferably where the information to be remembered is depressive, rather than neutral or pleasant, in content.
- Paired associate learning.
- Recognition memory.
- Semantic memory.
- Naming.
- Constructional praxis.
- Anomalous sentence repetition.
- Verbal letter fluency and category fluency.
- Executive function (abstraction, planning/organizing, set shifting, problem-solving).
- Attention (sustained, selective, divided).

Distinguishing Moderate from Severe Dementia

Understanding the severity of dementia for a given individual plays an important part in planning intervention and care. The CERAD studies (Welsh et al., 1991, 1992) demonstrated that performance on delayed recall tasks was not very useful in establishing the severity of dementia, since performance on delayed recall already showed floor effects in the early stages. For distinguishing between moderate and severe dementia, the best discriminators were verbal category fluency and constructional praxis. People with severe dementia can be assessed on the Severe Impairment Battery (Saxton et al., 1990), which permits identification of preserved areas of ability even in the very severe stages (Wild & Kaye, 1998). Similarly, Cockburn & Keene (2001) were able to identify elements of preserved memory ability in people with severe dementia using the Rivermead Behavioural Memory Test (Wilson et al., 1985).

Giving a Diagnosis

It is now fairly standard practice for carers to be told their relative's diagnosis, but the extent to which people with DAT are told of their own diagnosis remains very variable (Downs, 1999; Heal & Husband, 1998). The burden often falls on carers to decide whether to disclose. Carers may feel that they should disclose the diagnosis because the person has a right to know, or has asked for an explanation, or they may do so because the person asks an explicit question; alternatively, they may feel that disclosure would cause too much distress, or that the person is too cognitively impaired to understand, or that the news might result in a suicide attempt. In fact, although there is a risk of suicide, people with DAT do not attempt suicide at higher rates than those observed in the general population (Cohen & Eisdorfer, 1986). Professionals, too, may find it very difficult to speak honestly about the diagnosis, and may argue that it is not in the person's best interests to be told. However, as there is an increasing expectation of dialogue on an equal footing with professionals, it is likely that there will be an increasing trend for people to want to know (Goldsmith, 1996).

Certainly it is possible that disclosure could cause distress, and it is understandable that some carers may feel that witholding information is more compassionate. Failing to disclose, however, carries the implication that the person is unable to cope or to deal with difficult emotions. There are costs and risks attached to failing to disclose, including emotional distress, misunderstandings and marital discord. Furthermore, there are also possible benefits to disclosure, particularly in the earlier stages of DAT, since it may allow the person and the family to face the future in order to make decisions, settle financial and legal affairs and receive spiritual support (Cohen & Eisdorfer, 1986). Of course, the diagnostic process is characterized by uncertainty, and this does have to be taken into account. Both for this reason and for reasons connected with the psychological and social implications of attaching a label to the problem, practitioners may prefer to discuss the person's difficulties in terms of observable strengths and needs, for example referring to memory problems. In any case, if the intention is to give a diagnosis, then it is essential to do this in a sensitive manner (Downs, 1999) and to provide the appropriate back-up in terms of information, practical assistance, links with self-help and voluntary agencies, counselling and, where appropriate, psychological intervention for the person and family.

One issue often raised at the time of assessment is that of driving. Many people with early-stage dementia are able to continue to drive safely. The decision to give up driving when the appropriate time comes, however, can be very difficult for all concerned. McKenna (1998) provides a very clear account of the way in which neuropsychological assessment may contribute to an evaluation of fitness to drive, and the constraints on drawing firm conclusions. In cases of doubt, referral to a specialist driving assessment centre that offers driving assessments incorporating cognitive tasks, off-road vehicle handling and road tests may be helpful.

INTERVENTION IN DAT

The overall aims of intervention in DAT include optimizing functioning and well-being, slowing the progression of impairment, minimizing excess disability, enhancing self-efficacy and coping skills, combating threats to self-esteem, and preventing the development of a malignant social psychology in the person's support network or caregiving system. The concept of rehabilitation, implying as it does a focus on maximizing functioning across a whole range of areas, including physical health, psychological well-being, living skills and social relationships, therefore provides a unifying core concept around which to organize thinking about intervention in DAT (Cohen & Eisdorfer, 1986; Clare, 2000).

In order to begin to understand the particular psychological needs of the person with DAT, it is necessary to consider the role of cognition and emotion, personality and behaviour, life experience and preferred coping styles. There is a great deal of evidence to indicate that psychological distress is common in early-stage DAT, with high levels of anxiety and depression reported in many studies (Ross et al., 1998; Ballard et al., 1993; Burns, 1991; Wands et al., 1990). While subtle changes in behaviour and personality may result from an interaction of neurological and psychological factors (Hagberg, 1997; Hope, 1994; Teri et al., 1992; Petry et al., 1989), behavioural changes in many cases represent a manifestation of excess disability (Bleathman & Morton, 1994). Lack of social contact and environmental stimulation, perhaps resulting from loss of confidence, may contribute to lowered well-being (Woods & Britton, 1985).

Consideration of how the individual copes with the changes resulting from DAT is integral to a psychological understanding of DAT (Droes, 1997; Hagberg, 1997; Cottrell & Schulz, 1993; Woods & Britton, 1985). The development of adaptive coping strategies is important in maximizing well-being and minimizing excess disability, but the onset of DAT places major demands on coping resources. Furthermore, DAT most commonly arises at a time when the individual is negotiating development into later life, and is superimposed on the normative developmental tasks faced by the individual and family in relation to growing older, which may include reviewing one's life, achieving resolution of important themes or issues, accepting losses, and coming to terms with approaching death (Coleman, 1993, 1996). Recent studies of the phenomenological experience and coping strategies of people with early-stage DAT (Clare, 2002, 2003; Pearce et al., 2002) have demonstrated two key dimensions—the attempt to protect or maintain an existing or prior sense of identity, and the attempt to acknowledge and integrate the changes experienced in order to facilitate the development of a modified sense of identity. Understanding the current needs of each individual with respect to these tasks, and the way in which the individual perceives his/her situation, is invaluable in helping to determine what kinds of interventions may be appropriate at any given stage.

The range of psychosocial interventions that may be offered to individuals with DAT and their caregivers is considerable (for a review, see Kasl-Godley & Gatz, 2000). Approaches described in the literature include, for example, life review (Woods et al., 1992), reality orientation (Spector et al., 1998), reminiscence (Bender et al., 1998), self-maintenance therapy (Romero, 1999; Romero & Wenz, 2001), psychotherapy (Cheston, 1998; Sutton & Cheston, 1997; Knight, 1996; Hausman, 1992; Sinason, 1992), family therapy (Huckle, 1994), cognitive-behavioural therapy (Husband, 1999; Koder, 1998; Teri & Gallagher-Thompson, 1991), behavioural approaches (Bird, 2000), psychoeducational and support groups (Yale, 1995; 1999; Bourgeois et al., 1996; Brodaty & Gresham, 1989; Brodaty & Peters, 1991) and environmental modifications (Woods & Britton, 1985), as well as approaches that specifically target memory functioning. The emphasis here will be on the latter category; other approaches are discussed in detail by Bob Woods in Chapter 13, this volume. Before proceeding to a discussion of cognitive rehabilitation, however, the status of pharmacological treatments will be briefly considered.

Pharmacological treatments for DAT are now generally available, but as yet there is no agent that can either prevent the onset of DAT or provide a cure. The aim of the pharmacological treatments presently offered is to mitigate the symptoms of DAT, albeit for a limited period (Richards, 1996). Dysfunction in the cholinergic system provides the strongest association between DAT and neuronal loss, and acetylcholinesterase inhibitors have been the main focus of research (R.G. Morris, 1996). These may offer modest improvements in verbal learning and memory, psychomotor functioning and attention (Richards, 1996; Rogers et al., 1998a, 1998b; Rogers & Friedhoff, 1998; Corey-Bloom et al., 1998); such improvements might be reflected, for example, in a change of 2–3 points on a cognitive screening test such as the MMSE. It is suggested that this might represent at the most a saving of perhaps 6 months of deterioration (Bryson & Benfield, 1997). However, where improvements of one or two points on a cognitive test are evident, it is unclear to what extent this translates into meaningful differences in everyday life. If there is no improvement but performance remains stable, it is impossible to determine whether this is due to the drug or whether the same pattern would have been observed without the drug. Furthermore, there is a possibility that people who take the drug and later stop may show a precipitous decline in functioning once the drug is withdrawn, bringing them very rapidly back onto the trajectory of the untreated disorder. While the use of acetylcholinesterase inhibitors may provide modest benefits in controlled trials, the precise extent and nature of their effectiveness in any individual case is therefore difficult to determine, and side-effects remain a concern (Lovestone et al., 1997; Royal College of Psychiatrists, 1997).

In practice, it is evident that drug treatments are very limited in what they can offer at present. While rapid progress in the further development of approaches targeting the biological changes in DAT is to be expected, and more effective treatments are eagerly awaited, it is likely that psychosocial factors will remain an essential focus of intervention.

Cognitive Rehabilitation: Concept and Application

The goals of rehabilitation in DAT differ according to the needs of the individual and the severity of dementia. In the early stages, when impairments are predominantly in the cognitive domain, cognitive rehabilitation is particularly relevant, especially with regard to memory functioning. Since memory impairments are a defining feature of early-stage DAT and impact extensively on daily life and well-being (Bieliauskas, 1996), interventions targeting coping with memory difficulties are likely to have particular importance. Cognitive rehabilitation has been defined by Wilson (1997) as:

> ... any intervention strategy or technique which intends to enable clients or patients, and their families, to live with, manage, by-pass, reduce or come to terms with deficits precipitated by injury to the brain (p. 488).

The practice of cognitive rehabilitation incorporates a number of elements. Theoretical models in cognitive neuropsychology enable the identification of specific patterns of impaired and preserved functions, while experimental and clinical evidence derived from learning theory provides a basis for developing appropriate training methods. The resulting approach is often largely behavioural and goal-directed. Prigatano (1997) argues, however, that a behavioural approach is inadequate on its own, as it fails to take account of the patient's experiential world and emotional response to injury. Instead, he advocates an holistic approach, in which cognitive, emotional and motivational aspects of functioning are addressed together in an integrated manner, in acknowledgement of the complex inter-actions between them (Prigatano, 1997, 1999). This philosophy can be applied to cognitive rehabilitation in DAT. However, its expression in practical treatment approaches will need to differ somewhat from that seen in programmes for younger people with nonprogressive brain injury. Cognitive rehabilitation in DAT will require an understanding of the person's current level of awareness in order to work in a way that encourages development of ef-fective strategies and fosters personal adjustment and well-being for the person with DAT and his/her family carers, but is likely to be less confrontational and to place less emphasis on developing realistic awareness of impairments where this is limited or absent. Involving caregivers in the intervention process is essential, and this will require sensitivity to issues in family and marital relationships that may impact on the work (Quayhagen & Quayhagen, 1989, in press).

Theoretical Basis for Cognitive Rehabilitation of Memory in Early DAT

Theoretical justification for the use of cognitive rehabilitation in DAT derives from evidence regarding, first, the neuropsychology and neuroanatomy of memory impairments in DAT, which is presented by Becker & Overman (Chapter 6, this volume) and will be covered only briefly here, and second, the capacity of the person with DAT for new learning.

Consideration of memory systems in early-stage DAT shows that some subsystems are relatively preserved while others are severely impaired. In relation to long-term memory functions, episodic memory is usually severely impaired, while semantic and procedural memory may be relatively spared. This suggests, first, that there is scope for interventions aimed at improving memory functioning to build on those subsystems found to be intact, such as procedural memory. Second, compensatory methods and environmental adapta-tions may reduce the demands on explicit memory and substitute for impaired aspects of memory.

With regard to memory processes, Glisky (1998) points out that encoding, storage and retrieval are closely interrelated and difficult to separate. In general, however, the evidence suggests that the major difficulty in DAT lies in encoding, and that rates of forgetting are not significantly elevated (Christensen et al., 1998). This suggests that if appropriate help with learning designed to ensure adequate encoding can assist with getting information into the memory store, there is a reasonable likelihood of retention. Acknowledging the impairments in explicit memory, it is probable that such an approach would be most beneficial if reserved for small amounts of important information.

A review of the brain pathology observed in early-stage DAT suggests that while there are likely to be particular difficulties in linking new information with existing stored knowledge, it is possible that other brain areas may be able to take over this function if the right kind of assistance is provided at encoding (Glisky, 1998). This again suggests that the design of interventions should pay careful attention to providing strategies to ensure successful encoding. Additionally, since frontal lobe pathology affects strategic aspects of remember-ing and retrieval of stored information, it follows that people with DAT can be expected to have particular difficulty implementing strategies to help themselves remember (Bäckman, 1992). Interventions should therefore also incorporate ways of helping people with DAT to compensate for this difficulty and enhance the possibility of successful retrieval.

There is substantial experimental evidence to suggest that learning is possible in people with DAT (Woods, 1996b). Both classical and operant conditioning of responses has been demonstrated (Camp et al., 1993; Burgess et al., 1992) and people with DAT are capable of learning and retaining verbal information (Little et al., 1986). This suggests that people with DAT do have the potential to benefit from interventions targeting memory function.

Despite these positive findings, early studies in which a variety of training approaches were used produced few benefits or were interpreted negatively (see for example Yesavage, 1982; Zarit et al., 1982). Although in some cases the results could be regarded as indicating the possible value of cognitive rehabilitation as a component of early intervention, and as providing a challenge to researchers to find ways of enhancing the practical impact for those with mild DAT, some investigators concluded that there was little, if any, potential for memory improvement in DAT (Bäckman & Herlitz, 1996). Given that people with DAT appear to have the potential to learn and retain information, the question arises as to why many early experimental studies were unable to demonstrate effective facilitation of memory performance. This question has been addressed in the context of attempts to enhance performance by facilitating residual explicit memory functioning. Bäckman (1992) argues that DAT affects not only episodic memory but also the ability to make use of cognitive support for remembering. People with DAT, in contrast to healthy older adults, are impaired in their ability to use the kinds of methods that aid encoding and act as cues to facilitate retrieval. Bäckman (1992) notes that those studies that suggested that gains from memory training in DAT were small or nonexistent had generally required participants to use internal memory strategies, such as imagery or the organization of material, which in themselves require a considerable degree of cognitive effort and which are particularly difficult for the person with DAT to adopt.

The results obtained by Bäckman and colleagues indicate that when substantial support is provided both at encoding and at retrieval, termed "dual cognitive support", people with DAT can show improvements in episodic memory at all stages of severity (Bäckman, 1992). Studies attempting to enhance performance by encouraging organization of material and providing category cues indicated that people with DAT need more support than healthy older adults to enhance memory, and that the level of support required to produce an improvement increased as a function of increasing severity (Bäckman, 1996, 1992). That is, the person may need more guidance in encoding the material, and more learning trials, as well as extra prompts and cues for retrieval, compared to healthy older adults, and the amount of help required will increase as the severity of dementia increases. Previous studies failed to show benefits because they failed to provide support at both encoding and retrieval, and because they concentrated on patients with severe impairments rather than patients at earlier stages (Lipinska & Bäckman, 1997). In support of this view, a number of studies show beneficial effects of different types of cognitive support, and a number of guiding principles can be delineated (Herlitz et al., 1992); for example, memory performance is facilitated when multiple sensory modalities are involved at encoding (Karlsson et al., 1989) or where participants enact the target task (Bird & Kinsella, 1996), while, in accordance with the encoding-specificity principle, provision of retrieval cues that are compatible with conditions at encoding assists recall (R.G. Morris, 1996; Herlitz & Viitanen, 1991).

Bäckman & Herlitz (1996) argue that the ability to benefit from cognitive support in memory interventions relates to the way in which the person's knowledge structures are able to aid encoding and retrieval of episodic information. People with DAT show deficits in using semantic knowledge as an aid for episodic memory (Herlitz & Viitanen, 1991; Bäckman & Herlitz, 1990). However, people with early-stage DAT can benefit from semantic support when this is provided both at encoding and at retrieval, for example performance is facilitated when a semantic orientating task is used at encoding, followed by provision of category cues at retrieval (Lipinska & Bäckman, 1997; Bird & Luszcz, 1991, 1993). Results presented by Lipinska et al., (1994) indicate that participants performed better with self-generated than with experimenter-provided cues. Perlmuter & Monty (1989) emphasize that personalizing a task by allowing the participant to make choices about it increases perceived control and motivation, and consequently is likely to benefit performance.

A number of studies, then, demonstrate that elaboration and effortful processing can improve memory performance. It is essential, however, to consider the extent to which these effects might be harnessed to enhance functioning in real-life situations (Bird & Luszcz, 1991, 1993).

Clinical Interventions for Memory Problems in DAT

Reports of clinical interventions for memory problems in DAT provide valuable information about the suitability and effectiveness of specific rehabilitative techniques. Cognitive rehabilitation interventions are usually patient-driven and individually-designed. It is important to acknowledge that some investigators have reported positive results from general cognitive stimulation and cognitive training programmes for people with dementia (Quayhagen & Quayhagen, 1989, 2001; de Rotrou et al., 1999; Breuil et al., 1994; Moore et al., in press; Sandman, 1993). Despite the negative conclusions reached in the brain injury literature about the effectiveness of computerized cognitive remediation (Bird, 2000; Wilson, 1990; Ben-Yishay & Prigatano, 1990; Leng & Copello, 1990), there has also been a recent growth of interest in the use of computerized cognitive stimulation programmes for people with dementia (Butti et al., 1998; Hofmann et al., 1996). General cognitive stimulation programmes may, however, have more in common with the tradition of reality orientation (Spector et al., in press) than with cognitive rehabilitation. General stimulation and reality orientation programmes have been criticized on the grounds that it is not clear whether the observed small improvements in cognitive test scores translate into real-life clinical benefits (Bird, 2000). In addition, it is difficult to determine which elements of any such programme are responsible for observed improvements in particular domains. For these reasons, the present discussion will focus on individually-targeted interventions, where outcome has been assessed in relation to performance on targeted tasks rather than scores on cognitive tests, in an attempt to highlight specific techniques shown to be effective for at least some people with DAT.

Individually-targeted interventions for memory problems in DAT reported in the literature, as in the case of brain injury rehabilitation, can be grouped into three main categories: encouraging compensation through the use of external memory aids, provision of skills training to build on preserved memory ability, and facilitation of residual explicit memory functioning (Franzen & Haut, 1991). Each of these categories will be considered in turn.

Compensation using external memory aids.   Providing external support for remembering in the form of compensatory memory aids can help to reduce the demands on memory. The selection and introduction of external memory aids requires careful consideration. Aids should be targeted as specifically as possible, rather than simply providing a generalized reminder, the reason for which may be unclear to the person with DAT (Woods, 1996a). People with memory impairments are unlikely to start to use new memory aids spontaneously, and usually need training in their use, for example by means of prompting and fading of cues.

A number of studies with DAT patients have demonstrated improvements resulting from the use of various external memory aids or equivalent environmental support. In some cases these improvements have been maintained after the support has been withdrawn, while in other cases ongoing support has been required. Hanley (1986) trained in-patients with moderately advanced DAT to use a diary, reality-orientation board or personal notebook to find out personal information, although it is unclear to what extent the improvement was maintained. Bourgeois (1990, 1991, 1992) evaluated the effectiveness of memory wallets in enhancing conversational ability in a small sample of people with moderately advanced DAT, and reported significant improvements, with evidence of generalization to novel utterances. Benefits were maintained at 6 week follow-up, and for three individuals benefits were retained after 30 months. Clare et al. (2000) demonstrated that introduction of a memory aid could reduce repetitive questioning, with benefits maintained up to 6 months following the end of the intervention.

Developing technology offers increasing opportunities for identification of ingenious aids to remembering. An early example is provided by Kurlychek (1983), who used a digital watch set to beep every hour as a cue. Use of technology is now being extended beyond the realm of specific memory aids by developing computer and video equipment to monitor and control the environment of the person with dementia in order to support independent functioning (Marshall, 1999).

There is some evidence, therefore, that the use of compensatory aids may be beneficial. In view of the likely benefits of providing external support for remembering, and the potential for the development of new and more sophisticated forms of memory aid, this is clearly an area in which further research is indicated.

Skills training to optimize procedural memory functioning. The ability to perform everyday skills is particularly important in maintaining independence. Zanetti et al. (1994, 1997, 2001) used a training programme based on preserved procedural memory for rehabilitation of ADL skills in people with mild-to-moderate DAT. Training methods involved comprehensive prompting, with subsequent fading out of prompts. Preliminary results suggested this approach could be effective and produced some generalization of improvements to untrained tasks. Further evidence is provided by Josephsson et al. (1993), who used individualized training programmes for activities of daily living and showed improvements in three out of four participants, although only one maintained the gains 2 months later. An important feature of this study was the selection of tasks which were part of the patient's usual routine and which the patient was motivated to carry out. These studies show that rehabilitation strategies aimed at facilitating procedural memory offer promise in enabling people with early-stage DAT to maintain their skills and level of independence. Again, this is an area that warrants further research.

Facilitating residual long-term memory performance. Strategies for facilitating residual long-term memory performance are generally referred to as internal strategies. These have been categorized as implicit-internal or explicit-internal, depending on the extent to which they are thought to depend on implicit or explicit memory processes (Camp et al., 1993).

One important strategy for people with DAT, generally classified as implicit-internal, is expanding rehearsal. The expanding rehearsal method, termed "spaced retrieval" in the US literature, has been extensively used with people who have DAT. The act of retrieving an item of information is a powerful aid to subsequent retention under any conditions. In addition, the temporal sequencing of retrieval attempts affects the extent to which benefits are observed as a result of retrieval practice, with maximum benefit occurring when test trials are spaced at gradually expanding intervals (Landauer & Bjork, 1978). The expanding rehearsal pattern may be viewed as a shaping procedure for successively approximating the goal of unaided recall after a long delay (Camp & Stevens, 1990). An important aspect of this strategy is that it requires little cognitive effort, unlike many more elaborate mnemonic strategies. Experimental studies have demonstrated that expanding rehearsal can aid new learning in people with memory disorders following brain injury (Schacter et al., 1985). The method has been adapted for use in DAT (Camp et al., 2000; Camp, 1989), and a series of studies have demonstrated clear benefits in teaching face–name associations, object naming (Abrahams & Camp, 1993; Moffat, 1989), memory for object location, prospective memory assignments and use of memory aids (Camp, 1989). The approach has also been used to teach patients with advanced dementia living in residential settings to associate a cue with an adaptive behaviour as a means of reducing severe problem behaviours (Bird, 2000; Camp et al., 2000). A related method involves using instructional audiotapes containing biographical details to prompt rehearsal of information (Arkin,1992, 1998).

Explicit-internal strategies may be most applicable in real-life situations where support for remembering is not readily available. Strategies such as visual imagery mnemonics, chunking of information, the method of loci, the story method and initial letter cueing have been described in relation to the cognitive rehabilitation of memory disorders following brain injury, although some of these strategies may prove too difficult or demanding for many brain-injured patients (Wilson, 1995; Moffat, 1992). There is limited evidence for the success of strategies of this kind in DAT. People with DAT are likely to have difficulty both in learning an explicit mnemonic strategy of this kind and in remembering to use it appropriately (Woods, 1996a; Bäckman, 1992). It is, however, important to distinguish between the use of mnemonic strategies as a way of facilitating learning in specific tasks and the aim of developing spontaneous and independent use of the strategy in a wider sphere. The former is often a more appropriate goal in memory rehabilitation.

Successful use of a mnemonic strategy is reported by Hill et al. (1987). They describe a single case experiment in which a 66-year-old man with DAT was taught to use visual imagery to extend his retention interval for names associated with photographs of faces. When Bäckman et al. (1991) attempted to replicate the findings in a series of eight single-case studies, which included seven DAT patients, only one of the DAT patients showed training gains similar to those demonstrated by Hill et al. (1987). The authors concluded that the generalizability of the approach appears limited, but commented that there might be a subgroup of DAT patients who respond well to this form of memory training. Clare et al. (1999, 2000, 2001) demonstrated significant gains resulting from training with mnemonic strategies and expanding rehearsal in an errorless learning paradigm in a series of single-case designs, and reported long-term maintenance of treatment effects.

The evidence indicates that some approaches offer promise in facilitating residual long-term memory functioning, although gains may be circumscribed and not all patients may benefit. There is clearly scope for further development of appropriate methods that may provide assistance for people with early-stage DAT.

Effectiveness of Memory Rehabilitation

The above review highlights a number of specific methods that offer promise in facilitating memory functioning or development of compensatory behaviour. These include prompting and fading, expanding rehearsal, mnemonic or elaborative strategies, and ensuring effort-ful processing. The limitations on memory rehabilitation, even in early-stage DAT, must, however, be acknowledged (Bäckman, 1992). It is evident that the level of improvement achieved is generally modest. Individual variability is considerable; some people show no benefit from intervention, even in the early stages of the disorder, while others with ap-parently greater difficulties may improve considerably. Koltai et al. (2001) observed that, among the factors influencing outcome of cognitive rehabilitation, awareness of memory difficulties appeared to be important, and a relationship between higher levels of awareness and better outcome has been demonstrated in a prospective study (Clare et al., in press). Once again, this highlights the need to understand the phenomenological experience of the individual and target interventions accordingly.

There is at present no evidence to indicate whether memory rehabilitation has any long-term benefits in terms of reversing or arresting the progression of DAT; at best, there may be some slowing in the progression of the disease. Nonetheless, in the context of a progressive condition such as DAT, this is a highly desirable goal. A recent review of empirically validated treatments for older people (Gatz et al., 1998) identified memory therapy as a "probably efficacious treatment", a conclusion also supported by De Vreese et al. (2001). This indicates that further research is warranted to extend the evidence base, clarify outstanding questions, evaluate new methods, and develop clinically-relevant procedures.

SUMMARY AND CONCLUSIONS

Recent conceptual developments have emphasized the need to think broadly about DAT in terms of the interplay of biological and psychosocial variables, and this has important impli-cations for both assessment and intervention. Although detection and differentiation of DAT is complex, and the status of diagnostic classifications remains somewhat controversial, a neuropsychological assessment conducted within the context of a comprehensive multidis-ciplinary assessment can assist in identifying the presence of DAT and, more importantly, can contribute to developing the profile of the individual's strengths and needs that forms the basis for planning intervention and care. A review of the range of interventions available for people with DAT and their families and carers demonstrates that it is no longer possible to argue that nothing can be done. On the contrary, at any stage of DAT, appropriately-targeted interventions can provide some benefit, and cognitive rehabilitation approaches provide one important example of this. Interventions for DAT constitute a rapidly developing area, and future research can be expected to bring new hope for all those living with, and affected by, Alzheimer's disease.

REFERENCES

Abrahams, J.P. & Camp, C.J. (1993). Maintenance and generalisation of object naming training in anomia associated with degenerative dementia. *Clinical Gerontologist*, **12**, 57–72.

American Psychiatric Association. (1995). *Diagnostic and Statistical Manual of Mental Disorders*, 4th edn. Washington, DC: American Psychiatric Association.

Arendt, T. & Jones, G. (1992). Clinicopathologic correlations and the brain–behaviour relationship in Alzheimer's disease. In G.M.M. Jones & B.M.L. Miesen (eds), *Care-giving in Dementia: Research and Applications*. London: Tavistock/Routledge.

Arkin, S.M. (1992). Audio-assisted memory training with early Alzheimer's patients: two single subject experiments. *Clinical Gerontologist*, **12**, 77–96.

Arkin, S.M. (1998). Alzheimer memory training: positive results replicated. *American Journal of Alzheimer's Disease*, **13** (*March/April*), 102–104.

Bäckman, L. (1992). Memory training and memory improvement in Alzheimer's disease: rules and exceptions. *Acta Neurologica Scandinavica* (*suppl*), **139**, 84–89.

Bäckman, L. (1996). Utilizing compensatory task conditions for episodic memory in Alzheimer's disease. *Acta Neurologica Scandinavica* (*suppl*), **165**, 109–113.

Bäckman, L. & Herlitz, A. (1990). The relationship between prior knowledge and face recognition memory in normal aging and Alzheimer's disease. *Journal of Gerontology, Psychological Sciences*, **45**, P94–100.

Bäckman, L. & Herlitz, A. (1996). Knowledge and memory in Alzheimer's disease: a relationship that exists. In R.G. Morris (ed.), *The Cognitive Neuropsychology of Alzheimer-type Dementia*. Oxford: Oxford University Press.

Bäckman, L., Josephsson, S., Herlitz, A. et al. (1991). The generalisability of training gains in dementia: effects of an imagery-based mnemonic on face-name retention duration. *Psychology and Aging*, **6**, 489–492.

Ballard, C.G., Cassidy, G., Bannister, C. & Mohan, R.N.C. (1993). Prevalence, symptom profile, and aetiology of depression in dementia sufferers. *Journal of Affective Disorders*, **29**, 1–6.

Bender, M., Bauckham, P. & Norris, A. (1998). *The Therapeutic Purposes of Reminiscence*. London: Sage.

Ben-Yishay, Y. & Prigatano, G.P. (1990). Cognitive remediation. In M. Rosenthal, E.R. Griffith, M.R. Bond & J.D. Miller (eds), *Rehabilitation of the Adult and Child with Traumatic Brain Injury*. Philadelphia, PA: F.A. Davis.

Berrios, G.E. (1994a). Dementia and aging since the nineteenth century. In F.A. Huppert, C. Brayne & D.W. O'Connor (eds), *Dementia and Normal Aging*. Cambridge: Cambridge University Press.

Berrios, G.E. (1994b). Dementia: historical overview. In A. Burns & R. Levy (eds), *Dementia*. London: Chapman & Hall.

Bieliauskas, L.A. (1996). Practical approaches to ecological validity of neuropsychological measures in the elderly. In R.J. Sbordone & C.J. Long (eds), *Ecological Validity of Neuropsychological Testing*. Delray Beach, FL: GR Press/St Lucie Press.

Bird, M. (2000). Psychosocial rehabilitation for problems arising from cognitive deficits in dementia. In R.D. Hill, L. Bäckman & A.S. Neely (eds), *Cognitive Rehabilitation in Old Age*. Oxford: Oxford University Press.

Bird, M. (2001). Behavioural difficulties and cued recall of adaptive behaviour in dementia: experimental and clinical evidence. *Neuropsychological Rehabilitation*, **11**, 357–375.

Bird, M. & Kinsella, G. (1996). Long-term cued recall of tasks in senile dementia. *Psychology and Aging*, **11**, 45–56.

Bird, M. & Luszcz, M. (1991). Encoding specificity, depth of processing, and cued recall in Alzheimer's disease. *Journal of Clinical and Experimental Neuropsychology*, **13**, 508–520.

Bird, M. & Luszcz, M. (1993). Enhancing memory performance in Alzheimer's disease: acquisition assistance and cue effectiveness. *Journal of Clinical and Experimental Neuropsychology*, **15**, 921–932.

Blacker, D., Albert, M.S., Bassett, S.S. et al. (1994). Reliability and validity of NINCDS–ADRDA criteria for Alzheimer's disease. *Archives of Neurology*, **51**, 1198–1204.

Bleathman, C. & Morton, I. (1994). Psychological treatments. In A. Burns & R. Levy (eds), *Dementia*. London: Chapman & Hall.

Bourgeois, M.S. (1990). Enhancing conversation skills in patients with Alzheimer's disease using a prosthetic memory aid. *Journal of Applied Behavior Analysis*, **23**, 29–42.

Bourgeois, M.S. (1991). Communication treatment for adults with dementia. *Journal of Speech and Hearing Research*, **34**, 831–844.

Bourgeois, M.S. (1992). Evaluating memory wallets in conversations with persons with dementia. *Journal of Speech and Hearing Research*, **35** (*December*), 1344–1357.

Bourgeois, M.S., Schulz, R. & Burgio, L. (1996). Interventions for caregivers of patients with Alzheimer's disease: a review and analysis of content, process, and outcomes. *International Journal of Aging and Human Development*, **43**, 35–92.

Bowen, J., Teri, L., Kukull, W. et al. (1997). Progression to dementia in patients with isolated memory loss. *Lancet*, **349**, 763–765.

Bråne, G., Karlsson, I., Kihlgren, M. & Norberg, A. (1989). Integrity-promoting care of demented nursing home patients: psychological and biochemical changes. *International Journal of Geriatric Psychiatry*, **4**, 165–172.

Brayne, C. (1994). How common are cognitive impairment and dementia? An epidemiological viewpoint. In F.A. Huppert, C. Brayne & D.W. O'Connor (eds), *Dementia and Normal Aging*. Cambridge: Cambridge University Press.

Breuil, V., de Rotrou, J., Forette, F. et al. (1994). Cognitive stimulation of patients with dementia: preliminary results. *International Journal of Geriatric Psychiatry*, **9**, 211–217.

Brodaty, H. & Gresham, M. (1989). Effect of a training programme to reduce stress in carers of patients with dementia. *British Medical Journal*, **299**, 1375–1379.

Brodaty, H. & Peters, K. E. (1991). Cost-effectiveness of a training programme for dementia carers. *International Psychogeriatrics*, **3**, 11–22.

Bryson, H.M. & Benfield, P. (1997). Donepezil. *Drugs and Aging*, **10**, 234–239.

Burgess, I.S., Wearden, J.H., Cox, T. & Rae, M. (1992). Operant conditioning with subjects suffering from dementia. *Behavioural Psychotherapy*, **20**, 219–237.

Burns, A. (1991). Affective symptoms in Alzheimer's disease. *International Journal of Geriatric Psychiatry*, **6**, 371–376.

Burns, A. & Förstl, H. (1994). The clinical diagnosis of Alzheimer's disease. In A. Burns & R. Levy (eds), *Dementia*. London: Chapman & Hall.

Butti, G., Buzzelli, S., Fiori, M. & Giaquinto, S. (1998). Observations on mentally impaired elderly patients treated with THINKable, a computerized cognitive remediation. *Archives of Gerontology and Geriatrics (suppl)*, **6**, 49–56.

Camp, C.J. (1989). Facilitation of new learning in Alzheimer's disease. In G. Gilmore, P. Whitehouse & M. Wykle (eds), *Memory and Aging: Theory, Research and Practice*. New York: Springer.

Camp, C.J., Bird, M.J. & Cherry, K.E. (2000). Retrieval strategies as a rehabilitation aid for cognitive loss in pathological aging. In R.D. Hill, L. Backman & A.S. Neely (eds), *Cognitive Rehabilitation in Old Age*. Oxford: Oxford University Press.

Camp, C.J., Foss, J.W., Stevens, A.B. et al. (1993). Memory training in normal and demented elderly populations: the E–I–E–I–O model. *Experimental Aging Research*, **19**, 277–290.

Camp, C.J. & Stevens, A.B. (1990). Spaced retrieval: a memory intervention for dementia of the Alzheimer's type (DAT). *Clinical Gerontologist*, **10**, 58–61.

Carswell, A. & Spiegel, R. (1999). Functional assessment. In G.K. Wilcock, R.S. Bucks & K. Rockwood (eds), *Diagnosis and Management of Dementia: a Manual for Memory Disorders Teams*. Oxford: Oxford University Press.

Cheston, R. (1998). Psychotherapeutic work with people with dementia: a review of the literature. *British Journal of Medical Psychology*, **71**, 211–231.

Christensen, H., Griffiths, K., MacKinnon, A. & Jacomb, P. (1997). A quantitative review of cognitive deficits in depression and Alzheimer-type dementia. *Journal of the International Neuropsychological Society*, **3**, 631–651.

Christensen, H., Kopelman, M.D., Stanhope, N. et al. (1998). Rates of forgetting in Alzheimer dementia. *Neuropsychologia*, **36**, 547–557.

Clare, L. (2002). We'll fight it as long as we can: coping with the onset of Alzheimer's disease. *Aging and Mental Health*, **6**, 139–148.

Clare, L. (2003). Managing threats to self: awareness in early-stage Alzheimer's disease. *Social Science and Medicine*, **57**, 1017–1029.

Clare, L., Wilson, B.A., Breen, K. & Hodges, J.R. (1999). Errorless learning of face-name associations in early Alzheimer's disease. *Neurocase*, **5**, 37–46.

Clare, L., Wilson, B.A., Carter, G. et al. (2000). Intervening with everyday memory problems in early Alzheimer's disease: an errorless learning approach. *Journal of Clinical and Experimental Neuropsychology*, **22**, 132–146.

Clare, L., Wilson, B.A., Carter, G. et al. (2001). Long-term maintenance of treatment gains following a cognitive rehabilitation intervention in early dementia of Alzheimer type: a single case study. *Neuropsychological Rehabilitation*, **11**, 477–494.

Clare, L., Wilson, B.A., Carter, G., Ruth, I. & Hodges, J.R. (in press). Awareness in early-stage Alzheimer's disease: relationship to outcome of cognitive rehabilitation. *Journal of Clinical and Experimental Neuropsychology*.

Clarke, C., Sheppard, L., Fillenbaum, G. et al. & the CERAD Investigators. (1999). Variability in annual Mini-Mental State Examination score in patients with probable Alzheimer disease. *Archives of Neurology*, **56**, 857–862.

Cockburn, J. & Keene, J. (2001). Are changes in everyday memory over time in autopsy confirmed Alzheimer's disease related to changes in reported behaviour? *Neuropsychological Rehabilitation*, **11**, 201–217.

Cohen, D. & Eisdorfer, C. (1986). *The Loss of Self: a Family Resource for the Care of Alzheimer's Disease and Related Disorders*. New York: W.W. Norton.

Cohen, G. (1996). Memory and learning in normal ageing. In R.T. Woods (ed.), *Handbook of the Clinical Psychology of Ageing*. Chichester: Wiley.

Coleman, P.G. (1993). Adjustment in later life. In J. Bond, P.G. Coleman, & S. Peace (eds), *Ageing in Society: Introduction to Social Gerontology* (2nd edn). London: Sage.

Coleman, P.G. (1996). Identity management in later life. In R.T. Woods (ed.), *Handbook of the Clinical Psychology of Ageing*. Chichester: Wiley.

Corey-Bloom, J., Anand, R. & Veatch, J. for the ENA713 B352 Study Group. (1998). A randomised trial evaluating the efficacy and safety of ENA713 (rivastigmine tartrate), a new acetylcholinesterase inhibitor, in patients with mild to moderately severe Alzheimer's disease. *International Journal of Geriatric Psychopharmacology*, **1**, 55–65.

Cottrell, V. & Schulz, R. (1993). The perspective of the patient with Alzheimer's disease: a neglected dimension of dementia research. *Gerontologist*, **33**, 205–211.

Cox, S. & Keady, J. (eds) (1999). *Younger People with Dementia: Planning, Practice and Development*. London: Jessica Kingsley.

de Rotrou, J., Frambourt, A., de Susbielle, D. et al. (1999). La stimulation cognitive. In Fondation Nationale de Gérontologie (ed.), *La Maladie d'Alzheimer: Prédiction, Prévention, Prise en Charge. 10ème Congrès de la Fondation Nationale de Gérontologie*. Paris: Fondation Nationale de Gérontologie.

De Vreese, L.P., Neri, H., Fioravanti, M., Belloi, L. & Zanetti, O. (2001). Memory rehabilitation in Alzheimer's disease: a review of progress. *International Journal of Genatric Psychiatry*, **16**, 794–809.

Downs, M. (1999). How to tell? Disclosing a diagnosis of dementia. *Generations*, **23**(3), 30–34.

Droes, R.M. (1997). Psychosocial treatment for demented patients: overview of methods and effects. In B.M.L. Miesen & G.M.M. Jones (eds), *Care-giving in Dementia: Research and Applications*, Vol. 2. London: Routledge.

Feehan, M., Knight, R.G. & Partridge, F.M. (1993). Cognitive complaint and test performance in elderly patients suffering from depression or dementia. *International Journal of Geriatric Psychiatry*, **6**, 287–293.

Folstein, M.F., Folstein, S.E. & McHugh, P.R. (1975). "Mini-Mental State": a practical method for grading the cognitive state of patients for the clinician. *Journal of Psychiatric Research*, **12**, 189–198.

Fox, N.C., Warrington, E.K., Seiffer, A.L. et al. (1998). Presymptomatic cognitive deficits in individuals at risk of familial Alzheimer's disease: a longitudinal prospective study. *Brain*, **121**, 1631–1639.

Franzen, M.D. & Haut, M.W. (1991). The psychological treatment of memory impairment: a review of empirical studies. *Neuropsychology Review*, **2**, 29–63.

Gatz, M., Fiske, A., Fox, L. et al. (1998). Empirically validated psychological treatments for older adults. *Journal of Mental Health and Aging*, **4**, 9–45.

Gilliard, J. & Rabins, P.V. (1999). Carer support. In G.K. Wilcock, R.S. Bucks & K. Rockwood (eds), *Diagnosis and Management of Dementia: a Manual for Memory Disorders Teams*. Oxford: Oxford University Press.

Glisky, E.L. (1998). Differential contribution of frontal and medial temporal lobes to memory: evidence from focal lesions and normal aging. In N. Raz (ed.), *The Other Side of the Error Term*. Amsterdam: Elsevier North Holland.

Golding, E. (1989). *The Middlesex Elderly Assessment of Mental State*. Bury St Edmunds: Thames Valley Test Company.

Goldsmith, M. (1996). *Hearing the Voice of People with Dementia: Opportunities and Obstacles*. London: Jessica Kingsley.

Greene, J.D.W., Baddeley, A. & Hodges, J.R. (1996). Analysis of the episodic memory deficit in early Alzheimer's disease: evidence from the Doors and People Test. *Neuropsychologia*, **34**, 537–551.

Greene, J.D.W., Hodges, J.R. & Baddeley, A.D. (1995). Autobiographical memory and executive function in early dementia of Alzheimer type. *Neuropsychologia*, **33**, 1647–1670.

Gubrium, J.F. (1987). Structuring and destructuring the course of illness: the Alzheimer's disease experience. *Sociology of Health and Illness*, **9**, 1–24.

Hagberg, B. (1997). The dementias in a psychodynamic perspective. In B.M.L. Miesen & G.M.M. Jones (eds), *Care-giving in Dementia: Research and Applications*, Vol. 2. London: Routledge.

Hamilton, H.E. (1994). *Conversations with an Alzheimer's Patient: an Interactional Sociolinguistic Study*. Cambridge: Cambridge University Press.

Hanley, I. (1986). Reality orientation in the care of the elderly patient with dementia—three case studies. In I. Hanley & M. Gilhooly (eds), *Psychological Therapies for the Elderly*. Beckenham: Croom Helm.

Harvey, R.J. (1998). *Young Onset Dementia: Epidemiology, Clinical Symptoms, Family Burden, Support and Outcome*. London: Imperial College of Science and Technology & NHS Executive North Thames.

Hausman, C. (1992). Dynamic psychotherapy with elderly demented patients. In G.M.M. Jones & B.M.L. Miesen (eds), *Care-giving in Dementia: Research and Applications*, Vol. 1. London: Tavistock/Routledge.

Heal, H.C., & Husband, H.J. (1998). Disclosing a diagnosis of dementia: is age a factor? *Aging and Mental Health*, **2**, 144–150.

Henderson, A.S. & Sartorius, N. (1994). International criteria and differential diagnosis. In F. Huppert, C. Brayne & D.W. O'Connor (eds), *Dementia and Normal Aging*. Cambridge: Cambridge University Press.

Herlitz, A., Lipinska, B. & Bäckman, L. (1992). Utilization of cognitive support for episodic remembering in Alzheimer's disease. In L. Bäckman (ed.), *Memory Functioning in Dementia*. Amsterdam: Elsevier.

Herlitz, A. & Viitanen, M. (1991). Semantic organisation and verbal episodic memory in patients with mild and moderate Alzheimer's disease. *Journal of Clinical and Experimental Neuropsychology*, **13**, 559–574.

Heston, L.L., & White, J.A. (1991). *The Vanishing Mind: a Practical Guide to Alzheimer's Disease and Other Dementias*. New York: W.H. Freeman.

Hill, R.D., Evankovich, K.D., Sheikh, J.I. & Yesavage, J.A. (1987). Imagery mnemonic training in a patient with primary degenerative dementia. *Psychology and Aging*, **2**, 204–205.

Hodges, J.R. (1994). *Cognitive Assessment for Clinicians*. Oxford: Oxford University Press.

Hodges, J.R., Patterson, K., Ward, R. et al. (1999). The differentiation of semantic dementia and frontal lobe dementia (temporal and frontal variants of frontotemporal dementia) from early Alzheimer's disease: a comparative neuropsychological study. *Neuropsychology*, **13**, 31–40.

Hofmann, M., Hock, C., Kuhler, A. & Muller-Spahn, F. (1996). Interactive computer-based cognitive training in patients with Alzheimer's disease. *Journal of Psychiatric Research*, **30**, 493–501.

Hope, T. (1994). Personality and behaviour in dementia and normal aging. In F. Huppert, C. Brayne & D.W. O'Connor (eds), *Dementia and Normal Aging*. Cambridge: Cambridge University Press.

Huckle, P.L. (1994). Families and dementia. *International Journal of Geriatric Psychiatry*, **9**, 735–741.

Hughes, C., Berg, L., Danziger, W. et al. (1982). A new clinical scale for the staging of dementia. *British Journal of Psychiatry*, **140**, 566–572.

Huppert, F.A. (1994). Memory function in dementia and normal aging—dimension or dichotomy? In F.A. Huppert, C. Brayne & D.W. O'Connor (eds), *Dementia and Normal Aging*. Cambridge: Cambridge University Press.

Husband, H.J. (1999). The psychological consequences of learning a diagnosis of dementia: three case examples. *Aging and Mental Health*, **3**, 179–183.

Iliffe, S. (1997). Can delays in the recognition of dementia in primary care be avoided? *Aging and Mental Health*, **1**, 7–10.

Josephsson, S., Bäckman, L., Borell, L. et al. (1993). Supporting everyday activities in dementia: an intervention study. *International Journal of Geriatric Psychiatry*, **8**, 395–400.

Karlsson, I., Bråne, G., Melin, E. et al. (1988). Effects of environmental stimulation on biochemical and psychological variables in dementia. *Acta Psychiatrica Scandinavica*, **77**, 207–213.

Karlsson, T., Bäckman, L., Herlitz, A., Nilsson, L.-G., Winblad, B. & Osterlind, P.-O. (1989). Memory improvement at different stages of Alzheimer's disease. *Neuropsychologia*, **27**, 737–742.

Kasl-Godley, J. & Gatz, M. (2000). Psychosocial interventions for individuals with dementia: an integration of theory, therapy, and a clinical understanding of dementia. *Clinical Psychology Review*, **20**, 755–782.

Kay, D.W.K. (1991). The epidemiology of dementia: a review of recent work. *Reviews in Clinical Gerontology*, **1**, 55–66.

Kendrick, D. & Watts, G. (1999). *The Kendrick Assessment Scales of Cognitive Ageing*, 2nd edn. Windsor: NFER-Nelson.

Kitwood, T. (1996). A dialectical framework for dementia. In R.T. Woods (ed.), *Handbook of the Clinical Psychology of Ageing*. Chichester: Wiley.

Kitwood, T. (1997). *Dementia Reconsidered: the Person Comes First*. Buckingham: Open University Press.

Knight, B. (1996). *Psychotherapy with Older Adults*, 2nd edn. Beverly Hills, CA: Sage.

Koder, D.-A. (1998). Treatment of anxiety in the cognitively impaired elderly: can cognitive-behavior therapy help? *International Psychogeriatrics*, **10**, 173–182.

Koltai, D.C., Welsh-Bohmer, K.A. & Schmechel, D.E. (2001). Influence of anosognosia on treatment outcome among dementia patients. *Neuropsychological Rehabilitation*, **11**, 455–475.

Kurlychek, R.T. (1983). Use of a digital alarm chronograph as a memory aid in early dementia. *Clinical Gerontologist*, **1**, 93–94.

Landauer, T.K. & Bjork, R.A. (1978). Optimum rehearsal patterns and name learning. In K.M. Gruneberg, P.E. Morris & R.N. Sykes (eds), *Practical Aspects of Memory*. New York: Academic Press.

Leng, N.R.C. & Copello, A.G. (1990). Rehabilitation of memory after brain injury: is there an effective technique? *Clinical Rehabilitation*, **4**, 63–69.

Lezak, M.D. (1995). *Neuropsychological Assessment*, 3rd edn. New York: Oxford University Press.

Lipinska, B. & Bäckman, L. (1997). Encoding-retrieval interactions in mild Alzheimer's disease: the role of access to categorical information. *Brain and Cognition*, **34**, 274–286.

Lipinska, B., Bäckman, L., Mantyla, T. & Viitanen, M. (1994). Effectiveness of self-generated cues in early Alzheimer's disease. *Journal of Clinical and Experimental Neuropsychology*, **16**, 809–819.

Little, A. & Doherty, B. (1996). Going beyond cognitive assessment: assessment of adjustment, behaviour and the environment. In R.T. Woods (ed.), *Handbook of the Clinical Psychology of Ageing*. Chichester: Wiley.

Little, A.G., Volans, P.J., Hemsley, D.R. & Levy, R. (1986). The retention of new information in senile dementia. *British Journal of Clinical Psychology*, **25**, 71–72.

Lovestone, S., Graham, N. & Howard, R. (1997). Guidelines on drug treatments for Alzheimer's disease. *Lancet*, **350**, 232–233.

Marshall, M. (1999). Person centred technology? *Signpost*, **3**(4), 4–5.

McKenna, P. (1998). Fitness to drive: a neuropsychological perspective. *Journal of Mental Health*, **7**, 9–18.

McKhann, G., Drachman, D., Folstein, M. et al. (1984). Clinical diagnosis of Alzheimer's disease: report of the NINCDS–ADRDA Work Group under the auspices of Department of Health and Human Services task force on Alzheimer's disease. *Neurology*, **34**, 939–944.

Miller, E. (1996). The assessment of dementia. In R. Morris (ed.), *The Cognitive Neuropsychology of Alzheimer-type Dementia*. Oxford: Oxford University Press.

Moffat, N. (1989). Home-based cognitive rehabilitation with the elderly. In L.W. Poon, D.C. Rubin & B.A. Wilson (eds), *Everyday Cognition in Adulthood and Late Life*. Cambridge: Cambridge University Press.

Moffat, N. (1992). Strategies of memory therapy. In B.A. Wilson & N. Moffat (eds), *Clinical Management of Memory Problems*, 2nd edn. London: Chapman & Hall.

Molloy, D.W., Alemayehu, E. & Roberts, R. (1991). Reliability of a standardized Mini-Mental State Examination compared with the traditional Mini-Mental State Examination. *American Journal of Psychiatry*, **148**, 102–105.

Moniz-Cook, E., Agar, S., Gibson, G. et al. (1998). A preliminary study of the effects of early intervention with people with dementia and their families in a memory clinic. *Aging and Mental Health*, **2**, 199–211.

Moniz-Cook, E. & Woods, R.T. (1997). The role of memory clinics and psychosocial intervention in the early stages of dementia. *International Journal of Geriatric Psychiatry*, **12**, 1143–1145.

Moore, S., Sandman, C., McGrady, K. & Kesslak, P. (2001). Memory training improves cognitive ability in patients with dementia. *Neuropsychological Rehabilitation*, **11**, 245–261.

Morris, J.C. (1996). Classification of dementia and Alzheimer's disease. *Acta Neurologica Scandinavica (Suppl)*, **165**, 41–50.

Morris, R.G. (1996). The neuropsychology of Alzheimer's disease and related dementias. In R.T. Woods (ed.), *Handbook of the Clinical Psychology of Ageing*. Chichester: Wiley.

Morris, R.G. & McKiernan, F. (1994). Neuropsychological investigations of dementia. In A. Burns & R. Levy (eds), *Dementia*. London: Chapman & Hall.

Neary, D., Snowden, J.S., Bowen, D.M. et al. (1986). Neuropsychological syndromes in presenile dementia due to cerebral atrophy. *Journal of Neurology, Neurosurgery, and Psychiatry*, **49**, 163–174.

O'Brien, J., Ames, D., Chiu, E. et al. (1998). Severe deep white matter lesions and outcome in elderly patients with major depressive disorder: follow-up study. *British Medical Journal*, **317**, 982–984.

O'Brien, J., Desmond, P., Ames, D. et al. (1996). A magnetic resonance imaging study of white matter lesions in depression and Alzheimer's disease. *British Journal of Psychiatry*, **168**, 477–485.

O'Connor, D.W. (1994). Mild dementia: a clinical perspective. In F. Huppert, C. Brayne & D.W. O'Connor (eds), *Dementia and Normal Aging*. Cambridge: Cambridge University Press.

Pearce, A., Clare, L. & Pistrang, N. (2002). Managing sense of self: coping in the early stages of Alzheimer's disease. *Dementia*, **1**, 173–192.

Perlmuter, L.C. & Monty, R.A. (1989). Motivation and aging. In L.W. Poon, D.C. Rubin & B.A. Wilson (eds), *Everyday Cognition in Adulthood and Late Life*. Cambridge: Cambridge University Press.

Perry, R.J. & Hodges, J.R. (1999). Attention and executive deficits in Alzheimer's disease: a critical review. *Brain*, **122**, 383–404.

Petry, S., Cummings, J.L., Hill, M.A. & Shapira, J. (1989). Personality alterations in dementia of the Alzheimer type: a three-year follow-up study. *Journal of Geriatric Psychiatry and Neurology*, **2**, 203–207.

Pollitt, P.A. (1996). Dementia in old age: an anthropological perspective. *Psychological Medicine*, **26**, 1061–1074.

Prigatano, G.P. (1997). Learning from our successes and failures: reflections and comments on "Cognitive rehabilitation: how it is and how it might be". *Journal of the International Neuropsychological Society*, **3**, 497–499.

Prigatano, G.P. (1999). *Principles of Neuropsychological Rehabilitation*. New York: Oxford University Press.

Quayhagen, M.P. & Quayhagen, M. (1989). Differential effects of family-based strategies on Alzheimer's disease. *Gerontologist*, **29**, 150–155.

Quayhagen, M.P. & Quayhagen, M. (2001). Testing of a cognitive stimulation intervention for dementia caregiving dyads. *Neuropsychological Rehabilitation*, **11**, 319–332.

Rait, G., Walters, K. & Iliffe, S. (1999). The diagnosis and management of dementia in primary care: issues in education, service development, and research. *Generations*, **23** (3), 17–23.

Reifler, B.V. & Larson, E. (1990). Excess disability in dementia of the Alzheimer's type. In E. Light & B.D. Lebowitz (eds), *Alzheimer's Disease Treatment and Family Stress*. New York: Hemisphere.

Reisberg, B., Ferris, S.H., Leon, M.J. de & Crook, T. (1982). The global deterioration scale for assessment of primary degenerative dementia. *American Journal of Psychiatry*, **139**, 1136–1139.

Richards, M. (1996). Neurobiological treatment of Alzheimer's disease. In R. Morris (ed.), *The Cognitive Neuropsychology of Alzheimer-type Dementia*. Oxford: Oxford University Press.

Rogers, S.L. et al. & the Donepezil Study Group. (1998a). Donepezil improves cognition and global function in Alzheimer disease: a 15-week, double-blind, placebo-controlled study. *Archives of Internal Medicine*, **158**, 1021–1034.

Rogers, S.L. et al. & the Donepezil Study Group (1998b). A 24-week, double-blind, placebo-controlled trial of donepezil in patients with Alzheimer's disease. *Neurology*, **50**, 136–145.

Rogers, S.L. & Friedhoff, L.T. (1998). Long-term efficacy and safety of donepezil in the treatment of Alzheimer's disease: an interim analysis of the results of a US multicentre open label extension study. *European Neuropsychopharmacology*, **8**, 67–75.

Romero, B. (1999). Rehabilitative Ansätze bei Alzheimer-Krankheit: die Selbsterhaltungstherapie. In P. Frommelt & H. Grötzbach (eds), *Neurorehabilitation: Grundlagen, Praxis, Dokumentation*. Berlin: Blackwell Wissenschafts-Verlag.

Romero, B. & Wenz, M. (2001). Self-maintenance therapy in Alzheimer's disease. *Neuropsychological Rehabilitation*, **11**, 333–355.

Ross, L.K., Arnsberger, P. & Fox, P.J. (1998). The relationship between cognitive functioning and disease severity with depression in dementia of the Alzheimer's type. *Aging and Mental Health*, **2**, 319–327.

Roth, M., Huppert, F.A., Mountjoy, C.Q. & Tym, E. (1999). *The Revised Cambridge Examination for Mental Disorders of the Elderly*, 2nd edn. Cambridge: Cambridge University Press.

Roth, M. (1994). The relationship between dementia and normal aging of the brain. In F.A. Huppert, C. Brayne & D.W. O'Connor (eds), *Dementia and Normal Aging*. Cambridge: Cambridge University Press.

Royal College of Psychiatrists (1997). Interim statement on anti-dementia drugs: implications, concerns and policy proposals. *Psychiatric Bulletin*, **21**, 586–587.

Sabat, S.R. (1994). Excess disability and malignant social psychology: a case study of Alzheimer's disease. *Journal of Community and Applied Social Psychology*, **4**, 157–166.

Sabat, S.R. (1995). The Alzheimer's disease sufferer as a semiotic subject. *Philosophy, Psychiatry, and Psychology*, **1**, 145–160.

Sabat, S.R. & Harré, R. (1992). The construction and deconstruction of self in Alzheimer's disease. *Ageing and Society*, **12**, 443–461.

Sabat, S.R., Wiggs, C. & Pinizzotto, A. (1984). Alzheimer's disease: clinical vs. observational studies of cognitive ability. *Journal of Clinical and Experimental Gerontology*, **6**, 337–359.

Sandman, C.A. (1993). Memory rehabilitation in Alzheimer's disease: preliminary findings. *Clinical Gerontologist*, **13**, 19–33.

Saxton, J., Swihart, A., McGonigle-Gibson, K. et al. (1990). Assessment of the severely impaired patient: description and validation of a new neuropsychological test battery. *Psychological Assessment*, **2**, 298–303.

Schacter, D.L., Rich, S.A. & Stampp, M.S. (1985). Remediation of memory disorders: experimental evaluation of the spaced-retrieval technique. *Journal of Clinical and Experimental Neuropsychology*, **7**, 79–96.

Schneck, M.K., Reisberg, B. & Ferris, S.H. (1982). An overview of current concepts of Alzheimer's disease. *American Journal of Psychiatry*, **139**, 165–173.

Sevush, S. & Leve, N. (1993). Denial of memory deficit in Alzheimer's disease. *American Journal of Psychiatry*, **150**, 748–751.

Sinason, V. (1992). *Mental Handicap and the Human Condition: New Approaches from the Tavistock*. London: Free Association Books.

Sixsmith, A., Stilwell, J. & Copeland, J. (1993). "Rementia": challenging the limits of dementia care. *International Journal of Geriatric Psychiatry*, **8**, 993–1000.

Small, G.W., Rabins, P.V., Barry, P.P. et al. (1997). Diagnosis and treatment of Alzheimer disease and related disorders: consensus statement of the American Association for Geriatric Psychiatry, the Alzheimer's Association and the American Geriatric Society. *Journal of the American Medical Association*, **278**, 1363–1371.

Snaith, R.P. & Zigmond, A.S. (1994). *The Hospital Anxiety and Depression Scale*. Windsor: NFER-Nelson.

Spector, A., Orrell, M., Davies, S. & Woods, B. (2001). Can reality orientation be rehabilitated? Development and piloting of an evidence-based programme of cognition-based therapies for people with dementia. *Neuropsychological Rehabilitation*, **11**, 377–397.

Spector, A., Orrell, M., Davies, S. & Woods, R.T. (1998). *Reality Orientation for Dementia: a Review of the Evidence for Its Effectiveness* (Issue 4). Oxford: Update Software.

Spreen, O. & Strauss, E. (1998). *A Compendium of Neuropsychological Tests: Administration, Norms and Commentary*, 2nd edn. Oxford: Oxford University Press.

Storandt, M. & Hill, R.D. (1989). Very mild senile dementia of the Alzheimer type. II. Psychometric test performance. *Archives of Neurology*, **46**, 383–386.

Storandt, M., Morris, J.C., Rubin, E.H. et al. (1992). Progression of senile dementia of the Alzheimer type on a battery of psychometric tests. In L. Bäckman (ed.), *Memory Functioning in Dementia*. Amsterdam: Elsevier.

Sutton, L.J. & Cheston, R. (1997). Rewriting the story of dementia: a narrative approach to psychotherapy with people with dementia. In M. Marshall (ed.), *State of the Art in Dementia Care*. London: Centre for Policy on Ageing.

Teri, L. & Gallagher-Thompson, D. (1991). Cognitive-behavioral interventions for treatment of depression in Alzheimer's patients. *Gerontologist*, **31**, 413–416.

Teri, L., Truax, P., Logsdon, R. et al. (1992). Assessment of behavioral problems in dementia: the revised memory and behavior problems checklist. *Psychology and Aging*, **7**, 622–631.

Thompson, P., Inglis, F., Findlay, D. et al. (1997). Memory clinic attenders: a review of 150 consecutive patients. *Aging and Mental Health*, **1**, 181–183.

Tierney, M.C., Szalai, J.P., Snow, W.G. & Fisher, R.H. (1996). The prediction of Alzheimer disease. *Archives of Neurology*, **53**, 423–427.

Trenerry, M.R., Crosson, B., DeBoe, J. & Leber, W.R. (1989). Stroop Neuropsychological Screening Test. Odessa, FL: Psychological Assessment Resources.

van der Cammen, T.J.M., Simpson, J.M., Fraser, R.M. et al. (1987). The memory clinic: a new approach to the detection of dementia. *British Journal of Psychiatry*, **150**, 359–364.

van Hout, H., Vernooij-Dassen, M., Bakker, K. et al. (2000). General practitioners on dementia: tasks, practices and obstacles. *Patient Education and Counselling*, **39**, 219–225.

Vitaliano, P.P., Young, H.M. & Russo, J. (1991). Burden: a review of measures used among caregivers of individuals with dementia. *Gerontologist*, **31**, 67–75.

Wands, K., Merskey, H., Hachinski, V. et al. (1990). A questionnaire investigation of anxiety and depression in early dementia. *Journal of the American Geriatrics Society*, **38**, 535–538.

Welsh, K., Butters, N., Hughes, J. & Mohs, R. (1992). Detection and staging of dementia in Alzheimer's disease: use of the neuropsychological measures developed for the Consortium to Establish a Registry for Alzheimer's Disease. *Archives of Neurology*, **49**, 448–452.

Welsh, K., Butters, N., Hughes, J. et al. (1991). Detection of abnormal memory decline in mild cases of Alzheimer's disease using CERAD neuropsychological measures. *Archives of Neurology*, **48**, 278–281.

Whitehouse, P.J., Lerner, A. & Hedera, P. (1993). Dementia. In K.M. Heilman & E. Valenstein (eds), *Clinical Neuropsychology*. Oxford: Oxford University Press.

Wilcock, G.K., Bucks, R.S. & Rockwood, K. (1999). *Diagnosis and Management of Dementia: a Manual for Memory Disorders Teams*. Oxford: Oxford University Press.

Wild, K.V. & Kaye, J.A. (1998). The rate of progression of Alzheimer's disease in the later stages: evidence from the Severe Impairment Battery. *Journal of the International Neuropsychological Society*, **4**, 512–516.

Wilson, B.A. (1990). Cognitive rehabilitation for brain injured adults. In B.G. Deelman, R.J. Saan & A.H. van Zomeren (eds), *Traumatic Brain Injury: Clinical, Social and Rehabilitational Aspects.* Amsterdam: Swets & Zeitlinger.

Wilson, B.A. (1995). Management and remediation of memory problems in brain-injured adults. In A.D. Baddeley, B.A. Wilson & F.N. Watts (eds), *Handbook of Memory Disorders*, 1st edn. Chichester: Wiley.

Wilson, B.A. (1997). Cognitive rehabilitation: how it is and how it might be. *Journal of the International Neuropsychological Society*, **3**, 487–496.

Wilson, B.A., Cockburn, J. & Baddeley, A.D. (1985). *The Rivermead Behavioural Memory Test.* Bury St Edmunds: Thames Valley Test Company.

Woods, B., Portnoy, S., Head, D. & Jones, G. (1992). Reminiscence and life review with persons with dementia: which way forward? In G.M.M. Jones & B.M.L. Miesen (eds), *Care-giving in Dementia: Research and Applications*, Vol. 1. London: Tavistock/Routledge.

Woods, R.T. (1996a). Mental health problems in late life. In R.T. Woods (ed.), *Handbook of the Clinical Psychology of Ageing.* Chichester: Wiley.

Woods, R.T. (1996b). Psychological "therapies" in dementia. In R.T. Woods (ed.), *Handbook of the Clinical Psychology of Ageing.* Chichester: Wiley.

Woods, R.T. & Britton, P.G. (1985). *Clinical Psychology with the Elderly.* London: Croom Helm.

World Health Organization. (1992). *The ICD-10 Classification of Mental and Behavioural disorders: Clinical Descriptions and Diagnostic Guidelines.* Geneva: World Health Organization, Division of Mental Health.

Wright, N. & Lindesay, J. (1995). A survey of memory clinics in the British Isles. *International Journal of Geriatric Psychiatry*, **10**, 379–385.

Yale, R. (1995). *Developing Support Groups for Individuals with Early Stage Alzheimer's Disease: Planning, Implementation and Evaluation.* Baltimore, MD: Health Professions Press.

Yale, R. (1999). Support groups and other services for individuals with early-stage Alzheimer's disease. *Generations*, **23**(3), 57–61.

Yesavage, J.A. (1982). Degree of dementia and improvement with memory training. *Clinical Gerontology*, **1**, 77–81.

Yesavage, J.A., Brink, T.L., Rose, T.L. et al. (1983). Development and validation of a geriatric depression screening scale: a preliminary report. *Journal of Psychiatric Research*, **17**, 37–49.

Zanetti, O., Binetti, G., Magni, E. et al. (1997). Procedural memory stimulation in Alzheimer's disease: impact of a training programme. *Acta Neurologica Scandinavica*, **95**, 152–157.

Zanetti, O., Magni, E., Binetti, G. et al. (1994). Is procedural memory stimulation effective in Alzheimer's disease? *International Journal of Geriatric Psychiatry*, **9**, 1006–1007.

Zanetti, O., Zanieri, G., de Giovanni, G. et al. (2001). Effectiveness of procedural memory stimulation in mild Alzheimer's disease patients: a controlled study. *Neuropsychological Rehabilitation*, **11**, 263–272.

Zarit, S.H., Zarit, J.M. & Reever, K.E. (1982). Memory training for severe memory loss: effects on senile dementia patients and their families. *Gerontologist*, **22**, 373–377.

CHAPTER 13

Reducing the Impact of Cognitive Impairment in Dementia

Bob Woods

Dementia Services Development Centre, University of Wales Bangor, UK

Whilst in their early stages the dementias may be thought of as primarily "memory disorders", diagnostic definitions of a dementia in fact require "global" impairment of cognitive functions. In practice, this may mean memory plus one or two other areas of difficulty (American Psychiatric Association, 1994). The impact of a dementing disorder extends far beyond memory, and indeed many accounts now emphasize the importance of noncognitive features, such as depression, psychotic phenomena, behaviour problems and personality changes in contributing to the strain experienced by family caregivers and in reducing quality of life for the person with dementia. Interventions with people with dementia and their caregivers must, accordingly, have a broad focus if they are to be widely applicable.

Generally, dementing disorders are progressive, although the rate and pattern of change may vary greatly between individuals. This poses a particular difficulty for rehabilitation efforts, which need to be flexible enough to assist the person and caregivers in coping with and adjusting to both day-to-day fluctuations and longer-term deterioration. Maintaining function may be a valid target, rather than necessarily seeking improvements. Careful selection of targets for intervention that will make a real difference to the person's quality of life is also important, in order to maximize the usefulness of therapeutic input.

This chapter aims to outline broad psychosocial strategies for maximizing function in people with dementia, and to examine the evidence for their effectiveness and utility. The first section describes how the care environment might be adapted to support the person's cognitive abilities. Subsequent sections examine the two major cognitive approaches that have seen widespread use in the dementia care field—Reality orientation (RO) and reminiscence. Finally, the interplay between cognitive approaches and noncognitive features, specifically affect and behaviour problems, will be considered. Individually-tailored memory training programmes, using procedures such as spaced retrieval and errorless learning, which constitute a major and welcome development in this field, are considered by Clare in Chapter 12 (this volume).

The Essential *Handbook of Memory Disorders for Clinicians.* Edited by A.D. Baddeley, M.D. Kopelman and B.A. Wilson.
© 2004 John Wiley & Sons, Ltd. ISBN 0-470-09141-X.

THE CARE ENVIRONMENT

Environmental Design and Dementia

Lawton's "environmental docility" model (Parmelee & Lawton, 1990) suggests that persons with dementia are more likely than average persons to be shaped by and vulnerable to environmental contingencies, because of their lowered competence and function. Those with intact cognitive function are thought to be more able to shape the environment to suit their individual needs; those with dementia are much more vulnerable to the impact of their physical, social and interpersonal surroundings.

How can the care environment be designed to be more dementia-friendly? There has been great interest in this topic in recent years (Carr & Marshall, 1993). Potential environmental adaptations include simplifying the locating of important rooms and places through careful and clear signposting, reducing the number of irrelevant and distracting sources of stimuli, and making use of familiar, well-learned associations wherever possible. A small homely unit, with a few, consistent staff and many familiar items and possessions in the person's own room, should be much less inherently cognitively demanding than a large institution, with long corridors, many other residents and a frequently changing staff group. However, as Parmelee & Lawton (1990) indicate, there is little empirical research specifically evaluating design features, perhaps because of the methodological difficulties which would have to be overcome. It is not even established, for example, that reducing the size of the unit has beneficial effects; smaller units almost inevitably necessitate a higher staff:resident ratio, and this may be the crucial factor. Providing "wandering paths" which safely return the person to his/her starting point, and using colour, architectural and other features to distinguish areas within the unit have also not been adequately evaluated. Netten (1989, 1993) has examined the relationship between architectural complexity of residential homes and the ability of persons with dementia to find their way around; different factors were shown to operate in large, communal homes compared with those homes where residents lived together in small groups. Small group homes tended to assist orientation, with the presence of meaningful decision points acting as helpful landmarks.

There have been developments of specialized, small group-living environments for people with dementia internationally. In France, these are described as "cantou", a word meaning "hearth", reflecting that home is around the fireside (Ritchie et al., 1992). Typically there is one large communal room, with the residents' bedrooms and bathrooms and so on opening off the main room, avoiding confusing corridors and reducing the load on spatial memory. The kitchen area might typically be in a corner of the communal room, with food preparation a central interest and activity (in certain other countries this feature would be unacceptable to regulatory authorities). Ritchie et al. (1992) report that residents in the cantou units were more mobile and less dependent in daily activities, had better language skills and interacted more with other residents than residents in long-term hospital care. However, there were indications that these apparent benefits arose from differences in the patients admitted to the two types of care. Although there was considerable overlap in degree of dementia between the two settings, it appeared that the positive impact of the cantou became less evident at more severe levels of dementia.

In the UK, the "domus" units have been particularly influential. Lindesay et al. (1991) describe "the domus philosophy", which is aimed at tackling staff attitudes and fears which lead to poor quality of life in institutional settings for people with dementia. Emphasis is given to seeking to maintain the independence and preserved abilities of persons with dementia, through having an active role in the life of the domus, where the intention is to apply domestic rather than hospital standards of safety and hygiene. Dean et al. (1993) report a prospective evaluation of a domus unit for people with dementia. Patients were assessed in a longstay hospital ward prior to moving to the purpose-built domus (12 beds) and were then monitored at intervals during their first year of residence. Improvements were identified in cognitive function, self-care and communication skills; increased levels of activities and interactions were also observed. Some dramatic changes were observed: one patient spoke for the first time in 5 years within a week of moving to the domus. Skea & Lindesay (1996) report a further evaluation, involving a domus-type home and a community hospital ward offering enhanced care. Again, there are positive results favouring the domus unit, with an increase in both quantity and quality of interactions, and increases in residents' rated communication skills. Some less marked improvements were also noted on the enhanced-care hospital ward, compared with a traditional hospital unit. The improvements in quality of life in domus units do have a cost: staff–resident ratios are higher than in the hospital wards, and the costs are accordingly higher (Beecham et al., 1993) in contrast to the cantou units in France, which were established in part to lower the costs of care.

In Sweden, "group living homes" have been developed. These typically consist of a group of four flats in an ordinary housing block, in which eight people with dementia live, each having his/her own room and possessions, with 24 h staff cover for the unit as a whole (Wimo et al., 1991). A detailed evaluation of the Swedish group-living units by Annerstedt et al. (1993) compared a group of people with dementia moved from institutional care to such units with a control group who remained. Cognitive and mood changes favoured the group-living group over a 6 month period; although both groups declined over a full year, there were indications of this being less marked in the group-living residents.

The special care units described above involve a change in the pattern of care as well as changes to the physical structure and layout of the unit. Another study that has looked specifically at the impact of changing the care regime, and which included cognitive outcomes as well as outcomes relating to activity, mood and function, is reported from Sweden by Brane et al. (1989), evaluating "integrity-promoting care". This involved staff in a nursing home being trained and supported in implementing individualized care, with patients encouraged to participate more in decisions and activities. Staff were trained to allow more time to residents so that they could go at their own pace and not be rushed. Changes to the physical environment aimed at achieving a more home-like atmosphere, with domestic-style furnishing and personalized clothing and possessions, were also encouraged. Changes over the 3 month intervention period and at a follow-up 6 months later were compared with those of a control group in a second nursing home. Patients in the integrity-promoting care group were reported to have become less confused, anxious and distractible; there were also improvements in mood and motor performance. Many of the benefits remained at the follow-up evaluation.

Reducing Cognitive Load

If cognitive demands can be reduced on the person, their retained abilities may be used more effectively. Alberoni et al. (1992) have suggested that working with people with dementia individually, rather than in groups, would reduce the cognitive demands upon them and thus perhaps improve function. These researchers demonstrated that in group conversations, people with dementia have difficulty in remembering who said what, particularly when the group size was larger. They tended to use spatial location as a cue, with performance being particularly disrupted when group members changed places. It should be noted that these difficulties were elicited in relation to patients watching a videotape of a group conversation, rather than participating themselves. In an actual conversation with familiar people, the problems might not be so marked. Morris (1994) suggests that, because of these deficits, group therapies "can degenerate into a monologue between individual staff members and patients". This contention finds support from the finding of Woods et al. (1992), that in reminiscence sessions the majority of interactions taking place were between staff and patients; as would be predicted, they occurred more often between patients in a smaller group. Gibson (1994) similarly recommends small groups for people with dementia. In choosing whether to work with individuals or a small group, the advantages of working in groups—peer support, a social atmosphere, shared experiences—need to be weighed against their undoubted cognitive demands. Where groups are used they should be as small as possible, with members retaining the same seating position from session to session; background noise and distractions should be kept to a minimum, and care taken to ensure that only one person speaks at a time.

External Memory Aids

External memory aids reduce the level of demand on effortful, self-initiated cognitive processes and provide support for the person in cuing and prompting retrieval of information—key features of effective cognitive training approaches (Bäckman, 1992). Retrieval cues in dementia generally require a high degree of specificity in order to be effective; they also need to be salient and placed so that the person will encounter the cue at the relevant time. Nonspecific external aids, such as an alarm clock or a kitchen timer, serve only to remind the person that something is to be remembered, leaving him/her with the frustration of not recalling what it was that had to be done; a note of an appointment in a diary that is not consulted will not influence the person's behaviour. The effects of more specific aids have mainly been demonstrated through single-case studies; for example, a 68-year-old patient with a severe memory impairment successfully used a diary to prompt continuing awareness of personal information taught to her in daily individual sessions (Woods, 1983). Hanley & Lusty (1984) report a single-case study where an 84-year-old patient with dementia was able to achieve a higher level of orientation, using a watch and a diary as retrieval cues. Specific training was required in the use of the cues; without this, the patient did not spontaneously make use of them. During the training phase, the patient kept a far greater proportion of her "appointments" than previously, demonstrating an impact on everyday behaviour as well as on testing.

In a series of studies, Bourgeois (1990, 1992) has evaluated the effects of a prosthetic memory aid on conversational skills in people with dementia. The aid consisted of photographs and pictures of past and more recent events, important people in the person's life and so on, in a convenient, robust wallet or book format. The person's spouse and other visitors were encouraged to use the aid when talking with the person. The results suggest that its use was associated with less ambiguous utterances and more statements of fact. The quality of conversation was assessed by independent raters as being significantly improved with the use of the aid as a focus for conversation. The aid is also reported to have proved useful in improving the quality of interaction between pairs of people with dementia. Although the aid is described as a prosthesis, it appears to be effective in prompting a number of memories related to each item, rather than simply acting as a replacement memory store for the specific information contained therein.

External memory aids have been explicitly used by Josephsson et al. (1993) to reduce the load on the person's own memory and to support retrieval in daily living tasks. The performance of four patients with dementia was evaluated on tasks such as preparing and consuming a drink or snack. Signs on drawers and cupboards indicated the location of required items. Physical demonstrations of task components were provided for the patient to repeat. Verbal prompts and cues were also given. Improvements in task performance were shown by three patients; for two of these, continued environmental support and guidance were needed to maintain these gains. The remaining patient's lack of improvement was attributed to a high level of anxiety interfering with the learning process.

The need for staff input, at least initially, in reinforcing the use of the external aids is demonstrated by the RO literature on the effects of signposting on spatial orientation. In several studies where people with dementia have been trained to find locations in a hospital ward or nursing home, signposting alone had less impact than training to use the signposts and other landmarks in the environment (Hanley, 1981; Gilleard et al., 1981; Lam & Woods, 1986). Such signposts may be viewed as retrieval cues; certainly some people with dementia are capable of benefiting from them, with practice in their use, even though not using them spontaneously. Such a use of cues fits well with the conclusion of Bäckman (1992), that people with dementia require support at both the time of learning and at the time of retrieval for optimal performance.

REALITY ORIENTATION (RO)

This long-established psychosocial approach has been used with older people with dementia since the late 1950s, and an extensive literature, both evaluative and descriptive, is available (see for example Holden & Woods, 1995). Two major components of reality orientation (RO) are usually described. Twenty-four hour RO (or informal RO) involves a number of changes to the environment, with clear signposting of locations around the ward or home, extensive use of notices and other memory aids, and a consistent approach by all staff in interacting with the person with dementia. In its original form, staff undertaking 24-h RO were intended to offer orientating information in each and every interaction; more recently, a modification has been described where staff are trained to take a more reactive stance, orientating the person only in response to his/her requests (Reeve & Ivison, 1985; Williams et al., 1987). RO sessions (or RO classes) are structured group sessions, involving a small number of patients and staff, meeting regularly, often several times a week for half an hour or so. A wide variety of activities and materials are used to engage the patients with their surroundings, to maintain contact with the wider world and to provide cognitive stimulation. A typical session would go over basic information (such as names of those in the group, day, date, time and place), discuss a current relevant theme of interest, perhaps play a number or naming game, and finish with refreshments. Throughout there would be a tangible focus: a white-board for the current information; pictures or objects appropriate to the theme; personal diaries and notebooks for those able to record information for later use.

Although Holden & Woods (1995) identified over 20 studies meeting the criterion of reporting an evaluation of the effects of RO, in comparison with either no treatment or an alternative intervention, methodological weaknesses meant that only six could be included in a meta-analysis, which focused on randomized controlled trials (RCTs) of RO sessions (Spector et al., 1999a, 2000). This systematic review included studies where patients attended groups for at least 3 weeks, the minimum number of sessions being 10. From the six included RCTs there was a total of 125 patients, of whom 67 received RO and 58 were in control groups. All six studies utilized measures of cognitive function; the results overall were significantly in favour of an effect of RO on cognitive function (estimated effect size 0.59). Measures of behavioural function could be analysed from three studies, having a total of 48 patients (28 experimental, 20 control). In the individual studies the results on behavioural measures were insignificant, but the joint analysis indicated a significant effect of RO sessions in this domain also (estimated effect size 0.66).

Control groups used in the analysed studies included some form of "social therapy", to control for the effects of increased attention in half the studies and "no treatment" in the other half. There was no obvious difference in the results obtained depending on the nature of the control group, and it would appear that the effects observed are not simply attributable to an increase in staff attention and input to those in the experimental groups. The number and duration of RO sessions did not appear to influence the results; however, the severity of dementia of the patients included in each study could not be directly compared, and the amount of RO required for a therapeutic effect could potentially co-vary with severity. The effects reported are those immediately following the intervention. Longer-term follow-up has been attempted in a few studies, with conflicting results. Maintenance of any benefits is generally regarded as an important issue in RO studies, with the expectation that further input, perhaps less intensively, or as "booster" sessions, would almost certainly be required; this has yet to be thoroughly researched; 24 h RO may also have a part to play in the maintenance of improvements following RO sessions (Reeve & Ivison, 1985).

The exact nature of the cognitive improvements associated with RO remains unclear. Whilst it is clear that RO sessions are usually associated with increased scores on measures of verbal orientation, suggestions that more general cognitive improvements may occur are more controversial. Some studies suggest that only those orientation items specifically taught are learned; others that from a battery of cognitive tests, only the orientation items show improvement. More recent reports (e.g. Breuil et al., 1994; Zanetti et al., 1995) have tended to support the notion that more wide-ranging improvements in cognition may follow cognitive stimulation of this type.

Changes in function and behaviour have proved much more elusive than cognitive changes in individual studies; in general they have been the exception rather than the rule. This may reflect the small sample sizes in many studies, with the behaviour rating scales being used often appearing less sensitive to the small changes envisaged. In addition, an environment encouraging dependence (as many have been shown to do) may counteract any benefits from group sessions. It is also doubtful whether verbal orientation has any influence on many of the areas of function, such as feeding and dressing, which comprise much of the content of the behaviour rating scales typically used. It could be argued that direct training of a particular skill will be required to maximize the probability of behavioural change; several workers have shown this in relation to ward orientation—the person finding his/her way around the ward or home. Improvements in this domain have been shown in relation to specific training by Hanley et al. (1981) and associated with 24 h RO by Reeve & Ivison (1985) and

Williams et al. (1987). These studies have in common a demonstrable intervention in the person's living environment, the former through direct training, the latter two through the monitored evaluation of 24 h RO. The greatest range of behavioural improvement reported was evident in these studies. Holden & Woods (1995) conclude that behavioural changes appear to be more likely in studies where the implementation of the 24 h RO has been monitored to ensure that it has actually been carried out as planned. It cannot be assumed that training staff in the approach ensures its implementation (Hanley, 1984). Where the aim is for the patient to be better orientated around the ward or home, direct training for the patient, which can be simply monitored and evaluated, has much to commend it. Evidence of the effectiveness of simple training sessions in finding relevant locations on the ward or in the home is provided by a number of studies, including a small group study (five in each group), involving a comparison with no treatment (Hanley et al., 1981) and several single-case studies: Hanley (1981), reporting a series of eight single-cases; Gilleard et al. (1981), a series of six single-cases; and Lam & Woods (1986), one case. All the single-case studies utilized experimental designs allowing the effect of intervention to be clearly demonstrated. There is some evidence that clear signposting may add to the effectiveness of the training.

Twenty-four hour RO does not lend itself so readily to evaluation through RCTs, in view of the change of environment and regime it requires. However, there have been several comparison group studies (e.g. Zepelin et al., 1981; Williams et al., 1987) where the intervention takes place only in one of two units thought to be similar at baseline. Early studies tended to be disappointing, at least in terms of behavioural change. Indeed, Zepelin's study found a number of changes in behavioural function favouring an untreated control group over a 12 month period. However, this study also encountered a number of problems in relation to the reliability and comparability of the behavioural rating measures used. The modified 24 h RO approach adopted by Williams et al. in Australia appears more successful, being associated with cognitive and behavioural change. Interestingly, in Williams et al.'s (1987) study, cognitive changes were achieved with 24 h RO alone, without RO sessions.

Gatz et al. (1998), reviewing a range of psychological approaches in dementia, conclude that "reality orientation is probably efficacious in slowing cognitive decline". They point out, as do Holden & Woods (1995), the danger of RO being implemented without sufficient sensitivity, leading to possible frustration and distress in the patient (Dietch et al., 1989). This consideration has led the American Psychiatric Association in their 1997 Practice Guideline to suggest that the small gains associated with approaches such as RO do not justify the risk of negative effects. Certainly RO, as a general therapeutic programme, is now rarely encountered in practice, largely because of concerns that it was over-confrontational, tended to emphasize the patient's deficits rather than strengths, and did not focus sufficiently on clinically relevant treatment goals. What is the clinical significance of a change in a few points on a test of verbal orientation? Holden & Woods (1995) argue that there is much to be learned from the research on RO that could be applied in the framework of person-centred care. They suggest there is a need to identify individual goals specific to each patient, to recognize the possibility of learning and change, and to work with the patient on the areas of concern in a collaborative and empathic, rather than a controlling or confrontational, manner. They view an RO-type approach as having some role for selected patients in the context of their individual care plan.

The recent development of drugs which act on the cholinergic system by maintaining levels of acetylcholine (known to be depleted in Alzheimer's disease) has stimulated further interest in whether the impact of psychosocial approaches on cognition might be of a similar order to that of the pharmacological approach (Orrell & Woods, 1996). A major difficulty in making this comparison has been the relative lack of rigour of the research evaluating psychosocial interventions. Whilst double-blind RCTs of drug vs. placebo are standard in drug research, with sample sizes allowing adequate statistical power, and standardized assessment measures used, evaluations of RO, for example, have rarely incorporated assessors blind to treatment group, have had small samples and idiosyncratic outcome measures, and have not generally been adequately randomized or used a credible "placebo" control group. Some of these differences reflect the greater intrinsic complexity of evaluating psychosocial research, where the intervention simply cannot be as neatly packaged as a pill; others reflect the lack of priority and funding given to this area. Orrell & Woods determined to carry out a study of sufficient extent and quality to make a comparison with drug trials feasible. The development of this study is described by Spector et al. (2001). The intervention used has been developed primarily from a consideration of the evidence base reviewed for the systematic review described above, together with some features of reminiscence therapy (see below). It is designed to offer a group programme of 14 sessions, with an extensive cognitive input embedded in activities offering interest and enjoyment. Pilot groups led to the further development of the intervention programme and refinement of measures. An RCT comparing the intervention package with no treatment has been completed, involving 23 residential homes and day-centres, with assessments made by raters blind to group membership (Spector et al., 2003); 201 people with dementia participated, and the results indicated that significant cognitive changes (on the widely used ADAS–COG instrument) favouring the intervention group were evident. The effect size was almost identical to that obtained using the same measure in trials of the new "antidementia" drugs, although over a shorter time period, of 7 weeks rather than 6 months. Importantly, people with dementia in the intervention group also showed significant improvements in quality of life, suggesting that the implementation of this package is avoiding the negative features associated with the misuse of RO.

REMINISCENCE THERAPY

The use of past memories to establish a point of interest and contact has been often used in RO sessions, and has attracted much interest as an approach in its own right (Woods & McKiernan, 1995; Gibson, 1994). Reminiscence work with older people more generally developed from psychotherapeutic considerations, emphasizing the place of life-review in adaptation (Coleman, 1986; Bornat, 1994). Reminiscence has been used extensively with patients who are depressed as well as those with dementia; it should be recognized that the aims and techniques may need to be different in each case. Norris (1986) provides an excellent description of the practical application of a variety of reminiscence techniques.

Reminiscence work with people with dementia may have a variety of goals, including increasing communication and socialization, and providing pleasure and entertainment. It may take a variety of forms, and use a range of techniques. The use of memory triggers, such as photographs, objects, music and archive recordings, is a common feature of reminiscence work with people with dementia. In evaluating the impact of reminiscence therapy it is vital to specify the approach and procedures used.

Reminiscence work may be given a cognitive rationale. People with dementia often appear able to recall events from their childhood but not from earlier the same day. Accordingly, it may be sensible to tap into the apparently preserved store of remote memories. In fact, studies of remote memory suggest that recall for specific events is not relatively preserved—performance across the lifespan is depressed compared with age-matched controls. People with dementia, like all older people, recall more memories from earlier life (Morris, 1994). Some of the "memories" represent well-rehearsed, much-practised items or anecdotes or have particular personal and/or emotional significance for the person concerned. Morris points out there is an almost complete absence of autobiographical memories from the person's middle years; conceivably the resulting disconnection of past and present might contribute to the person's difficulty in retaining a clear sense of personal identity.

Outcome literature on reminiscence therapy in dementia is sparse, especially in relation to its impact on cognition. The Cochrane systematic review on reminiscence therapy for dementia (Spector et al., 1999b) identified only one suitable RCT, a comparison with RO and no treatment reported by Baines et al. (1987) in a residential home setting. Groups of residents having a moderate to severe degree of cognitive impairment met for 30 min a day, 5 days a week for 4 weeks, and a range of reminiscence aids were used. A variety of measures were used; cognitive (verbal orientation) and behavioural changes were analysed in the Cochrane review, both of which were not significant, although the behavioural scale slightly favoured treatment. However, it should be noted that the sample size was very small, with just five residents in each of the conditions compared. The study used a cross-over design, and it appeared that residents who took part in reminiscence following a period of RO did better than those participating in the interventions in the reverse order, compared with untreated controls. Staff involved in a reminiscence group acquired much more individual knowledge of the residents in the group than they did of residents in a control group who received no additional treatment. Residents were rated as deriving a great deal of enjoyment from the groups, both by staff taking part in the groups and by staff who saw the residents only outside the groups. Attendance at the reminiscence groups was consistently high.

At least one other RCT is available in the literature (Goldwasser et al., 1987). Twenty-seven nursing home residents with a diagnosis of dementia were randomly assigned to a reminiscence group, supportive group therapy or to a no-treatment control. The groups met for 30 min, twice a week for 5 weeks. No changes were evident on a cognitive measure (the Mini-Mental State Examination) or a measure of activities of daily living. There was a significant improvement on a depression scale for the reminiscence group compared with the other two conditions. However, Knight (1996) suggests that this may be largely due to their higher initial level of depression.

The evaluative literature on reminiscence is then inconclusive with regard to cognitive and behavioural change, perhaps because this has not been a major aim of work in this area. There has been perhaps more interest in whether reminiscence encourages communication and engagement in meaningful activity (see Woods & McKiernan, 1995) and, more recently, whether it has an impact on the person's observed well-being. For example, Brooker & Duce (2000) evaluated well-being in 25 people with dementia attending three different day-hospitals, using an observational method, dementia care mapping, developed by Kitwood & Bredin (1992). They showed that participation in reminiscence groups was associated with higher levels of well-being than other group activities or unstructured time. This study does not claim to show an enduring effect of reminiscence, but does show a clear benefit during the group session.

From a theoretical perspective, if autobiographical memory is, as seems likely, an important contributor to the person's sense of identity, which in turn contributes to the person's mood and well-being, then reminiscence work which aims to enhance the person's autobiographical memory may also have an effect on the person's affective state. In a recently completed study (Woods & Morgan, 2001), the impact of life-review work on people with dementia who had recently been admitted to residential care was evaluated. As the emphasis was on autobiographical memory, individual sessions were conducted, working chronologically through the person's life (approximately 10 sessions were held with each person). A life-story book was compiled for each person in the intervention group, with the assistance of relatives providing relevant photographs and information. The person with dementia exercised editorial control over the contents of the book, and he/she was encouraged to evaluate his/her memories and experiences and to place them in perspective and in the context of his/her life-course. Seventeen people with dementia participated, eight randomly allocated to the intervention group and nine to a no-treatment control group. Outcome measures included the Autobiographical Memory Interview (Kopelman et al., 1990) and the Geriatric Depression Scale (15 item version: Sheikh & Yesavage, 1986); a number of assessments were carried out by an assessor blind to group membership. The results showed a significant increase in autobiographical memory in the life-review group at the end of the treatment phase, compared with the control group. This improvement was maintained at a 6 week follow-up assessment. The intervention group also reported fewer symptoms of depression post-treatment, with continued improvement at follow-up. The average score of the life-review group fell outside the depressed range on this scale at follow-up, whilst that of the control group remained above the cut-off point for depression. Anecdotally, the impact of the life-story books was considerable, with participants proudly showing them to care staff and family, and apparently gaining a stronger sense of identity from the autobiographical memory prompts it provided.

The success of this small-scale study, which appears to be the first RCT to examine the effects of reminiscence work on autobiographical memory, emphasizes the need for careful distinctions to be made between different types of reminiscence work. Whilst the terms "reminiscence" and "life-review" have often been used interchangeably, Haight & Burnside (1993) suggest that life-review be used solely to describe an intervention where the therapist is seeking to assist the person in achieving a sense of integrity. This involves the person recalling and evaluating events and experiences throughout his/her life, usually in a one-to-one setting with the therapist, who acts as a therapeutic listener. Life-review therapy is much more likely to involve working through difficult and painful memories and experiences; it should be undertaken, like any other personal therapy, with the person's consent, with a clear aim, by properly trained and supervised workers.

Reminiscence, on the other hand, may be individual or group-based and may be structured or free-flowing. It may include general memories, rather than recall of specific events or experiences; themes and prompts are frequently used; evaluation of memories is not specifically encouraged; and the focus is on a relaxed, positive atmosphere. Sad memories may emerge, but support is available from the group leader and other members, or from the worker in individual work, to contain any distress or pain associated with such memories. Some caution is still required, taking into account Coleman's (1986) report of large individual differences in attitudes to reminiscence amongst older people and the need to avoid an intrusive approach that invades individuals' privacy. Particularly in a group setting, awareness of participants' life histories is important, to ensure that appropriate support can be given if events that have traumatic connotations for certain individuals are being raised by other members.

COGNITION, EMOTION AND BEHAVIOUR

There are then several procedures and techniques which may be used to enhance and maximize cognitive function in people with dementia. How helpful are these techniques in practice? Given that the person's cognitive abilities would be expected to continue to decline, are these approaches encouraging dementia care workers to make heroic, but ultimately hopeless, efforts to swim against the tide? There can be little question that efforts to generally reduce the cognitive load, to target the person's resources on areas of importance to him/her, to provide an environment where intact memory function is less important, will be of benefit to most people with dementia.

The social psychologist Tom Kitwood made a major contribution to the development of dementia care (Kitwood, 1997) in developing a person-centred model of dementia care, where the person's social environment is seen as central to the clinical picture observed. Environmental manipulations and adaptations may assist in reducing excess disability (disability beyond that necessitated by neuropathological changes). Excess disability may also be related to the person's emotional response to his/her predicament. Estimated rates of anxiety and depression in people with dementia are much higher than in the general population, with perhaps as many as 40% having symptoms of anxiety and/or depression (Cheston & Bender, 1999; Woods, 2001). Some success has been reported in reducing anxiety using progressive muscle relaxation (Suhr et al., 1999) and in depression through increasing participation in pleasurable activities (Teri et al., 1997).

Anxiety and depression may reduce cognitive performance; for example, the failure of one of the four people with dementia in the study reported by Josephsson et al. (1993) to show learning was attributed to high levels of anxiety. It is important that the effects of interventions on affective state as well as on cognition are monitored. In some situations having an impact on both may be possible, as in the life review study described previously.

There have been some suggestions that behavioural change is possible through the interventions described here, but there are clearly limitations to what may be achieved without individualized, tailored interventions (Woods & Bird, 1999). General programmes may help enrich an environment, so that there is more encouragement for the person to be independent, with more stimulation and generally a more positive approach. This may help reduce the probability of behaviour problems occurring, but when they do occur an individualized approach is essential.

CONCLUSION

Some issues seem to arise in relation to the approaches described in this chapter:

1. *How can family caregivers best be involved?*   Much of the work reported here is based in hospitals and residential and nursing homes, yet most people with dementia live at home. Training family caregivers to implement these approaches has not yet been given much attention (for review, see Brodaty, 1992). Some examples exist in the behavioural

literature (e.g. Green et al., 1986) and in the use of a prosthetic memory aid (Bourgeois, 1990) to enhance conversation. It is noteworthy that in the latter study, whilst independent raters confirmed improvements in conversational quality, the relatives involved did not perceive these changes. More attention needs to be given to developing approaches that family caregivers can make use of, without adding to their sense of strain, and which will target areas of value to both caregiver and care recipient. Families have the advantage of knowing the person for many years, and can often assist in holding and supporting the person's autobiographical memory (Cheston, 1998). A life-story book provides a tangible reminder of some important aspects of the person's life, and offers an opportunity for others to communicate to the person with dementia that he/she remains valued and worthy of attention and interest. The added dimension of the existing pattern of relationship may well complicate the application of approaches such as RO and reminiscence, and a good deal of creative work is needed to find ways of implementing useful techniques in the family home.

2. *What are the appropriate goals of intervention?* For example, is the emphasis placed on improved cognitive function justified, or should well-being and/or quality of life be the ultimate yardstick? If so, how should they be measured? The recent development of a number of quality-of-life scales is welcome in this respect (e.g. Brod et al., 1999). Measuring quality of life and related mood states, such as anxiety and depression, is progressing—largely driven by the requirements of pharmacological research. Bond (1999) suggests that there are, however, a number of radically different meanings of the concept "quality of life" emerging in the field, and some caution is required in taking at face value new assessment measures. The goals that are set in order to evaluate approaches to dementia care must be realistic but based on changes of importance and relevance to the individual with dementia:

> We need to break away from our preoccupation with treatment in the sense of cure and recovery, and be aware of the different types of goal that are feasible, and the value of some of the more limited goals in improving the patient's quality of life (Woods & Britton, 1985, p. 217).

3. *Are there negative effects associated with a particular approach?* Often, it seems that only positive results are published. RO has been most associated with misuse, but there may potentially be difficulties with other approaches if not used sensitively. Informed consent for people with more advanced dementia is often impossible. How can their wishes and preferences be properly taken into account? Can family members act as satisfactory proxies for the person with dementia?

4. *What works for whom?* No approach will be universally beneficial, of course. How can we identify what approach is most likely to be useful for a particular individual? Individual differences in response need to be studied in more detail. The weakness of group studies is that there is the danger of missing these individual differences in treatment response which are vitally important at the clinical level. A narrow focus on the person with dementia may mean that beneficial effects elsewhere in the system are not identified. Effects on caregivers—family or staff—may be important and worthwhile, and ultimately result in improved quality of care for the person with dementia.

There are no simple answers to the problems of providing good quality care for people with dementia; however, there are now a number of indications of approaches that can be incorporated sensitively and creatively within a framework of individualized care, that aims to meet the whole range of needs—social, physical and psychological—of the person with dementia.

Kitwood (1997) described how "personhood" might be recognized in people with dementia. This involved identifying indications that the person continued to function as a person, relating, interacting, feeling, choosing, acting in a purposeful manner. Psychological approaches need to be applied in a way that values and respects the individual as a person, taking account of the person's life-story, if they are to serve the best interests of the person with dementia and those who care for him/her.

REFERENCES

Alberoni, M., Baddeley, A., Della-Sala, S. et al. (1992). Keeping track of a conversation: impairments in Alzheimer's disease. *International Journal of Geriatric Psychiatry*, **7**, 639–646.

American Psychiatric Association (1994). *Diagnostic and Statistical Manual of Mental Disorders* (4th edn). Washington, DC: American Psychiatric Association.

American Psychiatric Association (1997). Practice guideline for the treatment of patients with Alzheimer's disease and other dementias of late life. *American Journal of Psychiatry*, **154**(5) (suppl), 1–39.

Annerstedt, L., Gustafson, L. & Nilsson, K. (1993). Medical outcome of psychosocial intervention in demented patients: one-year clinical follow-up after relocation into group living units. *International Journal of Geriatric Psychiatry*, **8**, 833–841.

Bäckman, L. (1992). Memory training and memory improvement in Alzheimer's disease: rules and exceptions. *Acta Neurologia Scandinavica* (suppl), **139**, 84–89.

Baines, S., Saxby, P. & Ehlert, K. (1987). Reality orientation and reminiscence therapy: a controlled cross-over study of elderly confused people. *British Journal of Psychiatry*, **151**, 222–231.

Beecham, J., Cambridge, P., Hallam, A. & Knapp, M. (1993). The costs of domus care. *International Journal of Geriatric Psychiatry*, **8**, 827–831.

Bond, J. (1999). Quality of life for people with dementia: approaches to the challenge of measurement. *Ageing & Society*, **19**, 561–579.

Bornat, J. (ed.) (1994). *Reminiscence Reviewed: Perspectives, Evaluations, Achievements*. Buckingham: Open University Press.

Bourgeois, M.S. (1990). Enhancing conversation skills in patients with Alzheimer's disease using a prosthetic memory aid. *Journal of Applied Behavior Analysis*, **23**, 29–42.

Bourgeois, M.S. (1992). *Conversing with Memory-impaired Individuals Using Memory Aids: a Memory Aid Workbook*. Bicester: Winslow.

Brane, G., Karlsson, I., Kihlgren, M. & Norberg, A. (1989). Integrity-promoting care of demented nursing home patients: psychological and biochemical changes. *International Journal of Geriatric Psychiatry*, **4**, 165–172.

Breuil, V., de Rotrou, J., Forette, F. et al. (1994). Cognitive stimulation of patients with dementia: preliminary results. *International Journal of Geriatric Psychiatry*, **9**, 211–217.

Brod, M., Stewart, A.L., Sands, L. & Walton, P. (1999). Conceptualization and measurement of quality of life in dementia: the dementia quality of life instrument (DQoL). *Gerontologist*, **39**, 25–35.

Brodaty, H. (1992). Carers: training informal carers. In T. Arie (ed.), *Recent advances in psychogeriatrics*, Vol. 2 (pp. 163–171). Edinburgh: Churchill Livingstone.

Brooker, D. & Duce, L. (2000). Wellbeing and activity in dementia: a comparison of group reminiscence therapy, structured goal-directed group activity and unstructured time. *Aging & Mental Health*, **4**(4), 354–358.

Carr, J.S. & Marshall, M. (1993). Innovations in long-stay care for people with dementia. *Reviews in Clinical Gerontology*, **3**, 157–167.

Cheston, R. (1998). Psychotherapeutic work with people with dementia: a review of the literature. *British Journal of Medical Psychology*, **71**, 211–231.

Cheston, R. & Bender, M. (1999). Brains, minds and selves: changing conceptions of the losses involved in dementia. *Ageing & Society*, **72**, 203–216.

Coleman, P.G. (1986). *Ageing and Reminiscence Processes: Social and Clinical Implications*. Chichester: Wiley.

Dean, R., Briggs, K. & Lindesay, J. (1993). The domus philosophy: a prospective evaluation of two residential units for the elderly mentally ill. *International Journal of Geriatric Psychiatry*, **8**, 807–817.

Dietch, J.T., Hewett, L.J. & Jones, S. (1989). Adverse effects of reality orientation. *Journal of American Geriatrics Society*, **37**, 974–976.

Gatz, M., Fiske, A., Fox, L.S. et al. (1998). Empirically validated psychological treatments for older adults. *Journal of Mental Health & Aging*, **4**(1), 9–46.

Gibson, F. (1994). What can reminiscence contribute to people with dementia? In J. Bornat (ed.), *Reminiscence Reviewed: Evaluations, Achievements, Perspectives* (pp. 46–60). Buckingham: Open University Press.

Gilleard, C., Mitchell, R.G. & Riordan, J. (1981). Ward orientation training with psychogeriatric patients. *Journal of Advanced Nursing*, **6**, 95–98.

Goldwasser, A.N., Auerbach, S.M. & Harkins, S.W. (1987). Cognitive, affective and behavioral effects of reminiscence group therapy on demented elderly. *International Journal of Aging & Human Development*, **25**, 209–222.

Green, G.R., Linsk, N.L. & Pinkston, E.M. (1986). Modification of verbal behavior of the mentally impaired elderly by their spouses. *Journal of Applied Behavior Analysis*, **19**, 329–336.

Haight, B.K. & Burnside, I. (1993). Reminiscence and life review: explaining the differences. *Archives of Psychiatric Nursing*, **7**, 91–98.

Hanley, I.G. (1981). The use of signposts and active training to modify ward disorientation in elderly patients. *Journal of Behaviour Therapy & Experimental Psychiatry*, **12**, 241–247.

Hanley, I.G. & Lusty, K. (1984). Memory aids in reality orientation: a single-case study. *Behaviour Research & Therapy*, **22**, 709–712.

Hanley, I.G., McGuire, R.J. & Boyd, W.D. (1981). Reality orientation and dementia: a controlled trial of two approaches. *British Journal of Psychiatry*, **138**, 10–14.

Holden, U.P. & Woods, R.T. (1995). *Positive Approaches to Dementia Care*, 3rd edn. Edinburgh: Churchill Livingstone.

Josephsson, S., Bäckman, L., Borell, L. et al. (1993). Supporting everyday activities in dementia: an intervention study. *International Journal of Geriatric Psychiatry*, **8**, 395–400.

Kitwood, T. (1997). *Dementia Reconsidered: the Person Comes First*. Buckingham: Open University Press.

Kitwood, T. & Bredin, K. (1992). A new approach to the evaluation of dementia care. *Journal of Advances in Health & Nursing Care*, **1**, 41–60.

Knight, B.G. (1996). Psychodynamic therapy with older adults: lessons from scientific gerontology. In R.T. Woods (ed.), *Handbook of the Clinical Psychology of Ageing* (pp. 545–560). Chichester: Wiley.

Kopelman, M., Wilson, B.A. & Baddeley, A. (1990). *The Autobiographical Memory Interview*. Bury St. Edmunds: Thames Valley Test Company.

Lam, D.H. & Woods, R.T. (1986). Ward orientation training in dementia: a single-case study. *International Journal of Geriatric Psychiatry*, **1**, 145–147.

Lindesay, J., Briggs, K., Lawes, M. et al. (1991). The domus philosophy: a comparative evaluation of a new approach to residential care for the demented elderly. *International Journal of Geriatric Psychiatry*, **6**, 727–736.

Morris, R.G. (1994). Recent developments in the neuropsychology of dementia. *International Review of Psychiatry*, **6**, 85–107.

Netten, A. (1989). Environment, orientation and behaviour: the effect of the design of residential homes in creating dependency among confused elderly residents. *International Journal of Geriatric Psychiatry*, **4**, 143–152.

Netten, A. (1993). *A Positive Environment? Physical and Social Influences on People with Senile Dementia in Residential Care*. Aldershot: Ashgate.

Norris, A. (1986). *Reminiscence*. London: Winslow Press.

Orrell, M. & Woods, R.T. (1996). Tacrine and psychological therapies in dementia—no contest? *International Journal of Geriatric Psychiatry*, **11**, 189–192.

Parmelee, P.A. & Lawton, M.P. (1990). The design of special environments for the aged. In J.E. Birren & K.W. Schaie (eds), *Handbook of the Psychology of Aging*, 3rd edn (pp. 464–488). San Diego, CA: Academic Press.

Reeve, W. & Ivison, D. (1985). Use of environmental manipulation and classroom and modified informal reality orientation with institutionalized, confused elderly patients. *Age & Ageing*, **14**, 119–121.

Ritchie, K., Colvez, A., Ankri, J. et al. (1992). The evaluation of long-term care for the dementing elderly: a comparative study of hospital and collective non-medical care in France. *International Journal of Geriatric Psychiatry*, **7**, 549–557.

Sheikh, J.I. & Yesavage, J.A. (1986). Geriatric Depression Scale (GDS): recent evidence and development of a shorter version. In T.L. Brink (ed.), *Clinical Gerontology: a Guide to Assessment and Intervention* (pp. 165–173). New York: Haworth.

Skea, D. & Lindesay, J. (1996). An evaluation of two models of long-term residential care for elderly people with dementia. *International Journal of Geriatric Psychiatry*, **11**, 233–241.

Spector, A., Orrell, M., Davies, S. & Woods, R.T. (1999a). Reality orientation for dementia (Cochrane Review). In *The Cochrane Library*, Issue 4. Oxford: Update Software.

Spector, A., Orrell, M., Davies, S. & Woods, R.T. (1999b). Reminiscence therapy for dementia (Cochrane Review). In The Cochrane Library, Issue 4. Oxford: Update Software.

Spector, A., Davies, S., Woods, B. & Orrell, M. (2000). Reality orientation for dementia: a systematic review of the evidence for its effectiveness. *Gerontologist*, **40**(2), 206–212.

Spector, A., Orrell, M., Davies, S. & Woods, B. (2001). Can reality orientation be rehabilitated? Development and piloting of an evidence-based programme of cognition-based therapies for people with dementia. *Neuropsychological Rehabilitation*, **11**, 377–397.

Spector, A., Thorgrimsen, L., Woods, B., et al. (2003). Efficacy of an evidence-based cognitive stimulation therapy programme for people with dementia. *British Journal of Psychiatry*, **183**, 248–254.

Suhr, J., Anderson, S. & Tranel, D. (1999). Progressive muscle relaxation in the management of behavioural disturbance in Alzheimer's disease. *Neuropsychological Rehabilitation*, **9**, 31–44.

Teri, L., Logsdon, R.G., Uomoto, J. & McCurry, S.M. (1997). Behavioral treatment of depression in dementia patients: a controlled clinical trial. *Journal of Gerontology*, **52B**, P159–P166.

Williams, R., Reeve, W., Ivison, D. & Kavanagh, D. (1987). Use of environmental manipulation and modified informal reality orientation with institutionalized confused elderly subjects: a replication. *Age & Ageing*, **16**, 315–318.

Wimo, A., Wallin, J.O., Lundgren, K. et al. (1991). Group living, an alternative for dementia patients: a cost analysis. *International Journal of Geriatric Psychiatry*, **6**, 21–29.

Woods, R.T. (1983). Specificity of learning in reality orientation sessions: a single-case study. *Behaviour Research & Therapy*, **21**, 173–175.

Woods, R.T. (2001). Discovering the person with Alzheimer's disease: cognitive, emotional and behavioural aspects. *Aging & Mental Health*, **5**(suppl 1), S7–S16.

Woods, R.T. & Bird, M. (1999). Non-pharmacological approaches to treatment. In G. Wilcock, K. Rockwood & R. Bucks (eds), *Diagnosis and Management of Dementia: a Manual for Memory Disorders Teams* (pp. 311–331). Oxford: Oxford University Press.

Woods, R.T. & Britton, P.G. (1985). *Clinical Psychology with the Elderly*. London: Croom Helm/Chapman Hall.

Woods, R.T. & McKiernan, F. (1995). Evaluating the impact of reminiscence on older people with dementia. In B.K. Haight & J. Webster (eds), *The Art and Science of Reminiscing: Theory, Research, Methods and Applications* (pp. 233–242). Washington, DC: Taylor & Francis.

Woods, R.T. & Morgan, S. (2001). Randomised-controlled trial of life review with people with dementia on entry to residential care. Paper presented at International Congress of Gerontology, Vancouver.

Woods, R.T., Portnoy, S., Head, D. & Jones, G. (1992). Reminiscence and life-review with persons with dementia: which way forward? In G. Jones & B. Miesen (eds), *Care-giving in Dementia* (pp. 137–161). London: Routledge.

Zanetti, O., Frisoni, G.B., DeLeo, D. et al. (1995). Reality orientation therapy in Alzheimer's disease: useful or not? a controlled study. *Alzheimer Disease and Associated Disorders*, **9**, 132–138.

Zepelin, H., Wolfe, C.S. & Kleinplatz, F. (1981). Evaluation of a year-long reality orientation program. *Journal of Gerontology*, **36**, 70–77.

CHAPTER 14

External Memory Aids and Computers in Memory Rehabilitation

Narinder Kapur

Southampton General Hospital and University of Southampton, UK

Elizabeth L. Glisky

University of Arizona, Tuscon, AZ, USA

and

Barbara A. Wilson

MRC Cognition and Brain Sciences Unit, Cambridge, and Oliver Zangwill Centre for Cognitive Rehabilitation, Ely, UK

> Feats can be performed with mnemonic devices that are marvellous and prodigious, but nevertheless it is a barren thing for human uses. It is not well contrived for providing assistance to memory in serious and business affairs (Sir Francis Bacon).

This chapter reviews external memory aids and computer-based resources in the management of patients with memory difficulties following brain disease or brain injury. We are concerned primarily with treatment interventions for memory-disordered people. Although various forms of memory aids and computer-based resources may be useful in the initial neuropsychological assessment and diagnosis of such people, these applications are outside the scope of this chapter. We focus mainly on adults who have suffered a brain insult, although we recognize that children with brain damage and those with memory loss related to psychiatric conditions might also benefit from external aids and computers.

Apart from drugs or other "physical" treatments for psychological management, there are several ways in which memory difficulties associated with neurological disease may be managed: general advice and counselling to provide information to patients and their carers about coping with memory difficulties; advice on the avoidance of exacerbating factors, such as alcohol, fatigue, stress, etc.; advice on simple changes to daily routines or to the environment; instruction in the use of specific cognitive strategies for encoding, rehearsing and retrieving information; and the use of external memory aids, computers, etc., to help improve everyday memory functioning. A number of self-help booklets and guides are

The Essential *Handbook of Memory Disorders for Clinicians.* Edited by A.D. Baddeley, M.D. Kopelman and B.A. Wilson.
© 2004 John Wiley & Sons, Ltd. ISBN 0-470-09141-X.

available which summarize such advice (Clare & Wilson, 1997; Kapur, 2001; Martyn & Gale, 1999)

Techniques to try to improve memory date back thousands of years (Herrmann & Chaffin, 1988). Memory *strategies* for improving memory have been well documented (Glisky, 1997; Gruneberg, 1992; McGlynn, 1990; Patten, 1990) but rather less attention has been paid to *external memory aids*. These act as a form of "prosthesis" for everyday memory functioning. Unlike the effects of novel cognitive strategies, they are rarely intended to change learning ability as such, although they may sometimes be as valuable or more valuable than conventional techniques for improving memory. Although cognitive-based memory strategies have a role to play in some aspects of memory rehabilitation, many memory-disordered patients may lack the motivation or prerequisite concentration/learning skills to acquire some of the strategies advocated, certainly those that are put forward in popular books on memory improvement. In a study by Park et al. (1990), psychologists involved in memory research indicated that simple external memory aids, such as writing things down on a note-pad, were among the techniques they themselves used most often for improving their memory. A survey of individuals of varying ages found that external memory aids were used more frequently than cognitive strategies to enhance prospective memory functioning (Long et al., 1999).

This chapter reviews the main types of external memory aids currently available, and assesses their suitability for use in clinical settings. More general reviews of memory rehabilitation, which include some discussion of memory aids, are available elsewhere (Glisky & Glisky, 2002; Harrell et al., 1992; Herrmann et al., 1992; Intons-Peterson & Fournier, 1986; Parente & Herrmann, 1996; Wilson, 1999a; Wilson & Evans, 2000; Wilson & Moffat, 1992).

At present, there is no detailed and widely accepted conceptual framework for considering the role of memory aids in neurological rehabilitation. The general importance of concepts in memory research has been emphasized by Tulving (2000). While there have been some promising attempts to develop conceptual frameworks to view aspects of memory rehabilitation (Bäckman & Dixon, 1992; Wilson & Watson, 1996), there is a need to develop new frameworks that take into account the range of cognitive strategies and of agents that can enhance memory functioning, and that also incorporate research findings from clinical and cognate sciences that influence memory functioning.

In this chapter, we shall deal with the following aids: environmental, stationery, mechanical, and electronic, together with computer-based resources. Some of the beneficial effects of memory aids can be considered in terms of the long-established distinction between experiential and knowledge memory (Nielsen, 1958), the subsequent distinctions between episodic and semantic memory (Tulving, 1972), and between memory for events and memory for facts (Warrington, 1986). Thus, aids may be used mainly to enhance event memory, or they may be more useful in knowledge acquisition and utilization. Often a specific memory aid can serve both purposes, and one function may merge into another.

In view of the relative paucity of research in the area of memory aids, we will add some general statements about their use and efficacy, based in part on our own clinical experience. We will review both novel memory aids and also the more obvious ways in which external memory aids may be useful in clinical settings. This allows us to provide a comprehensive overview of devices that can enhance memory functioning in neurological patients, and enables us to bring the wide range of memory aids within some form of coherent conceptual framework.

ENVIRONMENTAL MEMORY AIDS

Features of our environment shape our behaviour, both consciously and unconsciously. We respond (often automatically) to cues in our environment for many of our daily activities. Contextual support from environmental cues may be more critical for those with failing memory (Craik & Jennings, 1992). It makes sense to consider how our environment may be better designed and organized to enhance memory functioning. As in the case of visuospatial functions, where a distinction has been made between personal, peripersonal and extrapersonal space (Robertson & Halligan, 1999), it may be useful to divide environmental memory aids into two categories—proximal environmental and distal environmental memory aids. Memory aids that alter the personal make-up of the individual, such as wearable memory aids, are perhaps better considered along with other portable memory aids and are covered later.

Proximal Environmental Memory Aids

By proximal environment, we include such features as the design and contents of a room or vehicle and the design of equipment the individual uses in everyday domestic or work settings. Specific items that make up the proximal environment but which are not specific to a particular environment, such as clocks, are considered under "portable memory aids". Aspects of the proximal environment form a somewhat neglected area of scientific inquiry in relation to memory aids. Norman's (1988) excellent book remains a useful resource for considering some of the practical manifestations of poor ergonomic design in our everyday environment, and includes instances where poor design may result in memory lapses.

Changes to a work-place or home environment can be engineered to minimize a common memory lapse—forgetting to do something. Examples include leaving something beside the front door, attaching a message to a mirror in the hallway, and leaving around an empty carton of something that needs to be replaced. Simple changes to the design of an environment may act as a catalyst to such memory aids, for example items one has to take when leaving home or leaving the office could be located on an appropriate shelf near the exit itself. The shelf should be clearly labelled and within the horizontal and vertical limits of the person's visual field. Putting together two items may act as a visual reminder to carry out a particular action, for example a pill-bottle next to a toothbrush may remind a patient to take his medicine before cleaning his teeth. White boards, wall charts, etc., that allow messages to be displayed serve as useful memory aids. They can remind individuals to carry out an activity, and also act as a "knowledge board" to display important information, such as emergency telephone numbers. Moffat (1989) described the use of a simple flow chart of likely places to search to help a man who frequently lost items around the home. Sharps & Price-Sharps (1996) found that brightly coloured plates with internal dividers placed on a dining/kitchen table reduced memory lapses of elderly participants, who used the plates for items that might get lost, or for "things to do" messages. Thus, the plates served as message boards to improve event memory, or as semi-permanent storage devices to help remember where items were located.

Cars, mobile phones and other items may have alarm systems to remind the user to do something. In-built alarms or cut-off devices, as are found in some domestic appliances, help prevent event-memory lapses such as forgetting to carry out a certain activity. Voice-based messages to accompany or replace the actual alarm signal are sometimes helpful in order to tell the individual what the alarm means when it is activated.

A proximal environment, well-structured and organized, is less likely to result in memory lapses such as forgetting where something has been put (cf. Fulton & Hatch, 1991). As a basic principle, the items to be stored for later retrieval should be categorized, and separate shelves or storage units allocated to each category. Categories should be meaningful to the individual in question, and may have a number of subcategories, possibly reflected in the structure of the storage unit. Distinctive storage units should differ in features such as size, shape, colour and/or spatial position. They should be clearly labelled, and containers within the storage units should also be labelled. Labels should be in large print and may be of different colours, although black against white is often best for elderly or neurologically disabled people. If the storage units have to be retrieved according to sequence, then some form of alpha-numeric labelling will be of value. The prominence of a storage unit in a room will depend on how frequently the stored items are used, how important they are, and how often they tend to be forgotten. If possible, there should be some relationship between the contents and the visual features of the unit, for example a brown container for storing coffee, a white one for storing sugar, etc. Transparent storage boxes are preferable, as one can see at a glance what is inside and whether the contents need replenishing.

Orientation for time, place and current events will be helped by the presence of items such as clocks that display the day of the week and date, orientation boards, large windows at ground level to allow individuals to see the trees and therefore cues to indicate the time of year, etc. Regularity of routine activities may help improve knowledge such as orientation for time, for example if the tea trolley always comes at 11 am, this provides an anchor point for "confused" patients whose internal "clock memory" mechanisms are impaired.

In some circumstances, tactile memory aids may be useful in providing knowledge about the location of an item: when driving a car it is often impossible to look at the location of various switches. As Norman (1988) pointed out, the layout of such switches often pays little heed to their use in driving behaviour. If, as is often the case, switches of a similar design are in close proximity, or are particularly important to locate, it may be useful to attach a distinctive tactile cue, such as a Velcro pad, onto one of the switches. Similar applications may arise in other settings, such as finding switches in a room in the dark. There are electronic location devices to help locate objects. Thus if one cannot find one's car in the car park, pressing the alarm button an such a device will activate lights on the car.

Distal Environmental Memory Aids

By distal environment, we mean settings such as the layout of a building, shopping centres, the design of streets and towns, the design of transportation networks, and the people with whom we interact.

Wilson & Evans (2000) and Gibbs (2000) noted the emergence of "smart houses", where appliances are centrally controlled and include reminder functions that help prevent memory lapses, ensuring equipment is turned on or off. Future domestic and work environments may include electronic reminder and knowledge systems as an integral part of the environment. Refrigerators, one of the most commonly visited sites in a typical household, are already on the market with inbuilt reminder and internet facilities on the door! For memory-impaired people, family members and carers may act as reminders to carry out activities, such as taking medication. Dogu & Erkip (2000) point to some design features to be kept in mind if spatial orientation in a shopping complex is to be maximized. For similar observations relating to more general navigational activities, such as route finding, see Canter (1996), and for those relating to the specific needs of patients with dementia, see Passini et al. (1998, 2000).

Name badges and distinctive uniforms are obvious, but sometimes neglected, forms of memory aid to help memory-impaired people identify other residents and care staff. Simple labels help people know what to do in certain settings—as Norman (1988) has pointed out, we are all aware of doors where there is no indication whether to PULL or to PUSH. The carefully planned use of such signs (such as warning signs near stairs in homes for elderly people, road traffic warning signs, and so forth) can be of benefit as preventative measures. Other forms of visual cues may also help, such as cues on steps to alert someone who is visually impaired of the steps' existence.

In residential homes or hospitals for memory-impaired people, wall or floor markers indicating the direction to somewhere, together with clearly labelled rooms, may help residents to find their way about (cf. Elmstahl et al., 1997; Olsen et al., 1999). Alarms fitted to doors that activate when the door is opened help provide information to care workers on patients who are likely to wander out of the premises. It is useful for the therapist to carry out a "site visit" to a patient's residence to obtain a first-hand perspective of environmental features and how best to modify the environment so as to enhance everyday memory functioning.

PORTABLE EXTERNAL MEMORY AIDS

Stationery, Mechanical and Related Memory Aids

Stationery memory aids are the most commonly used and probably the most widely acceptable form of memory prostheses, for both the general population and for memory-impaired people. Such aids include self-adhesive POST-IT notes, notebooks, diaries, filofaxes, calendars/wall-charts (Gabriel et al., 1977) and address tags that enable lost items to be returned. Effectiveness may be improved by changing their distinctiveness and location. They should be readily visible and accessible, and also in close proximity to the to-be-remembered activity—thus, a note pad with a list of people to phone should be near the telephone, one that deals with groceries to buy could be on the refrigerator door, and a checklist for operating a piece of equipment should be kept near that equipment. Pencils/pens should form an integral part of the stationery memory aid. Diaries and filofaxes vary in the extent to which they incorporate "reminder" sections, and in some cases it may be appropriate to create distinctive sections dealing with separate categories, such as things to buy, people to meet, phone calls to make, etc.

POST-IT notes and similar items can be used as both general reminders and message-reminders. Thus, a blank POST-IT note placed near an item such as a telephone or television can be used as a cue to remind one to make a call or watch a programme. A POST-IT note that has a list of items to buy and is placed on the fridge door serves as a message-reminder. Memory aids such as dry-wipe boards may have a similar purpose. Diaries, filofaxes with TO DO lists, etc., may all serve as event memory aids.

Stationery items can also be used as permanent or temporary stores of knowledge. Thus, address books represent permanent stores of verbal knowledge, maps provide spatial/navigational knowledge, clocks convey knowledge of time and calendars contain temporal information. For "confused" patients, it may be useful to make up a bracelet that indicates essential orientation information, answers to questions repeatedly asked, and information (name, telephone number of current residence) for someone to use in case the patient becomes lost. Photographs of family members by the bedside may help those with severe memory impairment to retrieve both knowledge and event information relating to their loved ones.

Notebooks, diaries, organizers and similar items have been available for some time. Although they seem fairly straightforward to use with patients, their successful use, especially with the more severely impaired, requires some thought. One of the first systematic attempts to develop a coherent teaching method was described by Sohlberg & Mateer (1989b). They made up purpose-built notebooks with different sections and emphasized that these can be reduced or increased in number according to the patient. Their list of possible sections included Orientation, Memory Log, Diary, Things to Do, Transportation, Feeling Log, Names, and Today at Work.

A head-injured patient reported by Sohlberg & Mateer used a Memory Notebook with five sections—Orientation, Memory Log, Calendar, Things to Do and Transportation. Where note-books are especially designed for patients, page lay-out features such as colour coding, size of print, etc., should be carefully considered. In addition, because notebooks may need to be individualized, patients should be involved in their design early on (cf. Donaghy & Williams, 1998). Care-staff or family members also need to be made familiar with the memory aid.

Sohlberg & Mateer (1989b) divided their training into Acquisition, Application and Adaptation. We recommend combining these into two stages: (a) learning about the item and understanding its features; and (b) using it in everyday situations. Learning about the item involves going through the various sections, understanding what they are for and when they should be used, how to make and change entries, etc. One can test the subject's retention by usual question-and-answer techniques. Role rehearsal, involving practice of real-life examples, may be helpful. Use of direct feedback in such role rehearsal, perhaps also with video feedback, is important. Sohlberg & Mateer suggested that before patients can go on to the use of the notebook in real-life settings, they should have explicit knowledge of the book's features. In our experience, however, as long as there is accurate and successful use of the various notebook features, it does not really matter if the patient can provide explicit recall of particular features. Zencius et al. (1990) compared four memory improvement strategies in a group of six head-injured patients with memory difficulties—written rehearsal, oral rehearsal, acronym formation and memory notebook logging. Only the last technique was successful in increasing recall of target material. In a second study from the same centre (Zencius et al., 1991), four brain-injured patients were found, as a result of training in the use of memory notebooks, to show a more general improvement in memory that included both homework assignments and keeping appointments. Schmitter-Edgecombe et al. (1995) compared a 9-week period of notebook training with supportive therapy in the case of a group of memory-impaired patients who had suffered a severe head injury more than 2 years earlier. Their outcome measure included an index of everyday memory failures, and these were documented before treatment, immediately after treatment, and 6 months later. The authors found that, shortly after treatment, there was a significant benefit in favour of the notebook training group. At 6 months, this benefit was still present, but it no longer reached statistical significance. Some researchers (e.g. Burke et al., 1994; Fluharty & Priddy, 1993) have emphasized the importance of making the notebook acceptable to the patient, by individualizing it to particular patients. Other researchers have made important observations on how notebooks may best be introduced in the context of other changes to the patient's prosthetic environment (e.g. Schwartz, 1995; Wilson, 1999b) and on how they may be of more general benefit in tackling problems such as lack of insight and planning (Finset & Andresen, 1994).

A few mechanical memory aids, such as countdown kitchen timers, are available, although they have been largely overtaken by electronic equivalents. In addition, various types of pill-boxes and containers can be bought which are designed around the days of the week. Several studies have looked at the effectiveness of different medication reminders on patient compliance (Park & Kidder, 1996). Most studies have found that adherence to a medication schedule improves with the introduction of mechanical organizers—the design of the device should be simple and clear, ideally with separate compartments for different days of the week and for different times of the day; in addition, there should be some form of feedback to the patient, perhaps by use of a stationery memory aid, which provides information that the medication in question has actually been taken (McKenney et al., 1992; Nides et al., 1993; Park et al., 1991, 1992; Rehder et al., 1980; Szeto & Giles, 1997).

Electronic Organizers and Related Electronic Reminders

The most common form of commercially available electronic memory aids are electronic organizers. In recent years, these have become more compact, more sophisticated and more diverse in their functions, and also less expensive. In general, such devices can be useful as memory aids in five main ways:

1. An electronic diary to keep a record of appointments.
2. An alarm which provides auditory cues, with or without text information, at preset, regular or irregular times.
3. A temporary store for items such as shopping lists, messages, etc.
4. A more permanent store for information such as addresses, telephone numbers, etc.
5. In more expensive models, a communication device that can receive and send information, such as reminders and factual knowledge.

Electronic organizers range in size from pocket-sized to the size of a wallet/filofax—palmtop devices. Alarms can be set to sound at the same time as a stored message is displayed, and for some models multiple daily, weekly or monthly alarms can be set. Many electronic organizers can be interfaced to enable them to transfer data to computers, and for certain models add-on cards can be bought to store information and allow for specialized applications. Most models have back-up devices to safeguard against loss of stored information. Electronic organizers vary greatly in features which may or may not be applicable to the needs of neurological patients with memory impairment. The following features may be helpful to consider when selecting an electronic organizer for use with memory-impaired people.

General Features

The electronic organizer should be compact enough to fit into a shirt pocket or other handy place. Some of the more expensive electronic organizers may be too bulky to be carried around all of the time, although they could still be kept in a coat pocket or a briefcase.

Databank watches are available which have many of the functions of electronic organizers. While more compact and easier to carry around, they are more limited because of the fine motor control and visual acuity needed to operate them, limited storage capacity, and so forth.

Although batteries may need to be changed only once every few years, one needs to consider the motor dexterity involved in changing the battery and the simplicity of the instructions, in addition to the usual life of the battery and whether there is a back-up battery. Back-up batteries are useful especially where there is a large amount of stored data to be retained in the device's memory. Around 32K memory will usually suffice for most uses. More sophisticated organizers come with removable memory cards.

Patients should not have to consult the manual, but it helps if it is clear and not too intimidating in its length. Summarized forms of information, such as "Help Cards", are useful in that they provide a quick reference to turn to without having to refer to the manual. Those using the organizer as a data-gathering device in settings remote from their work-place will find it useful to be able to link up to a personal computer. In terms of cost, electronic memory aids are not routinely available in publicly-funded healthcare systems, but it is usually possible to buy a model with extensive alarm and text storage facilities for under £50/$75. The length and number of lines that can be displayed on screen is important. Obviously, the larger the screen the better, although the cost will rise with larger screens. At least 10 characters are usually needed on a single line for the minimum sorts of cue words required as reminders. In some cases, especially if there is limited screen space, it is important to train the patient to use key words or abbreviations in order to remember what to do.

The clarity of screen display is also important—some of the less expensive organizers have poor displays despite being useful in other ways. Clarity is a critical item for many neurological patients, especially older people who may have reduced visual acuity.

Since electronic organizers are designed for professionals or executives rather than for people with disability, there are usually keys which are superfluous when the device is used as a memory aid. These may serve as a distraction, especially if the patient has visual search problems, in which case redundant keys should be masked. The keys themselves should be clearly labelled and well laid out, and, if possible, operations should be executed by a single key press rather than by a sequence of keys. Keyboards that provide tone feedback when a key is pressed are desirable.

Voice organizers are available for those who find keyboard entry difficult because of tremor or other movement disorder. These have the same text storage and alarm features as most conventional electronic organizers, but rely on voice input. The device is "trained" to recognize the voice of the user, but even then occasional errors may occur. While current devices are compact, the input keys require a degree of motor control that may be outside the capacity of many neurological patients.

Entering, Storing and Retrieving Information

There are three basic operations that memory-impaired people need to learn: *entering* information; *reviewing* stored information; and *deleting* information from storage. It is useful to check whether these basic operations are simple or complicated for patients. Consider whether word-processing features are useful, for example if a phrase is entered frequently, can a code rather than the full phrase be entered?

In addition to a prospective memory feature giving an alarm (with or without an associated message), it is useful to have a general MEMO facility so that items can be stored which need to be done at some time, but not necessarily on a particular day or at a particular time. In less expensive organizers without such a MEMO facility, the telephone storage facility can be used instead.

While all electronic organizers have basic text storage devices that allow for both temporary and permanent stores of knowledge, some now come with the facility to offer advanced storage features, for example navigational information, the ability to store pictorial material such as photographs, and the ability to link to information resources on the Internet.

Alarm Features

Electronic organizers may be particularly useful as reminders in the following settings:

1. Instances where events may occur between thinking about doing something and remembering to do it (e.g. deciding in the morning to buy something later in the day). This is particularly important when intervening activities preoccupy the individual.
2. Situations where a long interval separates thinking about doing something and having to do it—if one makes an appointment for several months in the future.
3. When there is a high premium on very accurate, precise recall and where internal memory aids may be fallible (e.g. remembering to take a cake from an oven at a specific time).
4. Where multiple alarm reminders are required (e.g. having to take tablets several times a day).

There are essentially two types of alarm reminders, those with and those without a text message. The major virtue of electronic organizers is their ability to display text when an alarm goes off. Therefore, having an alarm with a simultaneous message display is a critical feature. This facility can be used for two main purposes—situations where something has to be done on a particular day and at a specific time, and those situations where it is important that certain things are done but which are not necessarily tied to a particular time. Some organizers emit a warning several minutes before the alarm sounds. For certain activities requiring initial preparation, such as having to go to a meeting, this can be useful. Alarms that can be set to occur at regular intervals, such as daily, weekly or monthly, may be helpful in contexts where activities need to be carried out repeatedly and at specific times.

Turning to research findings with electronic organizers, Azrin & Powell (1969) found that a pill container which sounded a tone at the time medication was to be taken, and which dispensed a tablet at the same time the tone was turned off, was better at inducing patient compliance than a simple alarm timer or a container that made no sound. Fowler et al. (1972) used a timer combined with a schedule card to help their patient stick to a daily routine in his rehabilitation programme. Naugle et al. (1988) worked with a man who consistently forgot to use stationery memory aids such as diaries and log books. They found an "alarm display" watch helped him remember rehabilitation activities. Although of benefit, the patient sometimes ignored the alarm, and sometimes turned it off without reading the message first. Further training in the use of the aid was then given. Giles & Shore (1989) used a PSION organizer to help their patient remember to do weekend domestic chores. This was more beneficial than a pocket diary. However, sometimes the alarm was not loud enough to be heard. Kapur (1995) described preliminary data on the use of an electronic organizer to help patients with head injury, multiple sclerosis and epilepsy. In general, an organizer proved to be useful both as a reminder and as a text storage device, but for one patient who was densely amnesic and was living at home, the electronic aid proved to be of little benefit. Van den Broek et al. (2000) found that for five memory-impaired patients who were provided with a voice-organizer, message-alarm reminder functions were effective in reducing memory lapses in two task settings—passing on a message they had been told 9 h earlier, and remembering to carry out specified domestic chores. Kim et al. (2000) reported that most brain-injured patients who had been trained to use a palm-top computer during their period of rehabilitation continued to use the device in everyday memory settings several years later. In a single-case study (Kim et al., 1999), one head-injured patient who used this device as an inpatient was better at remembering to attend therapy sessions and to take medication.

Wright et al. (2001) noted that, in a group of brain-injured patients, high-frequency users of organizers tended to prefer a standard keyboard organizer, whereas less frequent users preferred a more novel, penpad input system. In an earlier study involving elderly and younger participants from the general population, Wright et al. (2000) found that most participants preferred keyboard data entry to touch-screen data entry, and generally made fewer errors using the keyboard modality.

Speech Storage Devices

As memory aids, speech recording devices are useful when long messages need to be stored. They are also helpful for memory-disordered patients who have difficulty using an electronic organizer, possibly due to motor or visual impairment. As well as conventional tape recorders, digital "solid-state" recording devices have recently been introduced that can store up to several hours of speech. The attractive feature of these devices is the ability to store speech in discrete, labelled files that can be rapidly retrieved. Thus, different categories of messages or things to do can be readily stored and accessed.

Some memory-impaired people complain of difficulty in remembering telephone messages, and a few devices are available which automatically tape telephone conversations. Users of such devices should be aware that they need to inform the caller that the conversation is being taped! A few digital voice recorders have alarm features that can be tagged to stored messages, thus enabling the device to be used as an event memory aid.

The main function of these devices is to act as temporary or permanent stores of knowledge. They are of benefit in educational settings, such as listening to lectures, and are used for this purpose by many young patients with brain injury. Although at present they are not used as knowledge resources to the same extent as printed or visual electronic media, it is possible that in the future this may change with the enhanced storage and other features of recording devices.

There appear to be few formal research studies that have explored the use of conventional or newer recording devices as memory aids for brain-injured patients, apart from the study by Van den Broek et al. (2000) noted above, which successfully used a voice organizer for improving memory functioning in a group of memory-impaired patients.

Electronic Communication Devices

Electronic communication devices can be classified into fixed devices, such as standard corded telephones, or free-standing devices, such as cordless telephones, mobile phones and pagers. Laptop and palmtop computers that can access the Internet can also be classified as communication devices, and a number of mobile phones have additional functions similar to those found in electronic organizers, and so can be used to send text messages or pictures. We will mainly deal here with phone and paging systems for conveying verbal messages.

Telephones are available that allow storage and easy retrieval of frequently used numbers. Useful features can be found in most phones, such as the visual display of a number while it is being dialled and the ability to identify the caller. Fixed phones are currently available in some countries with a "photophone" feature—the face of the person to be called can be represented on a button that is programmed with the person's number. Mobile phones and pagers are available with vibration cues instead of a ringing tone. These are useful for people with auditory impairments. Pagers have similar call-signalling facilities, and some pagers are available with inbuilt alarm features.

Fixed telephones, mobile phones and pagers have a variety of reminder systems associated with them. These range from inbuilt alarms/message-alarms, which may be preset or can be set to signal at specified intervals or on a fixed date, through to alarm systems dependent on some other resource. Telephone-based reminding systems have in the past been shown to be useful in improving patient compliance with taking medication (Leirer et al., 1988, 1991) or keeping appointments (Morrow et al., 1999). In recent years, pagers have been employed to serve as more general reminder memory aids. Commercial paging companies in a number of countries offer reminder services, and a dedicated system for brain-injured patients has also been developed (Hersh & Treadgold, 1994; Wilson et al., 1997, 2001). Phones can also be used to activate devices elsewhere, and thus may help in settings where the individual has to remember to turn on equipment such as domestic appliances.

Most phones have enough storage capacity to store a large number of names and telephone numbers. Those that double-up as organizers have the usual text storage and retrieval facilities of organizers that were outlined above. The ability of both fixed and mobile phones to link up to the Internet has opened up a cornucopia of information resources that may act as knowledge memory aids.

Pagers can be useful as external memory aids, especially as reminders. Milch et al. (1996) found that a paging system used in a hospice environment was useful in improving compliance amongst residents in taking medication. In a single-case study, Aldrich (1998) used a dedicated paging system, NeuroPage, to help a head-injured patient remember to carry out a range of activities, such as getting up and dressing, making lunch, watching the news headlines, feeding the cat, and taking his medication. The pager led to a significant improvement in performance of these activities. After NeuroPage was withdrawn, some improvement was maintained, but this was task-dependent. Similar observations in a further single-case study with NeuroPage were made by Wilson et al. (1999). Wilson et al. (2001) carried out a large-scale study of 143 brain-damaged patients' use of NeuroPage. More than 80% of those who completed the 16 week trial were significantly more successful in carrying out everyday activities, such as self-care, taking medication and keeping appointments. For most patients, this improvement was maintained 7 weeks after returning the pager.

COMPUTER-BASED TECHNOLOGIES FOR ENHANCING MEMORY FUNCTION

While the distinction between desktop computers, laptop computers, palmtop computers and personal organizers is becoming increasingly blurred as a result of advances in technology, in the following sections we mainly deal with those applications where desktop computers have been used in memory rehabilitation. We also consider attempts to use virtual-reality devices to enhance memory functioning, since these invariably use computer-based technologies for their operation.

Exercises and Drills

Although evidence for restoration of function using exercises and drills has not been positive, advances in computer technology and the ready availability of relatively inexpensive hardware have revived interest in such methods (Bradley et al., 1993). The computer represents an ideal medium for presentation of repetitive exercises, and therapists have been attracted by the time-saving features of computer-delivered services. Proponents of the restoration approach to rehabilitation have eagerly adopted computers as "the ultimate drillmasters" (Gianutsos, 1992, p. 34) and have urged others to continue their use "... whatever the outcome" (Gianutsos, 1992, p. 29). However, evidence of beneficial effects of memory exercises has not been forthcoming, whether they are delivered by computer or in the more traditional pencil-and-paper format (Skilbeck & Robertson, 1992). For example, a study by Middleton et al. (1991) found no specific effects of 32 h of drill-orientated computer training of cognitive skills, including memory. Chen et al. (1997) found no major differences across a range of neuropsychological measures between two groups of head-injured patients, one that received computer-assisted cognitive rehabilitation and another that received more traditional rehabilitation. Skilbeck & Robertson (1992), in their review of computer techniques for the management of memory impairment, concluded that when appropriate controls are included in empirical studies, there is little evidence of positive outcome following computer drills.

Some investigators (e.g. Sohlberg & Mateer, 1989a) have suggested that attention may be more amenable to computer training than memory and that improvements in attentional processing might secondarily benefit memory performance. Although the evidence for restoration of function in the attentional domain is more promising than in the memory domain (Matthews et al., 1991; Robertson, 1990), it is, as yet, far from persuasive. For example, Sohlberg & Mateer (1987), in four single-case studies with brain-injured patients, demonstrated improved performance on the Paced Auditory Serial Addition Task (Gronwall, 1977) following computerized practice on other attention-demanding tasks. They also reported improved performance on the Randt Memory Test. Ben-Yishay et al. (1987) found that improved performance on computer training tasks (for attentional deficits) was associated with small gains on relevant neuropsychological tests. Gray et al. (1992) have reported long-term improvements in untrained attentional tasks as a result of computerized training (see also Sturm & Willmes, 1991). On the other hand, Wood & Fussey (1987) found no generalized improvements in attention after 20 h of computer practice, although performance on the specific training tasks did improve; Ponsford & Kinsella (1988) also reported negative results. No benefits for real-life functioning were indicated in any of these studies. Given the paucity and inconsistency of findings with respect to attention, no firm conclusions concerning computerized training of attentional deficits, or of its possible impact on memory, seem warranted (see Wood, 1992).

Exercises and drills have not proved useful for restoring general memory ability. Nevertheless, repetitive practice is probably essential for memory-impaired patients to improve on any specific task or to learn any specific information, and computers may be a useful medium for the repeated presentation of such materials. Because learning does not appear to generalize beyond the training task, it is important that practice is directed towards something relevant or useful in everyday life. Repetitive practice of meaningless lists of numbers, letters, shapes, or locations plays no beneficial role in memory rehabilitation (Glisky & Glisky, in press; Glisky & Schacter, 1989b; Wilson, 1991)

Mnemonic Strategies

There have been few reported attempts to test the effectiveness of computers with respect to the teaching of mnemonic strategies. In one study, Skilbeck (1984) used a microcomputer to teach a head-injured patient the pegword technique for learning short lists of items, such as shopping lists. The patient, who had sustained primarily left-hemisphere damage, learned the 10 pegs (i.e. one is a bun, two is a shoe, etc.) and was then provided with computer instructions concerning the interactive images that were to be formed for each to-be-remembered item and the pegword. The patient was able to use the visual imagery strategy to improve her verbal recall performance, relative to a straightforward repetition condition. However, there was no indication that she employed the strategy on her own. The technique thus enabled her to learn specific information relevant to her everyday functioning but did not improve her memory ability in any general sense.

A somewhat different use of a microcomputer for teaching mnemonic strategies was employed by Johnson (1990). In this study, a relatively high-functioning patient with a mild verbal memory impairment was allowed to experiment on the computer with different strategies for learning word lists. Although he did not adopt any of the presented strategies, he subsequently generated his own techniques after coming to realize the benefits of strategy use for his memory. This study implies that some form of generalized benefits of strategy learning may be possible, at least with mildly impaired patients.

The finding that mnemonic strategies are most useful for patients with relatively mild memory deficits (Benedict, 1989; Wilson, 1987) is consistent with the notion that the strategies rely on the use of residual memory processes. To the extent that memory is damaged rather than lost, residual skills may be tapped to facilitate the acquisition of new information. Such strategies, however, may not be as advantageous for patients with severe memory disorders, who lack the residual memory processes needed for their efficient use.

Evidence on the teaching and use of mnemonic strategies in rehabilitation suggests that the strategies may be beneficially employed by patients with mild-to-moderate disorders for the purposes of learning specific information important in their everyday lives. There is little indication, however, that strategy use generalizes beyond the training situation or that general improvements in memory functioning can be obtained. Repetitive use of strategies with meaningless laboratory materials therefore appears to be of little value (Wilson, 1991).

External Aids

The microcomputer has perhaps the greatest potential of any external aid for beneficial use by memory-impaired patients, although its capabilities have not been fully exploited (Ager, 1985; Harris, 1992). As an external aid, the computer has the power to act as a memory prosthesis, storing and producing on demand all kinds of information relevant to an individual's functioning in everyday life. It may also assist directly in the performance of tasks of daily living (see Cole & Dehdashti, 1990), acting as reminders for activities such as taking medication or meals (Flannery et al., 1997).

Progress in this area, however, has been slow for at least two reasons:

1. Early attempts to teach memory-impaired patients how to use even simple computing devices were not successful. Patients simply could not remember the commands needed to operate them (Wilson et al., 1989; Wilson & Moffat, 1984).
2. Until recently, computers have been too cumbersome to carry around and so their utility in everyday life has been somewhat limited (Harris, 1992; Vanderheiden, 1982).

Both of these problems, however, have been largely solved in the past few years and, although there are as yet few demonstrations of effective use of computers as external aids, there is reason for some optimism concerning the future use of computers by memory-impaired patients.

A series of successful studies employing microcomputers to assist memory-impaired people with tasks of daily living has been conducted by Kirsch et al. (1987, 1992). These investigators used the computer as an "interactive task guidance system", providing a series of cues to guide patients through the sequential steps of real-world tasks, such as cookie-baking and janitorial activities. In these studies, the computer acts solely as a compensatory device, providing the patient with step-by-step instructions for the performance of a task. Little knowledge of computer operation is required on the part of the subject, who merely responds with a single key-press to indicate that the instructions have been followed.

Another promising line of research was conducted by Cole and colleagues (Cole & Dehdashti, 1990; Cole et al., 1993). They designed highly customized computer interventions for brain-injured patients with a variety of cognitive deficits (see also Cole et al., 1988). Each intervention tried to help patients perform an activity of daily living they were able to accomplish prior to trauma but were now unable to perform without assistance. For example, a patient with severe memory and attentional deficits was able to use a customized text editor and software to construct things-to-do lists, take notes during telephone conversations, and carry out home financial transactions (cheque writing, deposits, withdrawals, mailings, etc.), activities that had become impossible since her injury. In this case, the computer was modified to simplify these tasks and to bypass the particular cognitive deficits that were problematic for the patient.

Memory-impaired patients have been able to learn how to use computers as word-processors; for example, Batt & Lounsbury (1990) constructed a simple flowchart with coloured symbols and simple wording that enabled a memory-impaired patient to use a word-processing package. The bypassing of confusing menus and the reduction of memory load enabled the patient to carry out the appropriate word-processing steps without difficulty and to operate the computer by himself (see also Glisky, 1995; Hunkin & Parkin, 1995; Van der Linden & Coyette, 1995).

In all of these studies, memory-impaired people used the computer to support some important activity of daily life. Hardware and software were modified so that problems were eliminated or reduced and only a few simple responses needed to be learned. The computer essentially served a prosthetic function, allowing brain-injured patients to perform activities that were otherwise impossible. These kinds of intervention require no assumptions concerning adaptation of the neural or cognitive mechanisms involved in memory, and in general they make no claims concerning restoration or changes in underlying mnemonic ability. Frequently, however, increases in self-confidence and self-esteem are observed in patients following successful computer experience (Batt & Lounsbury, 1990; Cole et al., 1993; Glisky & Schacter, 1987; Johnson, 1990). Whether these psychosocial changes are specifically attributable to computer use, as opposed to other non-specific features of training, has not been empirically documented.

The one negative feature of these interventions, from a clinical perspective, is their high cost and limited applicability. Design of customized systems requires time, money and expertise and each design may be useful only for a single patient. With continued development in this area, however, prototypical systems may become available that might serve a broader range of patients and be easily administered in the clinic.

Acquisition of Domain-specific Knowledge

In an effort to capitalize on the preserved memory abilities of amnesic patients, Glisky et al. (1986b) devised a fading-of-cues technique, called the "method of vanishing cues", which was designed to take advantage of patients' normal responses to partial cues to teach them complex knowledge and skills that might be used in everyday life. The training technique provides as much cue information as patients need to make a correct response and then gradually withdraws it across learning trials. The microcomputer serves essentially the role of teacher, presenting information and feedback in a consistent fashion, controlling the amount of cue information in accordance with patients' needs and prior responses, and allowing people to work independently at their own pace. Unlike interventions in which the computer is provided as a continuing prosthetic support, the goal of these interventions is to teach people the information that they need in order to function without external support (see Glisky, 1992b).

Using the method of vanishing cues, Glisky and colleagues successfully taught memory-impaired patients information associated with the operation of a microcomputer (Glisky et al., 1986a, 1986b; Glisky & Schacter, 1988b), the names of various business-related documents (Butters et al., 1993) and a number of vocational tasks, including computer data-entry

(Glisky, 1992a; Glisky & Schacter, 1987, 1989a), microfilming (Glisky & Schacter, 1988a), database management (Glisky, 1993) and word-processing (Glisky, 1995). Other researchers have demonstrated successful learning of a daily schedule (Heinrichs et al., 1992), basic items of orientation (Moffat, 1992), information pertaining to treatment goals, sections of a college course in sociology, and instructions for behaviour modification (Cotgageorge, personal communication).

There are, however, some caveats concerning the domain-specific learning approach. Although memory-impaired patients are able to learn considerable amounts of complex information, their learning may be exceedingly slow and may result in knowledge representations that are different from those of the general population. In particular, patients cannot always access newly acquired knowledge on demand or use it flexibly in novel situations. In other words, transfer beyond the training context cannot be assumed (Wilson, 1992), although it has been demonstrated under some conditions (Glisky, 1995; Glisky & Schacter, 1989a). It is therefore essential that all information relevant to the performance of a particular functional task be taught directly, so that the need for generalization is minimal (Glisky et al., 1994).

The problems of transfer and generalization are well known to rehabilitation specialists, and seem to plague all rehabilitation methodologies to some degree. The domain-specific learning approach assumes that transfer to new contexts is not automatic, and so the focus of the approach is on teaching information that is useful to memory-impaired people in their everyday lives. Other approaches, which are directed towards the restoration of general memory ability, assume that generalization does occur and that exercising memory is the key to that outcome. The material to be practised is viewed as irrelevant and consists generally of useless information, such as random digits, locations, words and so forth. Evidence suggests, however, that exercising memory does not improve basic memory ability, and so the procedure provides no benefits to patients whatsoever. The method of vanishing cues similarly requires extensive practice and repetition, but the purpose of practice is the acquisition of new meaningful and useful information. The technique has been found to be significantly more effective than simple repetition (Glisky et al., 1986b; Leng et al., 1991) and has enabled the learning of more complex knowledge than was previously thought possible.

The vanishing cues methodology was designed to capitalize on preserved abilities of amnesic patients in order to teach them knowledge and skills relevant in everyday life. Use of intact memory processes to compensate for those that have been disrupted or lost has often been suggested as an appropriate strategy for rehabilitation (Baddeley, 1992; Salmon & Butters, 1987); yet, as Baddeley has pointed out, few interventions of this type, other than the one used by Glisky and colleagues, have been attempted. It is likely that we still lack sufficient knowledge concerning the nature of the processes preserved in amnesia to take optimal advantage of them in rehabilitation. Nevertheless, this approach seems to be a promising one that may gain momentum as basic research provides additional information concerning processes and structures involved in normal memory.

Vocational Tasks

One area in which computers might serve a potentially important function is the workplace. Glisky (1992a, 1992b) has suggested that some vocational tasks requiring the use of a computer may present good opportunities for employment for memory-impaired patients for a number of reasons. First, patients are capable of procedural learning; they can acquire a fixed set of procedures, such as those required for data-entry or word-processing, and apply them in a consistent fashion over time. Second, computers in general require rather rigid adherence to a set of rules and can be counted on to be highly consistent, unlike their human counterparts. Once patients have learned the rules and their applications, they are less likely to be called upon to make online decisions or respond to novel circumstances. Third, many computer tasks lend themselves rather well to laboratory simulations, so that job training can be accomplished before patients enter the workplace. Glisky and colleagues have found that careful step-by-step training in the laboratory of all components of a task facilitates transfer to the real-world environment and allows the patient to enter the workplace with a high degree of confidence and skill (Glisky & Schacter, 1989a).

In general, computer jobs have been overlooked by rehabilitation and vocational specialists, perhaps because they seem too high-tech and complex and, therefore, beyond the capabilities of brain-injured patients. Yet even patients with quite severe memory impairments have been able to acquire the knowledge and skills needed to perform computer data-entry and word-processing tasks (Glisky, 1992a, 1995). It is worth keeping in mind, however, that all aspects of a task need to be taught explicitly and directly in order to minimize problems in generalization. Although transfer of work skills across changes in materials (Glisky, 1992a) and from a training to a work or home environment has been demonstrated (Glisky, 1995; Glisky & Schacter, 1989a), changes in the actual procedures may present serious difficulties.

Virtual Reality Technology

"Virtual reality" (VR) uses similar technology to that found in interactive computer games and simulators. VR provides a means of creating an artificial, computer-generated environment that the individual can explore, such as the inside of a building or an area within a neighbourhood. There are two types of VR, nonimmersive and immersive. Nonimmersive VR generally consists of conventional computer displays with control devices such as joysticks. Immersive VR is technically much more sophisticated and also much more expensive. The individual receives auditory, visual and tactile components of the computer-generated virtual environment through head-mounted displays and also through head and pressure emitting devices in clothing worn by the participant. Movements made by the subject are relayed back to computer systems that are part of the VR system, and these can amend the pattern of sensory stimulation accordingly, so that immersive VR is very much a two-way interaction between the individual and the system. This opens up a range of applications, including using items in the kitchen or similar everyday tasks (Gourlay et al., 2000).

More general reviews of VR in neuropsychological rehabilitation are provided elsewhere (e.g., Riva, 1997; Rose et al., 1996). For present purposes, we consider the relatively few studies that have so far attempted to apply VR to enhance memory functioning in neurological patients. Brooks et al. (1999) used nonimmersive VR to train an amnesic patient to find her way around a rehabilitation unit. This involved practice on a "virtual" route that had been programmed into a computer—the improvement on the VR task appeared to transfer to performance in the real-life environment of the rehabilitation unit. In a study of a group of patients with unilateral cerebrovascular lesions, Rose et al. (1999) used nonimmersive VR to study memory for spatial and object recognition. Participants either actively or passively explored the VR environment, in one case controlling movement through the environment by using a joystick, and in the other case simply passively viewing the journey through the virtual environment. Memory for spatial features of the VR environment was better in active compared to passive participants. However, memory for objects in the environment was better in passive compared to active control participants, but was the same in passive compared to active neurological patients.

THE APPLICATION OF MEMORY AIDS IN REHABILITATION SETTINGS

Factors to be considered in the use of memory aids in rehabilitation include general ones applicable to most forms of neuropsychological intervention and memory rehabilitation, and specific ones relating to the particular use of aids to overcome memory difficulties—a form of "compensatory memory training". In a critical review covering a number of areas of cognitive rehabilitation, Cicerone et al. (2000) offered useful guidelines that are relevant for the use of memory aids. They

> ...found evidence for the effectiveness of compensatory memory training for subjects with mild memory impairments compelling enough to recommend it as a Practice Standard. The evidence also suggests that memory remediation is most effective when subjects are fairly independent in daily function, are actively involved in identifying the memory problems to be treated, and are capable and motivated to continue active, independent strategy use (Cicerone et al., 2000, p. 1605).

General Factors

For any intervention to be effective and to be seen to be effective, some criteria need to be satisfied. These include:

1. The intervention needs to bring about meaningful changes in the patient's everyday memory functioning. How one defines "meaningful change" may vary from patient to patient, but the patient should be able to carry out more memory-related activities, with greater ease and success, and with less distress, than before the intervention.
2. The improvement in memory functioning should be permanent.
3. The improvement should have minimal side-effects.
4. The intervention should be cost-effective in terms of both money and time.
5. The intervention should be easy to administer by a third party.
6. The intervention should be applicable to a large number of patients, ideally across disease categories and severity of memory loss.
7. The intervention should be beneficial over and above any general "placebo" or incidental effects resulting from the treatment.

In individual patients, variables worth considering are:

1. Age, educational level, and premorbid knowledge and skills.
2. Any physical disability, such as sensory or motor loss.

3. The intactness or otherwise of nonmemory cognitive functions.
4. Supportive and possible negative influences that the family/carer may bring to bear on the therapeutic programme.
5. Current daily routine and the demands which this places on memory. Many memory functions, and in particular prospective memory, are better earlier than later in the day (Wilkins & Baddeley, 1978).
6. Any behavioural, attentional or motivational problems. On the one hand, memory aids may act as motivational cues to help with problems such as apathy, but the use of memory aids often requires some involvement of executive functions, such as initiation of behaviour, planning/organizational skills, problem-solving ability, focused attention, etc.

The severity and pattern of memory loss is a major factor, and it is important to pay particular attention to a number of areas:

1. Everyday memory symptoms as reported by the patient and by an informed observer, noting the patient's insight and concern about his/her memory difficulties.
2. Severity and pattern of anterograde memory loss.
3. Severity and pattern of retrograde memory loss, in particular the extent to which past knowledge and skills have been lost.
4. The extent to which new skill learning and implicit memory are preserved.

Specific Factors

There are a number of specific factors to be borne in mind when considering whether to encourage and train patients in the use of memory aids to help everyday memory:

1. How often and which type of memory aid has been used in the past? For example, many elderly people are accustomed to using simple diaries and are reluctant to change to electronic devices, no matter how much more effective they may be. Some patients need to be reassured that using memory aids will not lead to their becoming lazy or their brain wasting away through lack of use. They need to be reassured that using memory aids with other people around is nothing to be ashamed of, perhaps pointing out that such aids are increasingly used by the general population. Memory aids can be seen as status symbols and may enhance the self-esteem of memory-impaired people.
2. Although it is the principal duty of the clinician to find a memory aid simple to use and suitable for a particular patient, the patient should, if possible, be given a choice and be involved in any decisions.
3. A carer/relative needs to be closely involved in the process from the beginning, so as to encourage the use of the aid in domestic settings. In particular, if the aid is complicated to use, this person also needs to be taught to use it so that there is someone to turn to if problems arise in operating the aid.
4. Memory aids are often given to patients to use with little further or no intervention from the therapist. If only life were this simple. As Intons-Peterson & Newsome (1992) have pointed out, there are a number of cognitive processes involved in the use of even simple external memory aids. Thus, memory-impaired people need to be trained in the

"metamemory" skill of being able to identify situations where a memory aid will be useful, they must motivate themselves to use a memory aid, choose an aid that will be useful for the particular circumstances, and remember how to operate and use the memory aid effectively.

5. Memory-impaired people should be motivated to both learn to use the aid and to adapt daily routines and habits so as to incorporate the memory aid into such activities. Ideally, they themselves should formulate some of the reminders so that they are seen as self-cues rather than "nagging" from some external source.

For more complex aids such as electronic organizers, a specific training programme should be designed in which stages of learning a particular procedure are broken down into steps. Principles such as spaced rehearsal, graded reduction of support/vanishing cues and error-free learning, feedback and encouragement, and help-cards may be required in the teaching process. The training programme in the clinic should, as closely as feasible, mimic everyday uses of the memory aid, with concrete examples being drawn from the patient's daily routine. Training in the use of electronic organizers usually requires 4–6 sessions, and if these are provided weekly, homework can be set for the patient. The beginning of a therapy session can test long-term retention of what was learned in an earlier session. Finally, many effective interventions involve a particular combination of environmental, stationery, mechanical and electronic memory aids, as in the case described by Wilson (1999b). The challenge lies with the clinician to use his/her knowledge and experience to suggest and draw up a particular combination of treatment strategies.

CONCLUSIONS AND FUTURE DEVELOPMENTS

External memory aids are effective in improving everyday memory functioning, and this benefit is particularly evident in the area of prospective memory. Computer-related memory rehabilitation strategies remain largely task-specific in their benefit, but may be useful to the extent that they perform similar functions to external memory aids. The use of environmental cues, either to help navigational memory or to enhance man–machine interaction, is another area that is potentially beneficial to people with memory deficits.

While technological innovations may drive many of the developments in memory rehabilitation, advances in conceptual and clinical spheres are equally important. We do not yet have a comprehensive conceptual framework to consider the various strategies used to enhance memory functioning. If conceptual and empirical links could be made with other attempts to improve memory functioning, such as pharmacological agents and neural implants, rehabilitation might move forwards, especially if these attempts could be integrated into a theoretical framework that accounts for neural plasticity and recovery of memory function following neurological disease or injury (Robertson & Murre, 1999). In the clinical sphere, there may be a greater refinement in our understanding of which patients will benefit most from memory aids. Ideally, a patient's clinical and neuropsychological profile, together with factors such as specific memory needs, should be matched to the features of potential memory aids to inform the clinician of the particular memory aids, or combination of treatments, that will be of maximum benefit to the individual. Careful evaluation of the effectiveness of memory aids will require further advances in memory assessment procedures, in particular those that can reliably assess everyday memory functioning (see Glisky & Glisky, 2002).

The cost-effectiveness of memory aids needs to be considered, especially where computer-based aids or expensive electronic devices may perform functions that can be carried out by stationery memory aids or by less expensive electronic memory aids. Advances in technology may allow for the introduction of more sophisticated, cheaper and more user-friendly aids, and some memory aids may emerge that have been purpose-built for memory-impaired individuals. Future developments in external memory aids include:

1. The integration of multiple memory-related functions within a single electronic unit, which will carry out tasks currently performed by devices such as a personal organizer, mobile phone, e-mail/Internet facility, reminder/pager, etc.
2. Devices such as electronic organizers that more readily accept hand-written input via an adjacent note-pad, which permits infrared transfer of impressions made on paper.
3. Memory pens, which keep a record of what has been written and which allow this information to be transferred to another storage medium.
4. Reminders that have context-sensitive features, such that a message-alarm will activate when the individual engages in a related activity, or when other critical people are in the vicinity (Lamming et al., 1994).
5. Reminders that include a "task enactment–alarm" link, such that the alarm only turns off when the target activity has been carried out (cf. Azrin & Powell, 1969).
6. Wearable memory aids that integrate more naturally with the dress, habits and routines of patients (cf. Hoisko, 2000).
7. Devices that use wireless technology (such as the new "bluetooth" system) to convey information about the location of items.

It is too early to say which, if any, of these developments will have a major impact on the application of memory aids in clinical settings. If conceptual, empirical, biological and technological advances across disciplines are harnessed and harmonized in meaningful ways, and if clinicians and researchers focus their attention and resources on the application of resultant devices in clinical settings, there will be undoubted benefits for memory-impaired neurological patients in the years to come.

ACKNOWLEDGEMENT

N.K. is grateful to Pat Abbott for her help in preparing this chapter.

REFERENCES

Ager, A. (1985). Recent developments in the use of microcomputers in the field of mental handicap: implications for psychological practice. *Bulletin of the British Psychological Society*, **38**, 142–145.
Aldrich, F.K. (1998). Pager messages as self reminders: a case study of their use in memory impairment. *Personal Technologies*, **2**, 1–10.
Azrin, N. & Powell, J. (1969). Behavioral engineering: the use of response priming to improve prescribed medication. *Journal of Applied Behaviour Analysis*, **2**, 39–42.
Bäckman, L. & Dixon, R. (1992). Psychological compensation: a theoretical framework. *Psychological Bulletin*, **12**, 259–283.

Baddeley, A.D. (1992). Implicit memory and errorless learning: a link between cognitive theory and neuropsychological rehabilitation? In L. R. Squire & N. Butters (eds), *Neuropsychology of Memory*, 2nd edn (pp. 309–314). New York: Guilford.

Batt, R.C. & Lounsbury, P.A. (1990). Teaching the patient with cognitive deficits to use a computer. *American Journal of Occupational Therapy*, **44**, 364–367.

Benedict, R.B.H. (1989). The effectiveness of cognitive remediation strategies for victims of traumatic head injury: a review of the literature. *Clinical Psychology Review*, **9**, 605–626.

Ben-Yishay, Y., Piasetsky, E.B. & Rattok, J. (1987). A systematic method for ameliorating disorders in basic attention. In M. J. Meier, A. L. Benton & L. Diller (eds), *Neuropsychological Rehabilitation* (pp. 165–181). New York: Guilford.

Bradley, V.A., Welch, J.L. & Skilbeck, C.E. (1993). *Cognitive Retraining Using Microcomputers*. Hove: Erlbaum.

Brooks, B., McNeil, J., Rose, F. et al. (1999). Route learning in a case of amnesia: a preliminary investigation into the efficacy of training in a virtual environment. *Neuropsychological Rehabilitation*, **9**, 63–76.

Burke, J., Danick, J., Bemis, B. & Durgin, C. (1994). A process approach to memory book training for neurological patients. *Brain Injury*, **8**, 71–81.

Butters, M.A., Glisky, E.L. & Schacter, D.L. (1993). Transfer of learning in memory-impaired patients. *Journal of Clinical and Experimental Neuropsychology*, **15**, 219–230.

Canter, D. (1996). Wayfinding and signposting: penance or prosthesis? In D. Canter (ed.), *Psychology in Action* (pp. 139–155). San Diego, CA: Academic Press.

Chen, S., Thomas, J., Glueckauf, R. & Bracy, O. (1997). The effectiveness of computer-assisted cognitive rehabilitation for persons with traumatic brain injury. *Brain Injury*, **11**, 197–209.

Cicerone, K., Dalhberg, C., Kalmar, K. et al. (2000). Evidence-based cognitive rehabilitation: recommendations for clinical practice. *Archives of Physical Medicine and Rehabilitation*, **81**, 1596–1615.

Clare, L. & Wilson, B. A (1997). *Coping with Memory Problems*. Bury St Edmunds: Thames Valley Test Company.

Cole, E., Dehdashti, P., Petti, L. & Angert, M. (1988). Prosthesis ware: a new class of software supports the activities of daily living. *Neuropsychology*, **2**, 41–57.

Cole, E. & Dehdashti, P. (1990). Interface design as a prosthesis for an individual with a brain injury. *SIGCHI Bulletin*, **22**, 28–32.

Cole, E., Dehdashti, P., Petti, L. & Angert, M. (1993). Design parameters and outcomes for cognitive prosthetic software with brain injury patients. *Proceedings of the RESNA International '93 Conference*, **13**.

Craik, F.I.M. & Jennings, J.M. (1992). Human memory. In F.I.M. Craik & T.A. Salthouse (eds), *Handbook of Aging and Cognition* (pp. 51–110). Mahwah, NJ: Erlbaum.

Dogu, U. & Erkip, F. (2000). Spatial factors affecting wayfinding and orientation. A case study in a shopping mall. *Environment and Behaviour*, **32**, 731–755.

Donaghy, S. & Williams, W. (1998). A new protocol for training severely impaired patients in the usage of memory journals. *Brain Injury*, **12**, 1061–1076.

Elmstahl, S., Annerstedt, L. & Ahlund, O. (1997). How should a group living unit for demented elderly be designed to decrease psychiatric symptoms? *Alzheimer's Disease and Associated Disorders*, **11**, 47–52.

Finset, A. & Andresen, S. (1994). The process diary concept: an approach in training orientation, memory and behavioural control. In R. Wood & I. Fussey (eds), *Cognitive Rehabilitation in Perspective* (pp. 99–116). Hove: Erlbaum.

Flannery, M., Butterbaugh, G., Rice, D. & Rice, J. (1997). Reminding technology for prospective memory disability: a case study. *Pediatric Rehabilitation*, **1**, 239–244.

Fluharty, F. & Priddy, D. (1993). Methods of increasing client acceptance of a memory book. *Brain Injury*, **7**, 85–88.

Fowler, R.S., Hart, J. & Sheehan, M. (1972). A prosthetic memory: an application of the prosthetic environment concept. *Rehabilitation Counselling Bulletin*, **16**, 80–85.

Fulton, A. & Hatch, P. (1991). *It's Here . . . Somewhere*. Cincinnati, OH: Writers Digest Books.

Gabriel, M., Gagnon, J. & Bryan, C. (1977). Improved patient compliance through use of a daily drug reminder chart. *American Journal of Public Health*, **67**, 968–969.

Gianutsos, R. (1992). The computer in cognitive rehabilitation: it's not just a tool any more. *Journal of Head Trauma Rehabilitation*, **7**, 26–35.

Gibbs, W. (2000). As we may live. *Scientific American*, **283**, 26–28.

Giles, G.M. & Shore, M. (1989). The effectiveness of an electronic memory aid for a memory-impaired adult of normal intelligence. *American Journal of Occupational Therapy*, **43**, 409–411.

Glisky, E.L. (1992a). Acquisition and transfer of declarative and procedural knowledge by memory-impaired patients: a computer data-entry task. *Neuropsychologia*, **30**, 899–910.

Glisky, E.L. (1992b). Computer-assisted instruction for patients with traumatic brain injury: teaching of domain-specific knowledge. *Journal of Head Trauma Rehabilitation*, **7**, 1–12.

Glisky, E.L. (1993). Training persons with traumatic brain injury for complex computer jobs: the domain-specific learning approach. In D.F. Thomas, F.E. Menz & D.C. McAlees (eds), *Community-based Employment Following Traumatic Brain Injury* (pp. 3–27). Menomonie, WI: University of Wisconsin.

Glisky, E.L. (1995). Acquisition and transfer of word processing skill by an amnesic patient *Neuropsychological Rehabilitation*, **5**, 299–318.

Glisky, E.L. (1997). Rehabilitation of memory dysfunction. In T.E. Feinberg & M.J. Farah (eds), *Behavioral Neurology and Neuropsychology* (pp. 491–495). New York: McGraw-Hill.

Glisky, E.L. & Glisky, M.L. (1999). Memory rehabilitation in the elderly. In D. Stuss, G. Winocur & I. Robertson (eds), *Cognitive Neurorehabilitation* (pp. 347–361). Cambridge: Cambridge University Press.

Glisky, E.L. & Glisky, M.L. (2002). Learning and memory impairments. In P.J. Eslinger (ed.), *Neuropsychological Interventions*, (pp. 137–162). New York: Guilford.

Glisky, E.L. & Schacter, D.L. (1987). Acquisition of domain-specific knowledge in organic amnesia: training for computer-related work. *Neuropsychologia*, **25**, 893–906.

Glisky, E. L. & Schacter, D. L. (1988a). Acquisition of domain-specific knowledge in patients with organic memory disorders. *Journal of Learning Disabilities*, **21**, 333–339.

Glisky, E.L. & Schacter, D.L. (1988b). Long-term retention of computer learning by patients with memory disorders. *Neuropsychologia*, **26**, 173–178.

Glisky, E.L. & Schacter, D.L. (1989a). Extending the limits of complex learning in organic amnesia: computer training in a vocational domain. *Neuropsychologia*, **27**, 107–120.

Glisky, E.L. & Schacter, D.L. (1989b). Models and methods of memory rehabilitation. In F. Boller & J. Grafman (eds), *Handbook of Neuropsychology* (pp. 233–246). Amsterdam: Elsevier.

Glisky, E.L., Schacter, D.L. & Butters, M.A. (1994). Domain-specific learning and memory remediation. In M.J. Riddoch & G.W. Humphreys (eds), *Cognitive Neuropsychology and Cognitive Rehabilitation* (pp. 527–548). London: Erlbaum.

Glisky, E.L., Schacter, D.L. & Tulving, E. (1986a). Computer learning by memory-impaired patients: acquisition and retention of complex knowledge. *Neuropsychologia*, **24**, 313–328.

Glisky, E.L., Schacter, D.L. & Tulving, E. (1986b). Learning and retention of computer-related vocabulary in amnesic patients: method of vanishing cues. *Journal of Clinical and Experimental Neuropsychology*, **8**, 292–312.

Gourlay, D., Lun, K. & Liya, G. (2000). Telemedicinal virtual reality for cognitive rehabilitation. *Studies in Health Technology Informatics*, **77**, 1181–1186.

Gray, J.M., Robertson, I., Pentland, B. & Anderson, S. (1992). Microcomputer-based attentional retraining after brain damage: a randomised group controlled trial. *Neuropsychological Rehabilitation*, **2**, 97–115.

Gronwall, D. (1977). Paced auditory serial addition task: a measure of recovery from concussion. *Perceptual and Motor Skills*, **44**, 367–373.

Gruneberg, M.M. (1992). The practical application of memory aids. In M.M. Gruneberg & P. Morris (eds), *Aspects of Memory, vol. 1: Practical Aspects*, 2nd edn (pp. 168–195). Florence, KY: Taylor & Francis/Routledge.

Harrell, M. Parenté, F., Bellingrath, E.G. & Lisicia K.A. (1992). *Cognitive Rehabilitation of Memory*. Gaithersburg, MD: Aspen.

Harris, J.E. (1992). Ways of improving memory. In B.A. Wilson & N. Moffat (eds), *Clinical Management of Memory Problems*, 2nd edn (pp. 59–85). London: Chapman and Hall.

Heinrichs, R.W., Levitt, H., Arthurs, A. et al. (1992). Learning and retention of a daily activity schedule in a patient with alcoholic Korsakoff's syndrome. *Neuropsychological Rehabilitation*, **2**, 43–58.

Herrmann, D., Brubaker, B., Yoder, C. et al. (1999). Devices that remind. In F. Durso, R. Nickerson, R. Schvaneveldt et al. (eds), *Handbook of Applied Cognition* (pp. 377–407). Chichester: Wiley.

Herrmann, D.J. & Chaffin, R. (1988). *Memory in Historical Perspective*. New York: Springer-Verlag.

Herrmann, D.J., Weingartner, H., Searleman, A. & McEvoy, C. (1992). *Memory Improvement: Implications for Memory Theory*. New York: Springer-Verlag.

Hersh, N. & Treadgold, L. (1994). NeuroPage: the rehabilitation of memory dysfunction by prosthetic memory and cueing. *Neurorehabilitation*, **4**, 187–197.

Hoisko, J. (2000). Context-triggered visual episodic memory prosthesis. In *Proceedings of the Fourth International Symposium on Wearable Computers* (pp. 185–186). Atlanta, GA: IEEE Computer Society.

Hunkin, N.M. & Parkin, A.J. (1995). The method of vanishing cues: an evaluation of its effectiveness in teaching memory-impaired individuals. *Neuropsychologia*, **33**, 1255–1279.

Intons-Peterson, M.J. & Fournier, J. (1986). External and internal memory aids: when and how often do we use them, *Journal of Experimental Psychology: General*, **115**, 267–280.

Intons-Peterson, M.J. & Newsome, G.L. III (1992). External memory aids: effects and effectiveness. In D. J. Herrmann, H. Weingartner, A. Searleman & C. McEvoy (eds), *Memory Improvement: Implications for Memory Theory* (pp. 101–121). New York: Springer-Verlag.

Johnson, R. (1990). Modifying memory function: use of a computer to train mnemonic skill. *British Journal of Clinical Psychology*, **29**, 437–438.

Kapur, N. (1995). Memory aids in the rehabilitation of memory disordered patients. In A.D. Baddeley, B.A. Wilson & F.N. Watts (eds), *Handbook of Memory Disorders*, Ist edn (pp. 535–557). Chichester: Wiley.

Kapur, N. (2001). *Managing your Memory*, 2nd edn. Southampton: Wessex Neurological Centre, Southampton General Hospital.

Kim, H.J., Burke, D.T., Dowds, M.M. & George, J. (1999). Utility of a microcomputer as an external memory aid for memory-impaired head injury patient during inpatient rehabilitation. *Brain Injury*, **13**, 147–150.

Kim, H.J., Burke, D.T., Dowds, M.M. et al. (2000). Electronic memory aids for outpatient brain injury: follow-up findings. *Brain Injury*, **14**, 187–196.

Kirsch, N.L., Levine, S.P., Fallon-Krueger, M. & Jaros, L.A. (1987). The microcomputer as an "orthotic" device for patients with cognitive deficits. *Journal of Head Trauma Rehabilitation*, **2**, 77–86.

Kirsch, N.L., Levine, S.P., Lajiness-O'Neill & Schnyder, M. (1992). Computer-assisted interactive task guidance: facilitating the performance of a simulated vocational task. *Journal of Head Trauma Rehabilitation*, **7**, 13–25.

Lamming, M., Brown, P., Carter, K. et al. (1994). The design of a human memory prosthesis. *Computer Journal*, **37**, 153–163.

Leirer, V., Morrow. D., Pariante, G. & Doksum, T. (1988). Increasing influenza vaccination adherence through voice mail. *Journal of the American Geriatric Society*, **37**, 1147–1150.

Leirer, V., Morrow, D., Tanke, E. & Pariante, G., (1991). Elders' nonadherence: its assessment and medication reminding by voice mail. *Gerontologist*, **31**, 514–520.

Leng, N.R.C., Copello, A.G. & Sayegh, A. (1991). Learning after brain injury by the method of vanishing cues: a case study. *Behavioural Psychotherapy*, **19**, 173–181.

Long, T.E., Cameron, K.A., Harju, B.L. et al. (1999). Women and middle-aged individuals report using more prospective memory aids. *Psychological Reports*, **85**, 1139–1153.

Martyn, C. & Gale, C. (1999). *Forgetfulness and Dementia*. London: Dorling Kindersley.

Matthews, C.G., Harley, J.P. & Malec, J.F. (1991). Guidelines for computer-assisted neuropsychological rehabilitation and cognitive remediation. *Clinical Neuropsychologist*, **5**, 3–19.

McGlynn, S.M. (1990). Behavioural approaches to neuropsychological rehabilitation. *Psychological Bulletin*, **108**, 420–441.

McKenney, J., Munroe, W. & Wright, J. (1992). Impact of an electronic medication compliance aid on long-term blood pressure control. *Journal of Clinical Pharmacology*, **32**, 277–283.

Middleton, D.K., Lambert, M.J. & Seggar, L.B. (1991). Neuropsychological rehabilitation: microcomputer-assisted treatment of brain-injured adults. *Perceptual and Motor Skills*, **72**, 527–530.

Milch, R., Ziv, L., Evans, V. & Hillebrand, M. (1996). The effect of an alphanumeric paging system on patient compliance with medicinal regimens. *American Journal of Hospital and Palliative Care*, **13**, 46–48.

Moffat, N. (1992). Strategies of memory therapy. In B.A. Wilson & N. Moffat (eds), *Clinical Management of Memory Problems* (pp. 86–119). London: Chapman and Hall.

Moffat, N.J. (1989). Home-based cognitive rehabilitation with the elderly. In L.W. Poon, D.C. Rubin & B.A. Wilson (eds), *Everyday Cognition in Adulthood and Late Life* (pp. 659–680). Cambridge: Cambridge University Press.

Morrow, D., Leirer, V., Carver, L. et al. (1999). Repetition improves older and younger adult memory for automated appointment messages. *Human Factors*, **41**, 194–204.

Naugle, R., Naugle, C., Prevey, M. & Delaney, R. (1988). New digital watch as a compensatory device for memory dysfunction. *Cognitive Rehabilitation*, **6**, 22–23.

Nides, M., Tashkin, D., Simmons, M. et al. (1993). Improving inhaler adherence in a clinical trial through the use of the nebulizer chronolog. Chest, **104**, 501–507.

Nielsen, J. (1958). *Memory and Amnesia*. Los Angeles, CA: San Lucas Press.

Norman, D.A. (1988). *The Psychology of Everyday Things*. New York: Basic Books.

Olsen, R., Hutchings, B. & Ehrenkrantz, E. (1999). The physical design of the home as a caregiving support: an environment for persons with dementia. *Care Management Journals*, **1**, 125–131.

Parente, R. & Herrmann, D. (1996). *Retraining Cognition. Techniques and Applications*. Gaithersburg, MD: Aspen.

Park, D., Morrell, R., Frieske, D. et al. (1991). Cognitive factors and the use of over-the-counter medication organizers by arthritic patients. *Human Factors*, **33**, 57–67.

Park, D., Morrell, R., Frieske, D. & Kinkaid, D. (1992). Medication adherence behaviours in older adults: effects of external cognitive supports. *Psychology and Aging*, **7**, 252–256.

Park, D.C. & Kidder, D.P. (1996). Prospective memory and medication adherence. In M. Brandimonte, G. Einstein & M. McDaniel (eds), *Prospective Memory. Theory and Applications* (pp. 369–390). Mahwah, NJ: Erlbaum.

Park, D.C. Smith, A.D. & Cavanaugh, J.C. (1990). Metamemories of memory researchers. *Memory and Cognition*, **18**, 321–327.

Passini, R., Pigot, H., Rainville, C. & Tetreault, M.-H. (2000). Wayfinding in a nursing home for advanced dementia of the Alzheimer-type. *Environment and Behaviour*, **32**, 684–710.

Passini, R., Rainville, C., Marchand, N. & Joanette, Y. (1998). Wayfinding and dementia: some research findings and a new look at design. *Journal of Architecture and Planning Research*, **15**, 133–151.

Patten, B.M. (1990). The history of memory arts. *Neurology*, **40**, 346–352.

Ponsford, J.L. & Kinsella, G. (1988). Evaluation of a remedial programme for attentional deficits following closed head injury. *Journal of Clinical and Experimental Neuropsychology*, **10**, 693–708.

Rehder, T., McCoy, L., Blackwell, B., Whitehead, W. & Robinson, A. (1980). Improving medication compliance by counseling and special prescription container. *American Journal of Hospital Pharmacy*, **37**, 379–384.

Riva, G. (ed.) (1997). *Virtual Reality in Neuropsychophysiology: Cognitive, Clinical and Methodological Issues in Assessment and Rehabilitation*. Amsterdam: IOS Press.

Robertson, I. (1990). Does computerized cognitive rehabilitation work? A review. *Aphasiology*, **4**, 381–405.

Robertson, I. & Halligan, P. (1999). *Spatial Neglect: A Handbook for Diagnosis and Treatment*. Hove: Psychology Press.

Robertson, I.H. & Murre J (1999). Rehabilitation of brain damage: brain plasticity and principles of guided recovery. *Psychological Bulletin,* **125**, 544–575.

Rose, F., Brooks, B., Attree, E. et al. (1999). A preliminary investigation into the use of virtual environments in memory retraining after vascular brain injury: indications for future strategy? *Disability and Rehabilitation*, **21**, 548–554.

Rose, F., Johnson, D., Attree, E. (1996). Virtual reality in neurological rehabilitation. *British Journal of Therapy and Rehabilitation*, **3**, 223–228.

Salmon, D.P. & Butters, N. (1987). Recent developments in learning and memory: implications for the rehabilitation of the amnesic patient. In M.J. Meier, A.L. Benton & L. Diller (eds), *Neuropsychological Rehabilitation* (pp. 280–293). New York: Guilford.

Schmitter-Edgecombe, M., Fahy, J., Whelan, J. & Long, C. (1995). Memory remediation after severe closed head injury: notebook training vs. supportive therapy. *Journal of Consulting and Clinical Psychology*, **63**, 484–489.

Schwartz, S. (1995). Adults with traumatic brain injury: three case studies of cognitive rehabilitation in the home setting. *American Journal of Occupational Therapy*, **49**, 655–667.

Sharps, M. & Price-Sharps, J. (1996). Visual memory support: an effective mnemonic device for older adults. *Gerontologist*, **36**, 706–708.

Skilbeck, C. (1984). Computer assistance in the management of memory and cognitive impairment. In B.A. Wilson & N. Moffat (eds), *Clinical Management of Memory Problems* (pp. 112–133). London: Croom Helm.

Skilbeck, C. & Robertson, I. (1992). Computer assistance in the management of memory and cognitive impairment. In B. A. Wilson & N. Moffat (eds), *Clinical Management of Memory Problems,* 2nd edn (pp. 154–188). London: Chapman and Hall.

Sohlberg, M.M. & Mateer, C.A. (1987). Effectiveness of an attention training program. *Journal of Clinical and Experimental Neuropsychology*, **9**, 117–130.

Sohlberg, M.M. & Mateer, C.A. (1989a). *Introduction to Cognitive Rehabilitation.* New York: Guilford.

Sohlberg, M.M. & Mateer, C.A. (1989b). Training use of compensatory memory books: a three-stage behavioral approach. *Journal of Clinical and Experimental Neuropsychology*, **11**, 871–891.

Sturm, W. & Willmes, K. (1991). Efficacy of a reaction training on various attentional and cognitive functions in stroke patients. *Neuropsychological Rehabilitation*, **1**, 259–280.

Szeto, A. & Giles, J. (1997). Improving oral medication compliance with an electronic aid. *IEEE Engineering and Biology*, **16**, 48–54.

Tulving, E. (1972). Episodic and semantic memory. In E. Tulving & W. Donaldson (eds), *Organization of Memory* (pp. 381–403). New York: Academic Press.

Tulving, E. (2000). Concepts of memory. In E. Tulving & F. Craik (eds), *The Oxford Handbook of Memory* (pp. 33–43). New York: Oxford University Press.

Van den Broek, M.D., Downes, J., Johnson, Z. et al. (2000). Evaluation of an electronic memory aid in the neuropsychological rehabilitation of prospective memory deficits. *Brain Injury*, **14**, 455–462.

Van der Linden, M. & Coyette, F. (1995). Acquisition of word processing knowledge in an amnesiac patient: implications for theory and rehabilitation. In R. Campbell & M. Conway (eds), *Broken Memories*, (pp. 54–76). Oxford: Blackwell.

Vanderheiden, G.C. (1982). The practical use of microcomputers in rehabilitation. *Bulletin of Prosthetic Research*, **19**, 1–5.

Warrington, E.K. (1986). Memory for facts and memory for events. *British Journal of Clinical Psychology*, **25**, 1–12.

Wilkins, A.J. & Baddeley, A.D. (1978). Remembering to recall in everyday life: an approach to absentmindedess. In M. M. Gruneberg, P.E. Morris & R.N. Sykes (eds), *Practical Aspects of Memory* (pp. 27–34). London: Academic Press.

Wilson, B.A. (1987). *Rehabilitation of Memory.* New York: Guilford.

Wilson, B.A. (1991). Theory, assessment, and treatment in neuropsychological rehabilitation. *Neuropsychology*, **5**, 281–291.

Wilson, B.A. (1992). Memory therapy in practice. In B.A. Wilson & N. Moffat (eds), *Clinical Management of Memory Problems*, 2nd edn (pp. 120–153). London: Chapman and Hall.

Wilson, B.A. (1999a). Memory rehabilitation in brain-injured people. In D. Stuss, G. Winocur & I. Robertson (eds), *Cognitive Neurorehabilitation* (pp. 333–346). Cambridge: Cambridge University Press.

Wilson, B.A. (1999b). *Case Studies in Neuropsychological Rehabilitation* (Chapter 4). Oxford: Oxford University Press.

Wilson, B.A., Baddeley, A.D. & Cockburn, J.M. (1989). How do old dogs learn new tricks? Teaching a technological skill to brain injured people. *Cortex*, **25**, 115–119.

Wilson, B.A., Emslie, H.C., Quirk, K. & Evans, J. (2001). Reducing everyday memory and planning problems by means of a paging system: a randomised control crossover study. *Journal of Neurology, Neurosurgery, and Psychiatry*, **70**, 477–482.

Wilson, B.A., Emslie, H., Quirk, K. & Evans J. (1999). George: Learning to live independently with NeuroPage. *Rehabilitation Psychology*, **44**, 284–296.

Wilson, B.A., Evans, J., Emslie, H. & Malinek, V. (1997). Evaluation of NeuroPage: a new memory aid. *Journal of Neurology, Neurosurgery, and Psychiatry*, **63**, 113–115.

Wilson, B.A. & Evans, J. (2000). Practical management of memory problems. In G. Berrios & J. Hodges (eds), *Memory Disorders in Psychiatric Practice* (pp. 291–310). Cambridge: Cambridge University Press.

Wilson, B.A. & Moffat, N. (1984). Rehabilitation of memory for everyday life. In J.E. Harris & P.E. Morris (eds), *Everyday Memory: Actions and Absentmindedness* (pp. 207–233). London: Academic Press.

Wilson, B.A. & Moffat, N. (Eds.) (1992). *Clinical Management of Memory Problems*, 2nd edn. London: Croom Helm.

Wilson, B.A. & Watson, P. (1996). A practical framework for understanding compensatory behaviour in people with organic memory impairment. *Memory*, **4**, 465–486.

Wood, R.L. (1992). Disorders of attention: their effect on behaviour, cognition and rehabilitation. In B.A. Wilson & N. Moffat (eds), *Clinical Management of Memory Problems*, 2nd edn (pp. 216–242). London: Chapman and Hall.

Wood, R.L. & Fussey, I. (1987). Computer-based cognitive retraining: a controlled study. *International Disability Studies*, **9**, 149–153.

Wright, P., Bartram, C., Rogers, N. et al. (2000). Text entry on handheld computers by older users. *Ergonomics*, **43**, 702–716.

Wright, P., Rogers, N., Hall, C. et al. (2001). Comparison of pocket-computer memory aids for people with brain injury. *Brain Injury*, **15**, 787–800.

Zencius, A., Wesolowski, M. & Burke, W. (1990). A comparison of four memory strategies with traumatically brain-injured clients. *Brain Injury*, **4**, 33–38.

Zencius, A., Wesolowski, M., Krankowski, T. & Burke, W. (1991). Memory notebook training with traumatically brain-injured clients. *Brain Injury*, **5**, 321–325.

CHAPTER 15

Emotional and Social Consequences of Memory Disorders

Robyn L. Tate

Rehabilitation Studies Unit, University of Sydney, Australia

If memory, which makes up the very bones of thought, could be so isolated, and so selectively amputated from a man's mind, what was there to give his mind any human shape at all?... There would be for him nothing upon which he could build a past, or a future. And still more disturbing, he would be unable to form any human relationships. (Philip Hilts, 1995, p. 16, referring to H.M).

SETTING THE SCENE

In her book, *Case Studies in Neuropsychological Rehabilitation,* Wilson (1999) includes seven chapters describing patients with acquired memory disorders. The impact of the memory disorders on the lives of the seven individuals and their families is profound, and in all cases their lifestyles are changed irrevocably. Yet the emotional consequences of the memory disablement show considerable variability, even in the three individuals who suffer a pure amnesic syndrome, uncomplicated by the presence of additional cognitive impairments. The personal accounts of Jack, Alex and Jay provide rich insights into living with amnesia.

Jack comments: "Being continually made aware of mistakes, especially mistakes that I can't help but make, and being forced to challenge my own inability can result in personal humiliation... the feeling of indignation, frustration and fear from that incident has stayed with me" (Wilson, 1999, p. 41). Consequently, he avoids what he terms "high-risk" situations. An almost inevitable consequence of living with amnesia is the necessity for life to be simplified and routinized in order to minimize failures (Elliott, 1990). Alex ultimately made considerable achievements: employment, marriage, and becoming a father. These gains were not without cost, and his biggest problem was his low confidence: "Before I was more confident and sociable... This has changed... My confidence is down and that affects everything... Because I've got a bad memory it doesn't mean I'm intellectually

The Essential *Handbook of Memory Disorders for Clinicians.* Edited by A.D. Baddeley, M.D. Kopelman and B.A. Wilson.
© 2004 John Wiley & Sons, Ltd. ISBN 0-470-09141-X.

impaired. People talk down to me, they see the handicap, not the person" (pp. 64–66). For some people, the cognitive and physical effort involved in maintaining a lifestyle that approaches their premorbid expectations can strike at the very core of the person's identity and self-esteem (Meltzer, 1983). Jay assiduously refined compensatory strategies, elevating them into something of an art form. Yet in spite of his positive outlook and successful psychosocial reintegration, he has periods of feeling "very low and sad about his life. He was expecting to be a lawyer with a good income and has instead become a craftsman with just enough to live on" (p. 52). The mourning for personal losses, dashed hopes and expectations is a painful but necessary process to enable the person to rebuild his/her life in a different direction (Henderson, 1993).

In the original paper describing Jay (Wilson et al., 1997), the authors sought to understand why he should be so outstandingly successful in his use of compensatory strategies when his amnesia was so severe (screening score of 1/12 on the Rivermead Behavioural Memory Test) (Wilson et al., 1985). They point to "the combination of youth, intelligence, organized behaviour, determination, lack of additional cognitive deficits, and of course a fully supportive and imaginative family who worked with him at every stage of his problems" (p. 54). There is an increasing awareness that emotional and social factors are pivotal to rehabilitation success and, as in this case, override the severity of the initial impairments.

The first edition of this *Handbook* included a chapter by Prigatano (1995), entitled "Personality and Social Aspects of Memory Rehabilitation". He made the observation that memory rehabilitation does not occur in a vacuum, noting that half a century earlier such doyens of neuropsychology as Luria, Goldstein and Zangwill drew attention to the importance of personality factors, not only in shaping the symptom picture, but also potentially influencing the patient's adaptation to the permanent effects of such brain damage. Prigatano contrasted this perspective with "modern methods of memory rehabilitation (which) often emphasize cognitive strategies or mnemonic devices to aid the patient with only passing recognition of how emotional or motivational variables may influence treatment strategies and outcome" (p. 603). He concluded the chapter by calling for a more systematic consideration of social and personality factors in order to understand "how these variables interact and influence efforts . . . (regarding) various memory therapies" (p. 612). In the 7 years since the first edition of this *Handbook*, there is not a lot of evidence to suggest that either current clinical practice has changed or the detailed analytical work has been conducted. This chapter provides a detailed and comparative analysis of the social and emotional functioning of a selective group of individuals with circumscribed memory disorders in order to better understand this aspect of amnesia as a basis upon which to implement therapy programmes.

A CONCEPTUAL FRAMEWORK FOR STUDYING EMOTIONAL AND SOCIAL CONSEQUENCES OF MEMORY DISORDERS

Emotional and social consequences of acquired neuropsychological disorders in general, and memory disorders in particular, fall within the domain of psychosocial functioning. Emotional responses occur within the context of an individual's personality structure and their environment. Most authors make a distinction between underlying stable *traits*, which form the structure of the individual's personality, and transient fluctuations in emotional, affective and mood *states*, which occur in response to day-to-day events (Prigatano, 1992).

In the present chapter, "social" is conceptualized largely in World Health Organization (WHO) (1980, 2000) terms, referring to the person's everyday activities and participation in social roles.

One of the foci of this chapter is to examine emotional and social consequences of amnesia as outcomes, albeit outcomes that are not static and are determined by many intervening factors. Some of these are addressed by the WHO model (1980, 2000) of the consequences of illness or disease. It makes a tripartite distinction among impairments (abnormality or loss), disabilities (labelled "activity limitation" in the revised model), which refers to the restricting effects of impairments in functional performance and activities, and handicaps (labelled "participation restriction" in the revised model), referring to disadvantage arising from impairments and/or disabilities in the individual's performance of roles. The revised model includes a fourth component, contextual factors, involving both external (environmental) and internal (personal) influences on functioning.

This framework is helpful in understanding emotional and social consequences of memory disorders. For the present purposes, the nature and severity of the impairment (i.e. memory disorder) may result in a disability, in that the person is no longer able to engage in everyday activities previously taken for granted. Moreover, the impairments and/or disabilities may cause handicap if the person is no longer able to, or has difficulty in, resuming social roles, such as parent, employee, friend. Whereas a person might be able to minimize the effects of disability in one area of function (e.g. doing household chores) by the use of appropriate strategies (e.g. written lists for the housework schedule), he/she may be less able to compensate for aspects of memory impairment in other areas (such as raising a young child) and hence is significantly handicapped in the parenting area. The revised WHO model also recognizes that impairments, activity limitation (disabilities) and participation restriction (handicaps) are only some of the factors influencing outcome. Personal character (internal influences), together with the degree of emotional and practical support provided by family, friends and other people (external influences), play a crucial role in determining outcome. It is the sum total of all these factors and their interactions that contribute to social functioning, impact upon how a person feels about him/herself, his/her emotional responses to the situation, and thence the psychological adjustment to the amnesia.

It has long been recognized that nonmedical factors (in WHO terms, internal and external influences) affect outcomes. Within the neurological domain, specifically with reference to traumatic brain injury, Lishman (1973) made a distinction between "direct" and "indirect" factors. Direct factors were those directly related to the injury, such as locus and severity of lesion; indirect factors comprised a diverse range, including premorbid variables, environmental influences and emotional repercussions of the injury. It is important to recognize that emotional factors may play not only an "indirect" role but a "direct" role as well, when organic lesions are strategically placed. For example the limbic system is of central importance not only as the neural substrate for establishing new memories, but also in regulating emotions, mood and behaviour (Macchi, 1989). Additionally, the effects of orbital prefrontal lesions upon emotions, mood and behaviour can be so profound that the fundamental personality structure is altered (cf. Phineas Gage, described in MacMillan, 1996).

The component functions of the limbic system, as well as the interconnections between the limbic system and the frontal lobes, reinforce the intimate connection between the neural substrates of memory and emotions. Talland (1968) was among the first to recognize that amnesia was not restricted to memory processes alone, but was "regularly accompanied by abnormally reduced spontaneity, and usually also by some anomalies of affect"

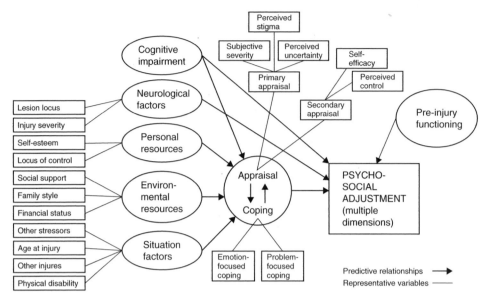

Figure 15.1 Model of psychosocial adjustment after closed head injury. Reproduced from Kendall & Terry (1996)

(p. 22), including lack of initiative. This was observed not only in patients with Korsakoff's syndrome but also in postencephalitic patients and those with ruptured aneurysms of the anterior communicating artery. Similarly, Schacter (1991; Schacter et al., 1990) has written extensively of the problems of unawareness of memory deficit in patients with amnesia. In many of these cases it can be difficult to disentangle the relative contribution of "direct" and "indirect" emotional factors in the resulting symptom picture. Hence, when considering emotional factors from the "indirect" perspective in people with acquired memory disorders, it is important to acknowledge the possibility of a "direct" contribution as well.

Lishman's (1973) conceptualization has received support from other authorities, including Gainotti (1993), Prigatano (1987) and, in its most developed form, by Kendall & Terry (1996). Their model (see Figure 15.1), also with specific reference to traumatic brain injury, is based on the theory of Lazarus & Folkman (1984) as this applies to stress and coping. This model forcefully asserts the central role played by psychosocial factors in influencing outcome or adjustment. A variety of factors are conceptualized as antecedent variables, comprising, in Lishman's (1973) terms, both direct (medical, neurological and neuropsychological) and indirect (demographic, personal and environmental) factors. The model is interactive and recursive in that a second group of factors is posited to intervene and thence mediate the influence of the antecedent variables upon adjustment. These mediating variables are cognitive appraisals and ensuing coping responses of the individual.

Kendall & Terry's (1996) model brings a refreshing perspective to the study of psychosocial consequences in that by including "person" factors, such as premorbid personality, coping style and postmorbid cognitive appraisals, it goes beyond the well-trodden path of focusing exclusively upon emotional well-being and social functioning. With some notable exceptions (e.g. Moore et al., 1989, 1991; Moore & Stambrook, 1995), research into the effects of cognitive appraisals has not featured strongly in the neurological rehabilitation literature to date. Yet their importance is underscored by the striking observation of a number of empirical studies regarding the apparent mismatch between the objective reality of patients' level of disability and their own appraisals of their degree of disability. Tate & Broe (1999) found, for example, that 27% of their traumatic brain injury group with moderate or severe disability as assessed by the Glasgow Outcome Scale (Jennett & Bond, 1975; Jennett et al., 1981) reported having "no" disability or handicap, whereas 14% of those who had made a good recovery reported experiencing "a lot" of disability/handicap. Consideration and understanding of the multitude of diverse factors enumerated in Kendall & Terry's model may also help to explain why Jay (Wilson, 1999; Wilson et al., 1997), described earlier in this chapter, has made such an outstandingly successful adjustment to his memory disorder, whereas other individuals with far less severe impairments experience continued failures and set-backs in their adaptation.

PSYCHOSOCIAL CONSEQUENCES OF MEMORY DISORDERS

There is a dearth of literature regarding the emotional and social consequences of amnesic conditions, and a number of authors have called for more specific and detailed study of this aspect of amnesia (Bachna et al., 1998; Prigatano, 1995; Schacter et al., 1990). There are good reasons to suspect that the broader literature that does exist, regarding the emotional and social functioning of people with *a range* of neuropsychological disorders, is not entirely applicable to the more selective group of individuals with pure memory disorders. First, it has been generally accepted that people with circumscribed memory disorders have their other neuropsychological functions intact, although, as will be argued later, this position is not so clear-cut. Nevertheless, those with fairly circumscribed memory disorders are well placed to harness their intelligence and other neuropsychological strengths and implement compensatory strategies to circumvent the memory disorders. This enables them to access a range of life options that otherwise would be unavailable or difficult to achieve—productive work, independent lifestyles and a regular social life. Second, the presence of other neuropsychological impairments in addition to memory disorder makes it difficult to attribute any emotional or social disturbance to the memory disorder itself, as opposed to some concomitant neuropsychological problem that the person may experience, such as aphasia, executive impairment, attention deficit and so forth. Despite these issues, the literature regarding emotional and social consequences for people with a range of neuropsychological problems is relevant and important, given that, as Wilson (1991) observes, the majority of adults who experience acquired memory disorder also have additional neuropsychological impairments.

Yet some common and, indeed, intriguing themes are evident among the few single case reports that are available regarding the emotional and social functioning of adults whose neuropsychological impairments are reported as being restricted to acquired disorders of memory. These include the well-known cases H.M., N.A. and S.S., whose salient psychosocial and medical features are presented in Table 15.1. The most famous case, H.M., was originally reported in Scoville & Milner (1957). He underwent bilateral resection of the hippocampus for the relief of intractable epilepsy and as a consequence was left with severe anterograde amnesia. He was evaluated psychiatrically in 1982 and 1992 and described briefly in Corkin (1984) and Corkin et al. (1997). Case N.A. sustained damage to the region

Table 15.1 Psychosocial consequences of memory disorders in selected single cases

	H.M. (Corkin, 1984; Corkin et al., 1997; Ogden, 1996)	N.A. (Kaushall et al., 1981)	S.S. (O'Connor et al., 1995)
Background			
Year of onset	1953	1960	1971
Age at onset	27	22	44
Cause of disorder	Neurosurgical resection of medial temporal lobe bilaterally for treatment of intractable epilepsy	Fencing foil penetrating dorsomedial nucleus of thalamus	Herpes simplex encephalitis
Premorbid work	Unemployed at time of operation, but previously process-type work	Radar technician in air force	President of optical physics firm
Presentation	Socially interactive, agreeable, cooperative	Relaxed, amiable, appropriate social graces	Pleasant and outgoing manner, conducts intelligent discourse
Initial cognitive test results (Wechsler Scales)			
Intelligence Quotient	112	99	136
Memory Quotient	67	64	<50 (WMS-R delay)
Social functioning			
Accommodation	Initially with parents, since age 54 in a nursing home	Lives with mother	Lives with wife and family
Use of transport	Unable to go anywhere unaccompanied	Drives to selected venues	No information
Instrumental activities of daily living	Limited information; requires prompt and assistance for showering routines	Appears to rely upon mother	No information
Work	When living at home assisted with domestic activities; attended rehabilitation workshop	Tidies house; small woodwork projects; attends outpatient day treatment centre weekly	Routine household chores under supervision of wife
Leisure activities	Cross word puzzles, reading newspapers and television	Collects memorabilia, goes for walks, assembles models	No information
Relationships with family	Angry outbursts when provoked, otherwise placid	Some conflict with mother	No information
Relationships with friends	No information, but no interest in sexual relationships	No close friends and no sexual relationships	No information

of the left dorsomedial thalamus as a result of an accidental injury with a miniature fencing foil (Teuber et al., 1968). This resulted in a severe memory disorder, particularly for verbal material. His social functioning has been carefully documented, both in the original report and in Kaushall et al. (1981). The case of S.S., who contracted herpes simplex encephalitis, was originally reported by Cermak (1976; Cermak & O'Connor, 1983). His residual impairment was an amnesic syndrome. The emotional functioning and personality structure of S.S. has been studied in detail by O'Connor et al. (1995).

Social Functioning

In the 20 years since his injury, case N.A., aged 42 at the time of the follow-up report, is described as having "a devastated life and isolated mental world" (Kaushall et al., 1981, p. 384). With reference to occupational activities, he has not returned to his previous work as a radar technician and spends most of his time tidying around the house, doing small woodworking projects and attending a hospital outpatient day treatment programme on a weekly basis. Although he takes a keen interest in his collections of memorabilia and goes for walks, his leisure activities are limited by his memory disorder. Television, for instance, is unsatisfying because he forgets the narrative during commercial breaks. In terms of interpersonal relationships, NA remains unmarried and has had virtually no sexual contact since the injury, or, it appears, intimate relationships outside family. He has no close friends and lives with his mother, with whom there is some degree of conflict. His communication and socializing skills are moderately handicapped given that, because of his memory impairment, he is unable to maintain a topic of conversation. Living skills, for the most part, show major restriction. NA does not appear to be able to travel independently around the community, having taken 4 years to learn to drive from his home to the hospital day treatment programme. He relies upon his mother to prepare the meals, and it seems that he would be unable to live in the community without such live-in support and supervision. On the positive side, however, his social skills are well preserved.

The other cases, H.M. and S.S., have similarly impoverished lifestyles dating from the time of their illnesses. Neither of these men engages in any type of productive work. Yet in spite of the large amount of spare time, there is little evidence of a well-developed avocational programme in lieu of work. They are isolated individuals, without the benefits of a social network. Even though, following hospital discharge, they live in the community, they are dependent upon such emotional and practical supports as are provided by family. When these are no longer available, as in the case of H.M., institutional care appears to be the only alternative.

Although it is difficult to compare individual cases with group studies, there is a suggestion in group studies examining other neurological conditions of sudden onset, such as stroke and traumatic brain injury, that many of these people may in fact have less disruption of their social roles than those with pure amnesia, in terms of occupational activity, interpersonal relationships and independent living skills (e.g. Anderson et al., 1995; Fleming et al., 1999; Flick, 1999; Ponsford et al., 1995; Raaymakers et al., 2000; Tate et al., 1989). This is in spite of the additional multiple neuropsychological and motor-sensory disabilities frequently experienced by the stroke and traumatic brain injury groups. It is counter-intuitive that people with fairly circumscribed memory disorders should experience lifestyles that are so extremely disrupted. It appears that case N.A., at least, does not use compensatory memory strategies to enhance his lifestyle. "NA has not developed, or taken an interest in, notekeeping or other mnemonic techniques. He stoutly maintains that note-taking and diary keeping are crutches that would prevent him from improving" (Kaushall et al., 1981, p. 385). Considering the model of Kendall & Terry (1996) presented earlier, however, the severity and nature of the impairment was only one factor contributing to outcome and psychosocial adjustment. A consideration of "person" factors (including the personality structure of the individual and the emotional responses to the situation) is necessary to understand the psychosocial effects of acquired memory disorders.

Personality Structure

In the context of conducting a psychometric study of the Minnesota Multiphasic Personality Inventory (MMPI) and its revised version, MMPI-2 (Butcher et al., 1989), Bachna et al. (1998) examined 10 individuals with circumscribed memory disorders. Two of the MMPI scales, Depression and Schizophrenia, showed significant elevations for the group as a whole, with more than 50% showing elevations on these scales. A literal interpretation of the elevated scales can be misleading, however, because of the preponderance of items that would likely be endorsed by persons with neurological conditions (see also Alfano et al., 1990). Items such as, "There is something wrong with my mind", rather than being indicative of psychiatric abnormality, represent an accurate interpretation of the effects of the impairments these individuals experience. Similar observations have been made about other instruments, such as the Symptom Checklist (Woessner & Caplan, 1995) and the Eysenck Personality Questionnaire (Tate, 2003).

One of the participants in the Bachna et al. (1998) study was case S.S. His MMPI results indicated significant emotional distress, with elevations on clinical scales indicative of depression and anxiety. The Rorschach test was also administered to explore "latent aspects of S.S.'s personality" (O'Connor et al., 1995, p. 49). The quantity of responses was low and additionally qualitative analysis indicated obsessional tendencies, as well as themes of deterioration and decay. The authors suggested that, whereas the latter may reflect a damaged sense of self as a result of his illness, the former may represent either "a lifelong personality pattern . . . [or] his attempt to organize and understand his unpredictable environment" (p. 50). The aberrant results of the MMPI and Rorschach may be explained on the basis of the effects of S.S.'s neurological damage. Hence, if the data are to be interpreted as showing pathology of his personality structure, this is secondary to the amnesic syndrome.

To these standardized results can be added the clinical observations made about H.M., whose personality is described as "placid, happy and uncomplaining" (Ogden, 1996, p. 54). It is also noted that his adjustment to all changes in relationships and circumstances has been smooth (Corkin, 1984), although whether this reflects maturity or is a function of his adynamia is a moot point. H.M. is described as being very compliant, to the extent that, "if he is asked to sit in a particular place, he will do so indefinitely" (Corkin, 1984, p. 251). The personality of N.A. is not described in any detail, although Kaushall et al. (1985) suggest that he has a stable personality structure, given his adjustment to life events, such as his mother's new partner, together with his intact social skills and "signs of continuing personality development" (p. 388). The earlier report (Teuber et al., 1968), however, commenting upon changes in NA's personality at assessments 6–7 years postinjury, also described some inertia-type behaviours, in that NA leads "a rather indolent life, mowing his lawn and performing other chores around the house and garden if, and only if, he is instructed to do so ('driven to it' according to his mother)" (p. 270). The later account (Kaushall et al., 1981) does not describe these types of behaviour or make reference to the comments of Teuber and colleagues. By contrast, they draw a distinction between N.A. and the personality changes in Korsakoff's syndrome patients who, as previously noted by Talland (1968), do exhibit signs of apathy, passivity and lack of initiative, and conclude that "there is no necessary association between amnesia and passivity" (p. 387). One possibility to account for the discrepancy in descriptions of N.A.'s personality profile pertains to the long-term process of adaptation of personality in living with amnesia.

These clinical observations, together with the test data from case S.S., raise many questions about the personality structure of amnesic individuals that warrant further investigation. To date, personality change from the premorbid state has not been examined in people with amnesia. Although the traumatic brain-injured group is one for which changes in personality are commonly reported, very few studies with that group have used standardized measures of personality, including ratings taken of the premorbid state soon after onset of injury. The few reports that are available have shown different patterns of results. Using the NEO Personality Inventory (Costa & McCrae, 1992), Kurtz et al. (1998) found a significant change (decrease) on only one scale, Extraversion, between premorbid and 6 month posttrauma ratings. Employing the Eysenck Personality Questionnaire—Revised (Eysenck & Eysenck, 1991), Tate (2003) found more extensive changes between premorbid and 6 month posttrauma ratings: significant decrease in Extraversion and increases in Neuroticism and Criminality, as well as Psychoticism at 12 months posttrauma. These data are interpreted as being changes in personality structure that are a direct consequence of the injury.

Other issues have been explored by the Boston group (Bachna et al., 1998; O'Connor et al., 1995). One of these pertains to the effect of the memory disorder on the development of personality over time. What is the effect of an individual being unable to incorporate and integrate new information and life experiences into the existing personality structure? Although Kaushall et al. (1981) gained the impression that N.A.'s personality was developing over time, this was not a finding for the more densely amnesic person, case S.S., when a standardized instrument, Measures of Personality Development (Hawley, 1980), was used. O'Connor and colleagues found that his emotional development was arrested at the time of onset of his illness, in that he had resolved conflicts appropriate to his maturational age at the time of onset of his illness (young adulthood), but not those thereafter (middle and older adulthood).

Bachna et al. (1998) also considered the role of memory processes in relation to the sense of self. They hypothesized that, if individuals with amnesia predominantly draw upon immediate memory as a reference point for their personality structure, then they will likely experience fluctuations in emotional states in response to changes in everyday events. By contrast, if they draw upon remote memories, then a much more stable profile will likely emerge. Their own data point to the latter alternative, but clearly this depends upon the nature of the memory disorder. What happens when the long-term store is difficult to access, as in case C.W. (Wilson et al., 1995; Wilson & Wearing, 1995)?

In 1985, at age 46, C.W., a famous and gifted musical scholar, contracted herpes encephalitis. This left him with the most severe episodic memory impairment reported to date, such that he is described as living in "a *moment* with no past to anchor it and no future to look ahead to" (Wearing, 1988, cited in Wilson & Wearing, 1995, p. 15). In addition, C.W. also has semantic memory impairments for both verbal and visual material, as well as a retrograde amnesia that extends back most of his life. With such devastating losses of personal knowledge, in addition to the inability to retain and build upon new memories, one can only speculate that his memory disorder must cut across his very sense of self. Articulate individuals, such as the psychologist Malcolm Meltzer (1983), who writes about the effect of his own (albeit comparatively less severe) memory disorder on his psyche, had such an experience:

> I felt to some extent that I had lost some of my identity. This was not total or extreme, but there were some questions in my mind about beliefs, values and purposes in life. In addition, I felt I had lost some of my cultural background when I had difficulty remembering some of the customs, traditions and beliefs of the groups to which I belonged. This produces a feeling of being somewhat alone" (p. 3).

Emotional Status

There is a substantial literature on the emotional distress encountered in other groups with acquired neurological conditions, such as stroke and traumatic brain injury, with anxiety and depression, in particular, commonly reported (e.g. Dennis et al., 2000; Gordon & Hibbard, 1997; Gordon et al., 2000; Hanks et al., 1999; Nelson et al., 1994; Satz et al., 1998; Wilson et al., 2000). The data are generally given a straightforward interpretation as being indirect consequences of the neurological event. The situation is much more complex with respect to the cases H.M., N.A. and S.S. in terms of both clinical presentation and aetiology.

Case S.S. did not resume his work as president of an optical physics firm developing laser technology following his illness, but lived at home with his family, doing household chores under the supervision of his wife. The authors contrast the demeanour of S.S., who presents as a well-adjusted individual, with his "dire circumstances", and they raise the question as to whether he has, in fact, a normal capacity for emotional experience: "Although he occasionally expresses concern about memory problems, he does so in an unemotional manner, and his mood varies little over time. In fact, his insight regarding his situation seems entirely superficial" (O'Connor et al., 1995, p. 48). As the authors expected, given his demeanour, S.S. did not endorse symptoms consistent with depression on scales such as the Beck Depression Inventory (BDI) (Beck et al., 1961), scoring 3.

These results suggest that S.S. is not depressed, at least not in an overt manner as assessed by instruments such as the BDI, and this is consistent with other anecdotal accounts. Case N.A. (Kaushall et al., 1981) does not manifest any of the responses indicative of emotional distress that one could reasonably expect, given his dramatically altered lifestyle: sadness, grief, depression, despair, frustration, irritability, poor self-esteem, loss of confidence, hopelessness. Rather, he "maintains a steadfastly optimistic, and sometimes unrealistic, view of his own life and progress" (p. 385). Similarly, the emotional functions of H.M. are described as "typically blunted, but he is capable of displaying the full range of emotions . . . There is no evidence of anxiety, major depression or psychosis" (Corkin et al., 1997, p. 3970). After his mother's death, the staff of the nursing home observed that his grief was mild, again suggesting that his emotional responses may be blunted. Ogden (1996, p. 54) further notes that, "it is surprising that H.M. does not react with some degree of confusion, frustration, or anger from continually facing the situation of not knowing where he is, what year it is, what new type of technology or development he is looking at, or who the people are who speak to him".

The common thread among these three cases of circumscribed amnesia is that the individuals do not admit to emotional distress, and their emotional responses appear to be attenuated. Yet the results of the O'Connor et al. (1995) study, using standardized instruments to evaluate the emotional functioning of case S.S., are inconclusive, in that on some scales (e.g. BDI) he does not endorse responses indicative of depressive symptomatology, but with other tests (e.g. MMPI) his profile indicates significant emotional distress, and specifically depression. The authors suggest three hypotheses to account for the test scores: first, that S.S. may have impaired insight, resulting in his failure to overtly endorse depressive symptomatology with face-valid instruments such as the BDI. A second hypothesis pertains to the presence of psychological denial as a protective mechanism to shield himself from the full knowledge of his situation. Goldstein (1939) had spoken of the catastrophic reaction that can occur in brain-injured people manifest as, in Gainotti's (1972, p. 42) memorable words, "the anxious, desperate reaction of the organism, confronted with a task it could not face". Finally, with respect to the MMPI results, O'Connor and colleagues point to situational factors (viz. item content of assessment instruments) that are related to the medical condition of S.S., rather than his psychological state, an issue noted in the previous section. To these possibilities needs to be added the method by which data are gathered, namely self-report instruments. Hermann (1982, cited in Schacter, 1991) observed that completing a self-report instrument is itself a memory task, and this could be a reason why memory-disordered individuals fail to reliably endorse items on checklists such as the Everyday Memory Questionnaire (Sunderland et al., 1983).

The aforementioned insight hypothesis of O'Connor et al. (1995) pertains to an organic explanation of these individuals' failure to endorse depressive symptomatology, when (in the opinions of researchers) they have every reason to be depressed given their altered life circumstances. The hypothesis is not only of theoretical importance but is also clinically relevant because it impacts upon management. A number of eminent rehabilitation clinicians (e.g. Ben-Yishay, 2000; Prigatano, 2000) maintain that awareness and insight are requisites for successful rehabilitation. Schacter et al. (1990) qualify the insight hypothesis when they observe that only certain groups of people with amnesia have impaired insight—viz. those with concomitant frontal dysfunction (e.g. patients with Korsakoff's syndrome, ruptured aneurysms of the anterior communicating artery, and closed head injury). Those with the so-called "pure amnesias" from circumscribed temporal and diencephalic lesions do not have problems with insight. In this latter category they give, as examples, cases H.M. and N.A., and also include encephalitic patients (cf. case S.S.). Yet, as Kopelman et al. (1998) observe, patient groups with impaired insight do not give "entirely random" responses on self-report measures of their memory competency. Although their temporal lobe group rated their memory performances worst of any group, nonetheless the frontal and diencephalic (mostly Korsakoff) groups endorsed significantly more severe responses than the normal control group.

These observations beg the question: what is meant by "insight"? Presumably it is more than mere awareness that a problem exists. As noted earlier, O'Connor et al. (1995) regarded case S.S.'s acknowledgement that he experienced memory problems as "entirely superficial". Schacter and colleagues (1990) made similar comments about case B.Z., a patient with a ruptured anterior communicating artery aneurysm, at the end of his "awareness training". Alternatively, perhaps it is not a *lack of insight* (i.e. anosognosia) that underlies the blunted emotional responses of these cases, but rather a *lack of concern* about their situation (i.e. anosodiaphoria), a distinction drawn by Babinski (1914, cited in McGlynn & Schacter,

1989). This would imply that these people have shallow and superficial emotional responses to many situations, not just to their own altered life circumstances, but also that their close relationships may be lacking in warmth, sensitivity and spontaneity. In none of the three cases, H.M., N.A. or S.S., are their interpersonal relationships described in sufficient detail to make informed comment, but the number of tantalizing comments peppered throughout the case descriptions suggests that this hypothesis is worthy of closer examination.

A Psychosocial Study of a Person with Amnesia—the Whole Picture

Background

The foregoing cases provide incomplete data from one or other psychosocial perspective: social functioning is well described in case N.A., but scarcely any details are available regarding his personality and emotional functioning; by contrast, the personality structure of case S.S. is documented in a detailed and standardized manner, but social functioning is described only in vague generalities. The following case of a person (who has requested that she be identified as Michelle), reported by Tate et al. (2001), focuses on the consequences of a relatively pure amnesia on each of social, personality and emotional functioning. The data are particularly instructive in that ratings on standardized personality instruments regarding her *premorbid* status were obtained from her father soon after the injury, and then compared with postinjury ratings at 6 and 12 months postinjury. Michelle and her family were recently interviewed at 6 years postinjury.

In 1994, at the age of 23, Michelle was allegedly assaulted during a robbery when an intruder broke into her home. She was stabbed in the region of her left eye with a long, narrow instrument and sustained a penetrating brain injury. The extent of the injury was well documented on magnetic resonance imaging some months later: "The path of the injury passes through the left frontal lobe, head of the left caudate nucleus inferiorly, genu of the internal capsule adjacent to the fornix anteriorly, third ventricle and right thalamus. There may also be a shorter second path a little more superiorly in the left frontal lobe".

On admission to the Lidcombe Hospital Brain Injury Rehabilitation Unit in Sydney, Australia, at 6 weeks postinjury, Michelle was confused, amnesic, tearful and agitated. Over subsequent weeks it became clear that her amnesic syndrome was not showing signs of substantial recovery. The initial neuropsychological examination was conducted between 2 and 3 months postinjury. From the outset, Michelle showed a relatively stable pattern of performances, with Table 15.2 providing the results of neuropsychological examinations. Her severe memory disorder, more pronounced for verbal material, was in the context of preserved IQ levels in the Average range, intact cognitive processing speed and, with the exception of generativity, good performances on tests of executive abilities. Her summary scores on the Wechsler Memory Scale at 4 years posttrauma may imply recovery of some aspects of memory, but in functional terms it is clear that Michelle continues to experience major difficulty in learning and retaining new information, as her scores on the Delayed Index (< 50) and relatively demanding learning tests, both verbal (Rey Auditory Verbal Learning Test) and visuospatial (Austin Maze), indicate. Behavioural evidence of frontal impairment came from early entries in the medical notes that documented her "lack of initative and poor insight", and need for prompting on self-care tasks. Neurological examination was essentially unremarkable, and she showed no motor-sensory impairments, apart from

Table 15.2   Test scores from serial neuropsychological examinations of Michelle

		2–3 Months postinjury	6 Months postinjury	1 Year postinjury	4 Years postinjury
NART		FSIQ 110	103	NA	NA
WAIS-R	Verbal IQ	92	85	93	NA
	Performance IQ	86	81	96	
	Full Scale IQ	88	82	94	
WMS-R	Attention/ Concentration	104	101	92	113
	Verbal Memory	51	68	75	94
	Visual Memory	72	88	91	106
	General Memory	<50	66	74	97
	Delayed Memory	<50	<50	<50	<50
WCST	Number of categories	6	6	6	NA
	Perseverative errors	9	4	8	
TMT	Part A (time, s)	45	42	36	42
	Part B	84	60	80	38
COWAT	Total correct	15	23	29	28
	Number of errors: (repeats/rule breaks)	5/2	9	3/7	3/1
Word fluency	Number correct	NA	18	33	NA
	Number of errors		3	2	
Design fluency	Number correct	NA	11	16	NA
	Number of errors		1	1	
SDMT	Written	NA	50	58	NA
	Oral		58	64	

Supplementary memory tests

RAVLT	
Trials 1–5	7^{+1}, 8, 8, 9, 6^{+2}
List B	5
Recall A	1^{+1}
Delay	3^{+1}
Recognition	12^{+9}
AM*	
Errors for trials 1–30 (Test abandoned at trial 30)	15, 12, 12, 9, 9, 9, 6, 6, 7, 5, 6, 6, 4, 5, 5, 4, 2, 5, 3, 2, 3, 2, 2, 2, 3, 2 ,4, 2, 2, 3

NART, National Adult Reading Test; FSIQ, Full Scale IQ; NA, not administered; WMS-R, Wechsler Memory Scale—Revised; WCST, Wisconsin Card Sorting Test; TMT, Trail Making Test; COWAT, Controlled Word Association Test; SDMT, Symbol-Digit Modality Test. RAVLT, Rey Auditory Verbal Learning Test; AM, Austin Maze.
* AM administered at 6 years posttrauma.

some cranial nerve abnormalities: a dilated left pupil, left IIIrd nerve palsy with ptosis, and partial IVth nerve palsy.

Social Outcome

At the time of her injury, Michelle had just completed a diploma in hotel management and was enrolled in a business administration course. She had previously done well at school, having completed her Higher School Certificate (12 years of education) at a selective high school. She was a single parent with a 5-year-old son and they lived with her parents.

At the 6 year follow-up, the nature and extent of changes in Michelle's social functioning (i.e. handicap or participation limitation) was assessed with the Sydney Psychosocial Reintegration Scale (SPRS) (Tate et al., 1999). This 12-item questionnaire, rated on a seven-point Likert-type scale, assesses functioning in three domains (occupational activities, interpersonal relationships and independent living skills). Total scores are in the range 0–72, with higher scores indicating better levels of reintegration. Her father's responses indicated major handicap (total score 31), particularly in the area of occupational activities (see Table 15.3). Michelle's self-report suggested a more favourable picture in all domains (total score 58).

Michelle has not had gainful employment since her injury, and is presently occupied in caring for her 11-year-old son, although she needs considerable support in her parenting role. She and her family are keen for her to pursue employment compatible with her memory disorder, but over the past 6 years this has been restricted to intermittent periods of work with voluntary community organizations. There has been a reduction in her leisure activities and she has not had a partner since the injury, neither does she have friends outside of the family whom she sees regularly. In terms of living skills, she requires prompts and reminders from other people about personal habits, such as dressing, and she is disorganized with respect to her personal effects and household duties. The severe difficulty she has in managing her finances (e.g. buys impulsively, orders goods which she cannot afford and then forgets she has purchased them) has been of major concern to her family, such that her sister now manages the finances for her. On the positive side, Michelle can drive independently anywhere and does not get lost, and socially she presents well, although she is over-familiar and will strike up conversations with strangers in the street, divulging intimacies, and hence is very vulnerable.

Issues of Insight

Michelle's level of insight was assessed by comparing her report of her memory functioning in everyday life with that of her father. Instruments comprised the Everyday Memory Questionnaire (EMQ) (Sunderland et al., 1983, 1984), Use of Memory Aids Questionnaire (Wilson, 1991) and the Effects of Neuropsychological Deficits Scale (ENDS) (Tate & Perdices, unpublished). The ENDS consists of 30 items rated on a five-point Likert-type scale from "extreme effect" to "no effect at all", examining both self-efficacy and the impact of neuropsychological disorder on 10 domains of everyday living. Scores are in the range 0–120, with higher scores indicating greater effect of neuropsychological impairments on everyday living. The results of these questionnaires are presented in Table 15.3.

Table 15.3 Scores on memory questionnaires regarding Michelle at 6 years postinjury

Instrument	Subscale	Informant ratings	Self-ratings
Sydney Psychosocial Reintegration Scale	Total score (range, 0–72)	31	58
	Occupational Activities (0–24)	5	15
	Interpersonal Relationships (0–24)	13	21
	Independent Living Skills (0–24)	13	22
Everyday Memory Questionnaire	Total score (Michelle) (range, 0–140)	38	31
	Total score (head-injured group)[1]	22	27
	Total score (control group)[1]	15	23
	Specific domains (Michelle):		
	Speech	13	10
	Reading and writing	7	2
	Faces and places	4	3
	Actions	2	7
	Learning new things	12	9
Use of Memory Aids Questionnaire	Total number of strategies used	13	13
Effects of Neuropsychological Deficits Scale	Total score (range, 0–120)	63	52
	Severity, now	Moderate	Moderate
	Severity, future	Moderate	Moderate
	Mean scores[2] on items for:		
	Impact on everyday activities	1.8	0.8
	Impact on the person	2.3	2.7
	Effort to avoid failures	3.0	2.5
	Help from others	3.5	3.0
	Reliance on aids	4.0	3.0
	Self-efficacy[3]	1.7	1.8

[1] Data from Sunderland et al. (1984).
[2] Mean scores: range 0–4 (0, "not at all" to 4, "extreme").
[3] Items for self-efficacy are reverse scored: 0, "extremely confident" to 4, "not at all confident".

On the EMQ, there was fairly good agreement between the ratings of Michelle and her father, although her father rated more memory failures. Her total scores indicated that she experiences more difficulty with memory than do the head-injured and control groups reported by Sunderland et al. (1984), their data also being included in Table 15.3. There was perfect agreement between Michelle and her father regarding the types of strategies she uses in everyday living to circumvent her memory difficulties. She uses 13 separate strategies, which is considerably more than the number reported in Wilson's (1991) survey of individuals with memory disorders (mean = 7.39, SD = 3.12). Some strategies are used more consistently and frequently than others, especially writing on her hand, use of a white board, wall calendar, and asking other people to remind her of things. Notably, in spite of intensive and specific rehabilitation efforts, Michelle does not use a memory notebook or other kind of permanent record. Her rehabilitation doctor, who continues to see her regularly, says that he has never seen her refer to any notes. There was some variability between responses from Michelle and her father on the ENDS, in terms of the effect upon

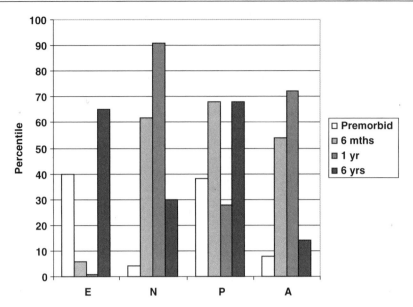

Figure 15.2 Michelle's scores on the Eysenck Personality Questionnaire—Revised. E, extraversion; N, neuroticism; P, psychoticism; A, addiction

everyday living for work, relationships and living skills, which her father considered was moderate, whereas Michelle's ratings suggested the impact was minor. Otherwise agreement was very good. She is concerned about her difficulties and frustrated by them, but they do not affect her emotionally in the sense of "getting her down". She has a lot of support from other people in dealing with her difficulties and relies heavily upon memory aids. Although it is unlikely that the severity of her memory problems will improve in the future, she is very confident about dealing with her difficulties.

Effect upon Personality, Self-concept and Self-esteem

Michelle's *premorbid* personality structure, as assessed by her father's endorsement of the Eysenck Personality Questionnaire—Revised (EPQ-R) (Eysenck & Eysenck, 1991) soon after Michelle's injury, showed a well-adjusted profile (see Figure 15.2). Scores on the E (Extraversion) and P (Psychoticism) scales were at the lower limits of the Average range, suggesting she was somewhat less sociable than her peers and more of a loner, as well as being a more sensitive and well-adjusted person. She had low addictive tendencies and was stable and even-tempered, experiencing low levels of emotionality on the N (Neuroticism) scale. No normative data are available for females for the C scale (Criminality). Following the injury, significant changes occurred on all scales, with data analysed using single-case methodology described in Ley (1972).[1] The changes were not, however, abnormal in a

---

[1] Using the stability coefficients reported in the EPQ-R manual, Michelle's scores between the premorbid and postinjury ratings were examined to determine whether any changes reflected a reliable change or were due to measurement error. The minimum difference (MD) required for the change in score between the two test occasions to be reliable was calculated using the following formula: $MD = z_{MD} \sqrt{(2 \times \sigma^2 (1 - r_{xx}))}$, where z_{MD} is the z score associated with a change in raw test scores of magnitude

Table 15.4 Test scores on personality examinations regarding Michelle at 6 years postinjury

Test	Subscale	Informant ratings	Self-ratings
Eysenck Personality	Extraversion	65	32
Questionnaire—	Neuroticism	30	9
Revised	Psychoticism	68	21
(percentiles)	Addiction	14	2
Tennessee Self-	Validity scales:	Not administered	
concept Scale	Inconsistency		50
(percentiles)	Self-criticism		2.5
	Faking Good		61
	Response Distribution		50
	Summary Scores:		
	Total Self-concept		50
	Conflict		8
	Self-concept Scales		
	Physical		61
	Moral		65
	Personal		46
	Family		9
	Social		75
	Academic/Work		34
	Supplementary Scores:		
	Identity		65
	Satisfaction		57
	Behaviour		65
Self-esteem	(Score range[1] 0–100)	Not administered	65
Inventory			
(raw score)			
Profile of Mood	Tension	3	2
States	Depression	8	18
(percentiles)	Anger	61	38
	Vigour	50	88
	Fatigue	34	72
	Confusion	13	21
Depression, Anxiety	Depression	Not administered	0
and Stress Scale	Anxiety		0
(raw score)	Stress		0

[1] High scores indicate high self-esteem.

clinical sense, with the exception of the E scale at 12 months postinjury (less than 1st percentile) and the N scale was also elevated (91st percentile). When recently reviewed at 6 years postinjury, an unexpected and most encouraging trend was evident in Michelle's EPQ-R ratings by her father, which were now indistinguishable from the premorbid level for all scales, except N, which was borderline. Her own evaluation differed (nonsignificantly) from her father's, with lower scores on all scales (see Table 15.4).

MD between test occasions, σ is the standard deviation of the normative sample, and r_{xx} is the test–retest correlation coefficient provided in the test manual. Given that scores could either increase or decrease over time, two-tailed tests of significance were used, and thus $z_{MD} = 1.96$.

At 6 years postinjury, Michelle completed a number of measures designed to examine her sense of identity and self-esteem, including the Tennessee Self-concept Scale (TSCS) (Fitts & Warren, 1996) and the Self-esteem Inventory (Coopersmith, 1981) (see Table 15.4). Scores on both instruments were mostly unremarkable, being within normal limits, although some interesting findings emerged from the TSCS. A very low score was obtained on one validity scale, Self-criticism (2.5 percentile). Michelle also showed a low Conflict score (8th percentile). Normally this, together with the low Self-criticism score, indicates defensiveness, but other interpretations may be hypothesized in the case of an individual with severe memory disorder. Limited awareness is an obvious contender, but Michelle's tendency to minimize emotional impact, or alternatively to simplify events to reduce the load on memory, are also possible explanations. The other relatively low score on the TSCS was that for Family (9th percentile). This was an unexpected result, given the extensive family support Michelle receives in terms of managing her memory disorder, which she herself also acknowledges. It may suggest she feels some degree of alienation from her family, given that the Family scale "reflects the individual's feelings of adequacy, worth and value as a family member" (Fitts & Warren, 1996, p. 23).

Effect upon Mood and Emotions

With respect to Michelle's emotional status, no premorbid ratings were undertaken because retrospective ratings of mood state are of questionable reliability. Postinjury ratings were made by her father, using the Profile of Mood States (POMS) (McNair et al., 1992). These were essentially unremarkable, as shown in Figure 15.3. Indeed, it is interesting to speculate that at 6 months postinjury the elevations on Fatigue and Confusion (88th and 84th

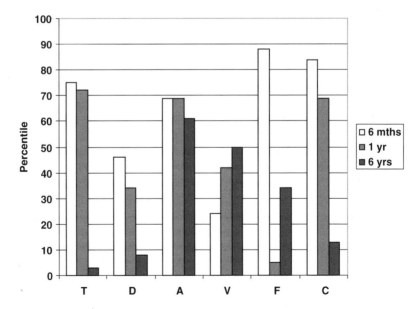

Figure 15.3 Michelle's scores on the Profile of Mood States. T, tension; D, depression; A, anger; V, vigour; F, fatigue; C, confusion

percentiles, respectively) and low score for Vigor (24th percentile) reflect organic-type aspects of the recovery process, whereas by 6 years postinjury, these had resolved (Fatigue, Confusion and Vigor at 34th, 13th and 50th percentiles, respectively). At this point, the (indirect) emotional sequelae (or lack thereof, in keeping with case S.S.) came to the fore, Tension and Depression being the 3rd and 8th percentiles, respectively (previously 75th and 46th percentiles at the 6 month postinjury assessment). It is noted, however, that no significant variation among the three assessments had occurred for Anxiety, ranging between the 61st and 69th percentiles. At the most recent interview (Table 15.4) Michelle's self-ratings on the POMS were in general agreement with those of her father, although her ratings on Vigor and Fatigue were somewhat higher.

Michelle's recent self-ratings on the Depression, Stress and Anxiety Scale (Lovibond & Lovibond, 1995) revealed no emotional distress. Her father says that her memory disorder does not make her unhappy, and he added that he would be unable bear it if Michelle were constantly emotionally distressed about her situation. Occasionally, there is the flicker of an emotional wound, but the effect dissipates quickly. Michelle's sister commented that Michelle has been unable to deal emotionally with some events. If the subject of her mother's death (which occurred 5 years previously, at 14 months postinjury) is brought up, "it is like it only just happened . . . her mood comes in blocks. Yesterday she was so distraught (about her finances) and an hour later she was fine. Ninety percent of the time she is very optimistic". Although Michelle's interpersonal interactions are entirely normal and appropriate in most situations, her family has noticed marked changes in her capacity to respond to another person's distress, such as when her young son falls and injures himself. She does not appear to know how to respond any more, is lost for words and actions, and does not show, in demonstrable terms, the empathy that typified her premorbid character.

CONCLUDING COMMENTS AND FUTURE DIRECTIONS

In the current chapter, a conceptual framework has been described within which emotional and social consequences of memory disorders have been examined. The essential component of that model was a distinction between direct and indirect effects of the causative neurological event. Available psychosocial data from four cases with fairly circumscribed memory disorders were discussed within the framework of the model. Michelle's psychosocial profile is a virtual composite of the famous cases, H.M., N.A. and S.S., and thus provides a good basis upon which to integrate the social and emotional consequences of memory disorders.

Like the other cases, the effects of Michelle's fairly circumscribed memory disorder have caused major disruption to her social functioning at virtually all levels, including instrumental activities of daily living, and without the support of her family she would be an isolated person, unable to live in the community. It is not possible to attribute this impoverished social functioning entirely to the amnesia, however, because these cases have additional neuropsychological, behavioural and/or emotional impairments. For example, H.M.'s other impairments include slight anomia, "clearly impaired" semantic and symbolic verbal fluency, as well as abnormal perception of internal states for pain and hunger (Corkin, 1984; Hebben et al., 1985). Additionally, he has behavioural abnormalities that are suggestive of a disorder of drive or, in Blumer & Benson's (1975) terminology, "pseudodepression": H.M. lacks initiative, rarely complains, and usually does not initiate conversations. The original report of N.A. (Teuber et al., 1968) documented similar inertia-type behaviours.

The most striking feature of these cases pertained to their emotional functioning, where a complex clinical picture emerged, predominantly characterized by an absence of emotional distress and diminished concern about their circumstances. It could reasonably be expected that, given their neuropsychological and social disabilities, these individuals would experience significant emotional distress at their losses. The accounts are noteworthy for the apparent absence of such distress. Although all individuals presented with a genial manner and had stable, even-tempered mood, cases H.M. and S.S. are described as having blunted affect, whereas case N.A. is described as "steadfastly optimistic". There is little additional qualitative comment about cases N.A. and S.S., but H.M. is further described as capable of showing the "full range" of emotions; occasionally, when stressed, he can be roused to anger "but as soon as he was distracted, his anger would dissipate immediately" (Corkin, 1984, p. 251). Michelle incorporates all these features—she presents with a pleasant, friendly and cooperative manner, her mood is characterized as being mostly happy and optimistic, and although she can become emotionally distressed, it is not sustained.

As was also observed in the other cases, Michelle appears to have insight into her memory disorder and its severity, but she tends to minimize its impact, which suggests that the issue here might be an interaction between diminished concern and impaired awareness rather than impaired awareness *per se*. Moreover, she does not display behaviours indicative of depression, loss of confidence, low self-esteem and so forth. Like case S.S., Michelle does not admit to any emotional distress in general when examined with standardized instruments. As the data from case S.S. indicates, however, the situation is ambiguous, in that emotional disturbance is revealed depending upon the standardized instrument used.

In the four cases reviewed here, there was a strong possibility of an organic (i.e. direct) component to the emotional dysfunction, given that the area of damage responsible for the memory disorder (i.e. limbic system) is likely to disrupt their emotional functioning also. O'Connor et al. (1995) suggest that limbic damage could interfere with the ability to derive meaning from emotional events and/or diminish the ability to express feelings. It is clear that a model such as that implied by many studies of other neurological groups, whereby emotional disturbance is conceptualized exclusively as a reaction to (i.e. indirect consequence of) the neurological event, is overly simplistic. In the context of amnesia, the direct factors are of two sorts: first, the emotional responses themselves, which showed some variety, including blunted affect, unconcern and unsustained emotional response; second, the memory variables are an important direct factor: if an individual is always living in "a moment", then there can be no context for an emotional response because the incident that caused emotional distress will not be remembered.

The foregoing does not imply that there is no functional (i.e. indirect) element to the emotional disturbance, such as presence of depression, but rather that the direct factors probably override indirect factors, making it difficult to identify their nature, severity and impact. In a recent interview with Michelle, when completing the Self-esteem Inventory, she omitted a response to one item: "I'm popular with persons my own age". When this was pointed out to her, she replied, "But I don't have friends my own age any more", whereupon her eyes welled up with tears. Her obvious and strong emotional distress was immediately extinguished when her attention was refocused on another matter. Clearly, more empirical study is required in order to understand better the behavioural and emotional responses in cases of fairly circumscribed memory disorders. The report of O'Connor et al. (1995) regarding case S.S. provides an excellent example of the type of specific, hypothesis-driven research that needs to be conducted, and results of such studies will directly inform clinical practice.

ACKNOWLEDGEMENTS

I am grateful to Michelle and her family, who have given permission to report on her experiences. I also thank Ms Kim Ferry, Clinical Neuropsychologist from the Brain Injury Rehabilitation Unit at Liverpool Hospital, Sydney, for data from Michelle's most recent neuropsychological assessment. Discussions with Dr Michael Perdices and his comments on an earlier version of this work were of great benefit, and the support of the Rehabilitation Studies Unit has enabled me to prepare this chapter in a most conducive environment.

REFERENCES

Alfano, D.P., Finlayson, M.A.J., Stearns, G.M. & Neilson, P.M. (1990). The MMPI and neurologic dysfunction: profile configuration and analysis. *Clinical Neuropsychologist*, **4**, 69–79.

Anderson, C.S., Linto, J. & Stewart-Wynne, E.G. (1995). A population-based assessment of the impact and burden of caregiving for long-term stroke survivors. *Stroke*, **26**, 843–849.

Bachna, K., Sieggreen, M.A., Cermack, L. et al. (1998). MMPI/MMPI-2: comparisons of amnesic patients. *Archives of Clinical Neuropsychology*, **13**, 535–542.

Beck, A.T., Ward, C.H., Mendelson, M. et al. (1961). An inventory for measuring depression. *Archives of General Psychiatry*, **4**, 53–62.

Blumer, D. & Benson, D.F. (1975). Personality changes with frontal and temporal lobe lesions. In D.F. Benson & D. Blumer (eds), *Psychiatric Aspects of Neurologic Disease* (pp. 151–170). New York: Grune and Stratton.

Ben-Yishay, Y. (2000). Postacute neuropsychological rehabilitation: a holistic perspective. In A.-L. Christensen & B.P. Uzzell (eds), *International Handbook of Neuropsychological Rehabilitation* (pp. 127–135). New York: Kluwer.

Butcher, J.N., Dahlstrom, W.G., Graham, J.R. et al. (1989). *Manual for the Restandardized Minnesota Multiphasic Personality Inventory: MMPI-2: an Interpretive and Administrative Guide*. Minneapolis, MN: University of Minnesota Press.

Cermak, L.S. (1976). The encoding capacity of a patient with amnesia due to encephalitis. *Neuropsychologia*, **14**, 311–326.

Cermak, L.S. & O'Connor, M. (1983). The anterograde and retrograde retrieval ability of a patient with amnesia due to encephalitis. *Neuropsychologia*, **21**, 213–234.

Coopersmith, S. (1981). *SEI: Self-Esteem Inventories*. Palo Alto, CA: Consulting Psychologists Press.

Corkin, S. (1984). Lasting consequences of bilateral medial temporal lobectomy: clinical course and experimental findings in H.M. *Seminars in Neurology*, **4**(2), 249–259.

Corkin, S., Amaral, D.G., Gonzalez, G. et al. (1997). H.M.'s medial temporal lobe lesion: findings from magnetic resonance imaging. *Journal of Neuroscience*, **17**(10), 3964–3979.

Costa, P.T. & McCrae, R.R. (1992). *NEO PI-R. Professional Manual. Revised NEO Personality Inventory (NEO PI-R) and NEO Five-factor Inventory (NEO-FFI)*. Odessa, FL: Psychological Assessment Resources.

Dennis, M., O'Rourke, S., Lewis, S. & Warlow, C. (2000). Emotional outcomes after stroke: factors associated with poor outcome. *Journal of Neurology, Neurosurgery, and Psychiatry*, **68**, 47–52.

Elliott M. (1990). Coping with a memory loss—a personal perspective. *Cognitive Rehabilitation*, **8**, 8–10.

Eysenck, H.J. & Eysenck, S.B.G. (1991). *Manual of the Eysenck Personality Scales (EPS Adult)*. London: Hodder & Stoughton.

Fitts, W.H. & Warren, W.L. (1996). *Tennessee Self-Concept Scale, TSCS:2*. Los Angeles, CA: Western Psychological Services.

Fleming, J., Tooth, L., Hassell, M. & Chan, W. (1999). Prediction of community integration and vocational outcome 2–5 years after traumatic brain injury in Australia. *Brain Injury*, **13**, 417–431.

Flick, C.L. (1999). Stroke outcome and psychosocial consequences. *Archives of Physical Medicine and Rehabilitation*, **80**, S21–S26.

Gainotti, G. (1972). Emotional behaviour and hemispheric side of lesion. *Cortex*, **8**, 41–55.

Gainotti, G. (1993). Emotional and psychosocial problems after brain injury. *Neuropsychological Rehabilitation*, **3**, 259–277.

Goldstein, K. (1939). *The Organism. A Holistic Approach to Biology, Derived from Pathological Data in Man.* New York: American Books.

Gordon, W.A., Haddad, L., Brown, M. et al. (2000). The sensitivity and specificity of self-reported symptoms in individuals with traumatic brain injury. *Brain Injury*, **14**, 21–33.

Gordon, W.A. & Hibbard, M.R. (1997). Poststroke depression: an examination of the literature. *Archives of Physical Medicine and Rehabilitation*, **78**, 658–663.

Hanks, R.A., Temkin, N., Machamer, J. & Dikmen, S.S. (1999). Emotional and behavioral adjustment after traumatic brain injury. *Archives of Physical Medicine and Rehabilitation*, **80**, 991–997.

Hawley, G. (1980). *Measures of Personality Development.* Odessa, FL: Psychological Assessment Resources.

Hebben, N., Corkin, S., Eichenbaum, H. & Shedlack, K. (1985). Diminished ability to interpret and report internal states after bilateral medial temporal resection: case HM. *Behavioural Neurosciences*, **99**, 1031–1039.

Henderson, P. (1993). My life a routine. *Journal of Cognitive Rehabilitation*, **11**, 32–34.

Hilts, P.J. (1995). *Memory's Ghost. The Strange Tale of Mr M and the Nature of Memory.* New York: Simon and Schuster.

Jennett, B. & Bond, M.R. (1975). Assessment of outcome after severe brain damage. A practical scale. *Lancet*, i, 480–484.

Jennett, B., Snoek, J., Bond, M.R. & Brooks, N. (1981). Disability after severe head injury: observations on the use of the Glasgow Outcome Scale. *Journal of Neurology, Neurosurgery, and Psychiatry*, **44**, 285–293.

Kaushall, P.I., Zetin, M. & Squire, L.R. (1981). A psychosocial study of chronic circumscribed amnesia. *Journal of Nervous and Mental Disease*, **169**, 383–389.

Kendall, E. & Terry, D.J. (1996). Psychosocial adjustment following closed head injury. *Neuropsychological Rehabilitation*, **6**, 101–132.

Kopelman, M.D., Stanhope, N. & Guinan, E. (1998). Subjective memory evaluations in patients with focal frontal, diencephalic, and temporal lobe lesion. *Cortex*, **34**, 191–207.

Kurtz, J.E., Putman, S.H. & Stone, C. (1998). Stability of normal personality traits after traumatic brain injury. *Journal of Head Trauma Rehabilitation*, **13**(3), 1–14.

Lazarus, R.D. & Folkman, S. (1984). *Stress, Appraisal and Coping.* New York: Springer.

Lishman, W.A. (1973). The psychiatric sequelae of head injury: a review. *Psychological Medicine*, **3**, 304–318.

Ley, P. (1972). *Quantitative Aspects of Psychological Assessment. An Introduction.* London: Duckworth.

Lovibond, S.H. & Lovibond, P.F. (1995). *Mannual for the Depression, Anxiety and Stress Scale*, 2nd edn. Sydney: Psychology Foundation.

Macchi, G. (1989). Anatomical substrate of emotional reactions. In F. Boller & J. Grafman (eds), *Handbook of Neuropsychology, vol 3, section 6: Emotional Behavior and Its Disorders* (pp. 283–303). Amsterdam: Elsevier.

MacMillan, M. (1996). Phineas Gage: a case for all reasons. In C. Code, C.-W. Eallesch, Y. Joanette & A.R. Lecours (eds), *Classic Cases in Neuropsychology* (pp. 243–262). Hove: Psychology Press.

McNair, D.M., Lorr, M. & Droppleman, L.F. (1992). *POMS Manual: Profile of Mood States.* San Diego, CA: Educational and Industrial Testing Service.

McGlynn, S. & Schacter, D.L. (1989). Unawareness of deficits in neuropsychological syndromes. *Journal of Clinical and Experimental Neuropsychology*, **11**, 143–205.

Meltzer, M. (1983). Poor memory: a case report. *Journal of Clinical Psychology*, **39**(1), 3–10.

Moore, A.D. & Stambrook, M. (1995). Cognitive moderators of outcome following traumatic brain injury: a conceptual model and implications for rehabilitation. *Brain Injury*, **9**, 109–130.

Moore, A.D., Stambrook, M. & Peters, L.C. (1989). Coping strategies and adjustment after closed head injury: a cluster analytic approach. *Brain Injury*, **3**, 171–175.

Moore, A.D., Stambrook, M. & Wilson, K.G. (1991). Cognitive moderators in adjustment to chronic illness: locus of control beliefs following traumatic brain injury. *Neuropsychological Rehabilitation*, **1**, 185–198.

Nelson, L.D., Cicchetti, D., Satz, P. et al. (1994). Emotional sequelae of stroke: a longitudinal perspective. *Journal of Clinical and Experimental Neuropsychology*, **16**, 796–806.

O'Connor, M.G., Cermak, L.S. & Seidman, L.J. (1995). Social and emotional characteristics of a profoundly amnesic postencephalitic patient. In R. Campbell & M.A. Conway (eds), *Broken Memories: Case Studies in Memory Impairment* (pp. 45–53). Oxford: Blackwell.

Odgen, J.A. (1996). *Fractured Minds. A Case-study Approach to Clinical Neuropsychology*. New York: Oxford University Press.

Ponsford, J.L., Olver, J.H. & Curran, C. (1995). A profile of outcome: 2 years after traumatic brain injury. *Brain Injury*, **9**, 1–10.

Prigatano, G.P. (1987). Psychiatric aspects of head injury: problem areas and suggested guidelines for research. In H.S. Levin, J. Grafman & H.M. Eisenberg (eds), *Neurobehavioral Recovery from Head Injury* (pp. 215–231). New York: Oxford University Press.

Prigatano, G.P. (1992). Personality disturbances associated with traumatic brain injury. *Journal of Consulting and Clinical Psychology*, **60**(3), 360–368.

Prigatano, G.P. (1995). Personality and social aspects of memory rehabilitation. In A.D. Baddeley, B.A. Wilson & F.N. Watts (eds), *Handbook of Memory Disorders*, Ist edn (pp. 603–614). Chichester: Wiley.

Prigatano, G.P. (2000). A brief overview of four principles of neuropsychological rehabilitation. In A.-L. Christensen & B.P. Uzzell (eds), *International Handbook of Neuropsychological Rehabilitation* (pp. 115–125). New York: Kluwer.

Raaymakers, T.W.M. on behalf of the MARS Study Group (2000). Functional outcome and quality of life after angiography and operation for unrupted intracranial aneurysms. *Journal of Neurology, Neurosurgery, and Psychiatry*, **68**, 571–576.

Satz, P., Forney, D.L., Zaucha, K. et al. (1998). Depression, cognition and functional correlates of recovery outcome after traumatic brain injury. *Brain Injury*, **12**, 537–553.

Schacter, D.L. (1991). Unawareness of deficit and unawareness of knowledge in patients with memory disorders. In G.P. Prigatano & D.L. Schacter (eds), *Awareness of Deficit after Brain Injury. Clinical and Theoretical Issues* (pp. 127–151). New York: Oxford University Press.

Schacter, D.L., Glisky, E. & McGlynn, S. (1990). Impact of memory disorders on everyday life. Awareness of deficits and return to work. In D.E. Tupper & K.D. Cicerone (eds), *The Neuropsychology of Everyday Life* (pp. 231–257). Norwell, MA: Kluwer.

Scoville, W.B. & Milner, B. (1957). Loss of recent memory after bilateral hippocampal lesions. *Journal of Neurology, Neurosurgery, and Psychiatry*, **20**, 11–21.

Sunderland, A., Harris, J.E. & Baddeley, A.D. (1983). Do laboratory tests predict everyday memory? A neuropsychological study. *Journal of Verbal Learning and Verbal Behavior*, **22**, 341–357.

Sunderland, A., Harris, J.E. & Baddeley, A.D. (1984). Assessing everyday memory after severe head injury. In J.E. Harris & P.E. Morris (eds), *Everyday Memory, Actions and Absent-mindedness* (pp. 191–206). London: Academic Press.

Talland, G.A. (1968). Some observations on the psychological mechanisms impaired in the amnesic syndrome. *International Journal of Neurology*, **7**, 21–30.

Tate, R.L. (2003). Impact of pre-injury factors on outcome after severe traumatic brain injury: does posttraumatic personality change represent an exacerbation of premorbid traits? *Neuropsychological Rehabilitation*, **13**, 43–64.

Tate, R.L. & Broe, G.A. (1999). Psychosocial adjustment after traumatic brain injury: what are the important variables? *Psychological Medicine*, **29**, 713–725.

Tate, R., Hodgkinson, A., Veerabangsa, A. & Maggiotto, S. (1999). Measuring psychosocial recovery after traumatic brain injury: psychometric properties of a new scale. *Journal of Head Trauma Rehabilitation*, **14**(6), 543–557.

Tate, R.L., Lulham, J.M., Broe, G.A. et al. (1989). Psychosocial outcome for the survivors of severe blunt head injury: the results of a consecutive series of 100 patients. *Journal of Neurology, Neurosurgery, and Psychiatry*, **52**, 1128–1134.

Tate, R.L., Veerabangsa, A., & Hodgkinson, A. (2001). Where there's a will, there's a way. The functional consequences of amnesia. *Brain Impairment* (abstr), **2**(1), 59–60.

Teuber, H.-L., Milner, B. & Vaughn, H.G. (1968). Persistent anterograde amnesia after stab wound of the basal brain. *Neuropsychologia*, **6**, 267–282.

Wilson, B.A. (1991). Long-term prognosis of patients with severe memory disorders. *Neuropsychological Rehabilitation*, **1**, 117–134.

Wilson, B.A. (1999). *Case Studies in Neuropsychological Rehabilitation*. New York: Oxford University Press.

Wilson, B.A., Baddeley, A.D. & Kapur, N. (1995). Dense amnesia in a professional musician following herpes simplex virus encephalitis. *Journal of Clinical and Experimental Neuropsychology*, **17**, 668–681.

Wilson, B.A., Cockburn, J. & Baddeley, A.D. (1985). *The Rivermead Behavioural Memory Test*. Bury St Edmunds: Thames Valley Test Company.

Wilson, B.A., J.C. & Hughes, E. (1997). Coping with amnesia: the natural history of a compensatory memory system. *Neuropsychological Rehabilitation*, **7**, 43–56.

Wilson, B.A. & Wearing, D. (1995). Prisoner of consciousness: a state of just awakening following herpes simplex encephalitis. In R. Campbell & M.A. Conway (eds), *Broken Memories: Case Studies in Memory Impairment* (pp. 14–30). Oxford: Blackwell.

Wilson, J.T.L., Pettigrew, L.E.L. & Teasdale, G.M. (2000). Emotional and cognitive consequences of head injury in relation to the Glasgow outcome scale. *Journal of Neurology, Neurosurgery, and Psychiatry*, **68**, 204–209.

Woessner, R. & Caplan, B. (1995). Affective disorders following mild to moderate brain injury: interpretive hazards of the SCL-90-R. *Journal of Head Trauma Rehabilitation*, **10**(2), 78–89.

World Health Organization (1980). *International Classification of Impairments, Disabilities and Handicaps. A Manual of Classification Relating to the Consequences of Disease*. Geneva: World Health Organization.

World Health Organization (2000). *ICIDH-2. International Classification of Functioning, Disability and Health. Prefinal Draft*. Geneva: World Health Organization.

Author Index

Page numbers in **bold** refer to complete chapters and page numbers in *italics* refer to figures and tables

Subject Index

Page numbers in **bold** refer to complete chapters and page numbers in *italics* refer to figures and tables